The Childbearing Family: A Nursing Perspective

The Childbearing Family: A Nursing Perspective

MARY ANN MILLER, R.N., M.S.N.
Assistant Professor, School of Nursing, The University of Pennsylvania, Philadelphia

DOROTHY A. BROOTEN, R.N., M.S.N.
*Associate Professor, Department of Baccalaureate Nursing, College of Allied Health Sciences
Thomas Jefferson University, Philadelphia*

Illustrated by Donna Nicolo, B.S.N.

LITTLE, BROWN AND COMPANY, BOSTON

To Elizabeth Miller,
without whom half of this book would not have been possible

To Gary Brooten,
whose love and support made the other half possible

To Lisa and Lars,
the most patient, understanding, and important children in the
world

Preface

THE EXPANSION AND COMPLEXITY of today's nursing practice demand the soundest of basic foundations for the practitioner. We have written this book to satisfy the need expressed by our many students, as well as observed by us, for a textbook on nursing care of the childbearing family—one that builds on the knowledge of the natural, social, and behavioral sciences which the undergraduate and graduate student brings to each clinical course.

We have not treated this specialty as an isolate but rather have identified principles that are common to all nursing practice. We have organized the material to provide a basic foundation in this area of nursing, to answer the student's "whys" without needless repetition of facts, to provide understanding as well as a challenge not only for students but for current practitioners as well. It is our hope, therefore, that more classroom time can be profitably spent discussing alternative approaches to providing nursing care for new parents, their babies, and their families and discussing relevant research and its application in clinical situations.

In this regard, the text begins with a consideration of the history of, and the current practices in, the care of the childbearing family, basic concepts of human sexuality, and a thorough review of female and male reproductive systems. A complete presentation of the options available to a couple during their reproductive years is given in the chapter on contraception, infertility, and therapeutic abortion. Aspects of the entire reproductive process are presented with their physiological and psychological bases and their related nursing implications. The importance of the nursing process, the family concept, and the role of the father is emphasized throughout the text.

We wish to alert our readers that occasionally in the text the nurse is referred to as "she." The term is used only for editorial convenience and does not reflect in any way our philosophy concerning men in nursing or, more specifically, male nurses practicing in the specialty.

We would like to pay special tribute to Donna Nicolo, our illustrator, for her invaluable services and for the tremendous amount of energy and skill she brought to her work. We would also like to acknowledge the efforts of many others who helped so much in the preparation of this text: Pauline Holt and Patricia Yost, for typing the manuscript; David Przestrzelski, for proofreading and critical comment; Marsha Whinston, for many hours in the library; JoAnn Jamann, for technical assistance; the Public Relations Departments of Thomas Jefferson University and Pennsylvania Hospital; Colonel Skinner of Booth Maternity Center; representatives of Mead Johnson Laboratories; and the publishers and authors who gave their permission for selected illustrations.

We would also like to acknowledge the efforts of the staff of Little, Brown and Company, especially Sarah Boardman and Kathy O'Brien, who demanded, queried, and encouraged p.r.n. If it had not been for the support we received from our families, friends, colleagues, and students, the book would never have become a reality. We thank all of you.

M. A. M.

D. A. B.

Philadelphia

Contents

The Childbearing Family: A Nursing Perspective

Chapter 1 Trends in Childbearing

BROADLY INTERPRETED, *obstetrics* refers to all aspects of reproduction and the childbearing process—conception and contraception, pregnancy, labor, the postpartum period, and whatever pathology may be involved. It extends from an understanding of intrauterine development to an appreciation of the consequences of world population growth. The practice of health care personnel working within this discipline is aimed at the ideal that every pregnancy end in a healthy mother, baby, and family unit. Since this is not always a possibility, health care personnel try to prevent deviations from health or at least recognize them at an early stage and prevent undesirable consequences or minimize their ill effects as much as possible. As a result, they promote the optimal physical and emotional well-being for each member of the family unit.

HISTORICAL PERSPECTIVE

In order to appreciate the present trends in childbearing, one should have some understanding of their historical precedents. The term *obstetrics* is derived from the Latin verb *obstare,* meaning to protect or to stand by. *Obstetrix* referred to the midwife or the woman who stood by the expectant mother and gave her aid. Actually *midwifery,* rather than *obstetrics,* was the most widely used term until the latter part of the nineteenth century in both the United States and Great Britain. In England today the two words are used synonymously.

Historically, most women were delivered with the assistance of midwives whose knowledge was based purely on experience. When complications developed, medicine men or priests were called upon to pray over the mother. It is not surprising that childbirth was associated with mystery and superstition.

In the ancient Greek, Roman, Hindu, and Egyptian cultures, Hippocrates and others began to write the theory of obstetrics. Although medieval times saw a decline in the progress of obstetrical knowledge and practice, midwives continued to perform deliveries. Women gave birth while sitting on special stools or obstetrical chairs (Figure 1-1).

From the seventeenth to nineteenth centuries further advances were made in the science of obstetrics. The first modern cesarean section was performed, puerperal fever was described, and obstetrical forceps and the use of chloroform as an anesthetic were introduced. Even greater strides have been taken in the twentieth century. Between 1900 and 1910, antepartal care became an organized part of the medical and nursing supervision of mothers. Statistics began to be compiled and groups were established to study and to remedy high infant and maternal mortality. In 1912

Figure 1-1. Birth chair used by early midwives. The chair was folded and carried on the midwife's back as she went from house to house assisting with deliveries. (Courtesy of Thomas Jefferson University, Philadelphia, Pa.)

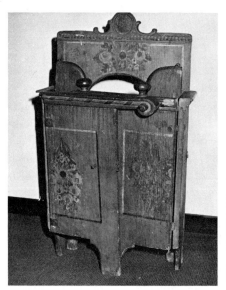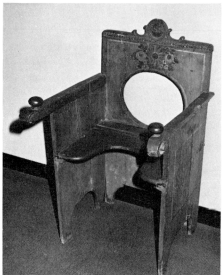

the Children's Bureau was established by the United States government to conduct research and provide education to promote the health and welfare of children of all ages. In the 1920s, the Frontier Nursing Service was established in Kentucky and the Margaret Sanger Research Bureau was founded for planned parenthood and infertility research and assistance.

During the 1930s, a part of the Social Security Act, administered by the Children's Bureau, extended services for infant care to local areas. Maternity clinics, prenatal classes, premature care centers, and "well baby" clinics were established. Public health nursing services were provided for pregnant women. Improvements during the 1940s and 1950s, which had a dramatic effect in lowering maternal mortality, included the development of blood transfusions, antibiotics, the increased number of hospital deliveries, and the rising standards of hospital care.

MATERNAL AND INFANT CARE PROGRAMS

In the past decade the number of neighborhood prenatal clinics has increased, high-risk clinics have been established, and programs have been developed for pregnant women who are unable to afford medical care. In 1963 in the United States, Maternal and Infant Care (MIC) programs were funded under Title V of the Social Security Act, with the purpose of providing health care to high-risk pregnant women and, following delivery, to their newborn infants. The projects have been set up in large and middle-size cities and in rural areas where there are few doctors in private practice or where clinics are overcrowded. Federal funding meets up to 75 percent of the operating costs. The woman, depending on her financial situation and overall physical condition, receives care without cost or pays only a portion of it.

Populations served by these programs have reported decreases in maternal and infant mortality, in premature births, in low birth weight babies, and in the number of pregnant women delivering without prenatal care. The number of women returning for postpartum and family planning visits has increased, as has the number of women seeking prenatal care early in pregnancy.

Communities, in addition to establishing MIC programs, have developed increasing numbers of neighborhood health centers. These centers include on their staffs nonprofessionals from the community, who are able to contribute its perspective when the needs of the consumers are considered and appropriate services are planned.

Other factors have also resulted in better services for pregnant women and reduced mortality and morbidity for them and their babies. Improved methods of anesthesia and analgesia, more sophisticated use of x-ray and ultrasonic diagnostic tools, and generally improved standards of living and sanitation have all played a part in these advances. Better education of health personnel has resulted in specialized training for physicians and nurses. Nurse midwives, as well as clinical nurse specialists, are being increasingly utilized.

VITAL STATISTICS

Birth Rate and Fertility Rate

Statistics often provide clues regarding the magnitude of certain problems or trends in population growth. The birth rate is always of interest to those predicting the need for obstetrical personnel. This rate has shown rather steady decreases during the last decade (Table 1-1). There is some evidence to suggest that the decline in the birth rate in the United States may be approaching a reversal [7]. This is based on the rapidly rising proportions of young women who have not yet had any children.

Maternal Mortality

A statistic which is of particular concern is that of maternal mortality (Table 1-2). Since the 1940s there has been a marked decrease in maternal mortality in the United States, Canada, and most of Western Europe. Over the last 20 years there has been a decline of 80 percent in maternal deaths in the United States. Many factors are responsible for the tremendous fall in the maternal death rate. Most of them have already been mentioned: use of blood transfusions, antibiotics, better standard of living, better education of health practitioners, and more widely available antepartal care.

Maternal deaths resulting from the childbearing process (pregnancy, delivery, post partum) are stated in terms of the number of deaths per 100,000 live births (Table 1-3). Many of these deaths are caused by preeclampsia/eclampsia, hemor-

Table 1-1. Birth Rate in the United States per 1000 Population

1940	1945	1950	1955	1960	1965	1970	1972	1973
19.4	20.4	24.1	25.0	23.7	19.4	18.4	15.6	15.0

Source: U.S. National Center for Health Statistics. *Vital Statistics of the United States.* Washington, D.C. (published annually).

Table 1-2. Maternal Mortality in the United States (per 100,000 Live Births) from Deliveries and Complications of Pregnancy, Childbirth, and the Puerperium

Deaths	1940	1950	1960	1965	1968	1970	1971[a]	1972[a]
Maternal deaths	376.0	83.3	37.1	31.6	24.5	21.5	20.5	24.0
White deaths	319.8	61.1	26.0	21.0	16.6	14.4	—[b]	—[b]
Nonwhite deaths	773.5	221.6	97.9	83.7	63.6	55.9	—[b]	—[b]

[a]Preliminary.
[b]Not available.
Source: Modified from U.S. National Center for Health Statistics. *Vital Statistics of the United States.* Washington, D.C. (published annually).

rhage, or infection. Heart disease is not officially recognized as a statistical category among the causes of maternal mortality, but it is related to a significant number of maternal deaths. Maternal mortality varies with the age of the woman. Increased age is also often related to the number of previous pregnancies; the effects of the two appear to be additive. The increased incidence of hypertension and a greater tendency to uterine hemorrhage are causative factors. Maternal mortality also tends to increase in the very young pregnant women, who are more subject to a variety of complications. The optimal age for childbearing seems to be between 20 and 24 years of age.

One of the most serious problems in maternity care in the United States is the markedly higher maternal mortality among nonwhite women and those in rural areas. These women often receive care which may be inferior in quantity as well as quality. Since few health personnel choose to practice in rural and poverty areas, deliveries may not be properly attended. Pregnant women who live in urban poverty areas may have their care provided in great measure by large institutions, and that care may be depersonalized as a result. This may, in itself, discourage early and

Table 1-3. Maternal Mortality in the United States (per 100,000 Live Births) by Age, Race, and Cause of Death

Age/Cause	1957–1958			1967–1968		
	White	Nonwhite	Total	White	Nonwhite	Total
All ages	26.9	108.3	39.2	18.1	66.6	26.3
Under 20	18.0	60.0	27.5	13.0	35.3	19.2
20–24	13.0	55.5	19.5	10.1	45.5	15.4
25–29	20.0	98.5	30.0	13.5	66.0	20.3
30–34	37.5	180.5	56.5	28.7	109.8	41.3
35–39	66.5	272.0	94.5	51.2	179.0	72.7
40–44	109.5	382.5	147.5	100.1	250.2	126.8
All causes	26.9	108.3	39.2	18.1	66.6	26.3
Infection	3.0	8.5	4.0	3.4	7.2	4.0
Preeclampsia/eclampsia	6.5	31.5	10.0	3.0	13.5	4.8
Hemorrhage	5.5	19.5	7.5	2.7	7.3	3.5
Ectopic pregnancy	1.5	10.5	3.0	1.0	7.4	2.1
Abortion	3.0	21.0	6.0	2.3	13.4	4.2
Other	7.5	19.5	9.0	5.7	18.0	7.8

Source: Statistical Bulletin of the Metropolitan Life Insurance Company, Vol. 53. New York, June 1972.

Table 1-4. Fetal Mortality in the United States per 1000 Live Births (Fetal Deaths [Stillbirths] for Which Period of Gestation Was 20 Weeks [or 5 Months] or More, or Was Not Stated)

Deaths	1950	1960	1965	1968	1970	1971	1972
Fetal deaths	19.2	16.1	16.2	15.8	14.2	—[a]	—[a]
White deaths	17.1	14.1	13.9	13.8	12.4	—[a]	—[a]
Nonwhite deaths	32.5	26.8	27.2	25.6	22.6	—[a]	—[a]

[a]Not available.
Source: Modified from U.S. National Center for Health Statistics. *Vital Statistics of the United States.* Washington, D.C. (published annually).

regular attendance, although there may also be other problems with lack of transportation, inadequate baby sitting arrangements, fear, lack of understanding about the necessity of care, or long waiting periods. Lower socioeconomic status may be accompanied by poor living standards, poor nutrition, or increased stress, any of which can increase a woman's chances of a complicated pregnancy. It does not take much thought to conclude that many of the above factors can be easily remedied by interested health personnel.

Perinatal Mortality

Perinatal mortality is the sum of the fetal and neonatal death rates, or the number of stillborn infants and neonatal deaths per 1000 total births.

A fetal death (or stillbirth) is said to have occurred when the period of gestation is 20 weeks or more or the fetus weighs 500 grams or more and is born without any sign of life—no heartbeat, respiration, or movement. (The loss of a fetus up to 20 weeks of gestation or weighing less than 500 grams is referred to as a spontaneous abortion—see page 422.) This death rate (per 1000 live births), which is related to the quality of care before and during birth, is still high (Table 1-4). Improvements in prenatal care and fetal monitoring may significantly reduce the fetal death rate in the future.

Neonatal death rates are relatively high, although significant reductions have occurred (Table 1-5). More than half of the neonatal deaths (deaths of live-born infants up to 28 days of age) occur during the first day of life, which emphasizes the importance of careful observation and accurate assessment of the newborn's condition. Premature birth remains the most frequent cause of neonatal death; central nervous system injuries, whether from hypoxia or trauma, and congenital malformations are also significant factors.

Table 1-5. Neonatal Mortality in the United States per 1000 Live Births (Infants under 28 Days Old, Exclusive of Fetal Deaths)

Deaths	1940	1950	1960	1965	1968	1970	1971[a]	1972[a]
Neonatal deaths	28.8	20.5	18.7	17.7	16.1	15.1	14.3	13.7
White deaths	27.2	19.4	17.2	16.1	14.7	13.8	12.9	12.3
Nonwhite deaths	39.7	27.5	26.9	25.4	23.0	21.4	20.8	20.6

[a]Preliminary.
Source: Modified from U.S. National Center for Health Statistics. *Vital Statistics of the United States.* Washington, D.C. (published annually).

Table 1-6. Infant Mortality in the United States per 1000 Live Births (Infants under 1 Year Old, Exclusive of Fetal Deaths)

Deaths	1940	1950	1960	1965	1968	1970	1971[a]	1972[a]
Infant deaths	47.0	29.2	26.0	24.7	21.8	20.0	19.2	18.5
White deaths	43.2	26.8	22.9	21.5	19.2	17.8	16.8	16.3
Nonwhite deaths	73.8	44.5	43.2	40.3	34.5	30.9	30.2	29.0

[a]Preliminary.
Source: Modified from U.S. National Center for Health Statistics. *Vital Statistics of the United States.* Washington, D.C. (published annually).

Infant Mortality

The infant death rate (calculated per 1000 live births) includes deaths of infants under one year of age, exclusive of fetal deaths. This rate is decreasing gradually, as can be seen in Table 1-6. Most infant deaths occur during the neonatal period.

GENETIC COUNSELING

Recent accomplishments in genetic counseling have helped to reduce infant mortality and morbidity. Refinements in chromosome studies and in biochemical and tissue culture methods have greatly improved our ability to diagnose, treat, and advise families on genetic matters. From a sample of amniotic fluid, it is possible to detect all major chromosomal abnormalities and well over 30 inborn errors of metabolism. With this information, couples at risk can be better informed when they decide whether or not to have children. They may choose to conceive, have the amniotic fluid of the fetus tested for abnormalities, and then choose to continue the pregnancy or not, depending on the results. This advance has enabled couples who in the past would not have chosen to have children to go through the childbearing process.

Genetic counseling has had other benefits as well. Serious problems in interpersonal relationships between a couple are averted by informing them that a genetic trait is an unfortunate coincidence of parental genotype and is not related to habit, conduct, or misconduct. This information should help to dispel guilt feelings; the knowledge that all persons are carriers for a variety of disorders likewise lessens their anxiety. This knowledge also helps to decrease in the extended family any hostility or feelings that the couple should not bear children.

For purposes of counseling, a genetic history is taken. The age, sex, and past and present health of the father, mother, siblings, and all close relatives of the couple are recorded, and a pedigree chart is compiled. The age at death and cause of death are noted for those relatives who have died. It is also important to record how the diagnosis of cause of death was made (e.g., biopsy, clinical examination, or biochemical test) and the age of onset of the genetic disorder in each family member. (Siblings may not yet be affected because they are too young.) Based on this information, the couple is counseled by reviewing its special problems and explaining the genetic prognosis and the alternatives open to them.

Birth defect monitoring systems are in effect in Canada, Great Britain, Finland, Sweden, Norway, Hungary, and Israel. Recently, the United States has begun establishing such a system. Data on approximately 230 different kinds of birth defects will be collected from one million births per year in 1200 short-term hospitals in the United States. The information will be computerized and reported quarterly by the Center for Disease Control in Atlanta. This system should enable the detection of any unusual pattern in the occurrence of birth defects, such as regional outbreaks that might be linked to drugs, viral infections, radiation, pollutants, or other environmental causes. It is hoped that such patterns can be detected in time to minimize the risk of these birth defects' reaching epidemic proportions.

FETAL MONITORING

In addition to monitoring the incidence of birth defects, in the last two decades health care personnel have become increasingly experienced in monitoring and evaluating the status of the unborn. Fetal maturity can be measured by obtaining a sample of amniotic fluid and testing for the lecithin-sphingomyelin (L/S) ratio, fat cell content, and creatinine and bilirubin levels. Maturity can also be determined by using ultrasonic examination to measure the biparietal diameter of the fetal head. Functioning of the fetoplacental unit can be ascertained by testing estriol levels in a 24-hour collection of the woman's urine or by using the oxytocin challenge test. During labor, fetal monitoring equipment can be used to follow the well-being of the fetus.

NEONATAL INTENSIVE CARE UNITS

After birth, the newborn continues to be observed very carefully. Recent changes in the care of high-risk neonates have resulted in the development of intensive care nurseries. This organized intensive care has led to a decrease in mortality among the neonates and fewer serious handicapping conditions among the surviving infants [6]. The development of a number of medical subspecialties, such as neonatology and perinatology, has provided highly prepared and highly skilled personnel to care for high-risk infants in these intensive care units.

Because such skilled personnel are still limited in number and because such units require rather expensive equipment, it has been strongly recommended that the sites for neonatal intensive care units be chosen carefully and that each one be large enough for efficient and effective service. Unnecessary duplication and uneven distribution have been a problem, and little consideration has been given to actual community needs [4]. Regionalization obviously would ensure better use of available resources. Its lack of fragmentation would also increase our knowledge about the relationship of the methods of treatment to the outcome of this type of care.

Since nurses are responsible for making the majority of observations and carrying out most of the treatment for infants in these units, it is essential that these nurses are adequately prepared and that they have a high degree of clinical expertise. The same degree of preparation is necessary for nurses who work in the obstetrical intensive care units that are being established for the treatment of high-risk pregnant women.

THE FAMILY CONCEPT IN CHILDBEARING

More attention is now being paid to the response of the total family to the pregnancy experience. The expectant father is just beginning to receive the attention he deserves. He or a close friend or relative is encouraged to become involved in childbirth preparation classes. He is an essential member of the health team, giving emotional and physical support to the woman during pregnancy and labor (Figure 1-2). He should be permitted to accompany the woman to the delivery room, where they share in the birth of their baby. In some instances he may even participate in the actual delivery. He should be able to be present when the baby is fed in the hospital and to participate in the infant's care. If there are other children in the family, they should be able to visit their mother during this time. Anxiety levels are kept at a minimum for both mother and children when such visits are possible.

Rooming-in is a desirable option for many families. This arrangement permits parents to see and care for their baby whenever they want. Usually visitors are limited; the father is encouraged to help care for and feed the infant (after he washes his hands and puts on a gown). Policies regarding rooming-in vary from hospital to hospital. In some hospitals the baby remains with the mother for 24 hours a day; in others he is returned to the nursery during the night. In some institutions the physical plant is specifically designed to accommodate mothers who desire rooming-in. In other hospitals existing facilities can usually be easily modified to provide this service.

Some obstetricians are consenting to do deliveries in the home, where the mother can readily receive emotional support from the father and other family members during the birth process. Home deliveries are usually less expensive than hospital

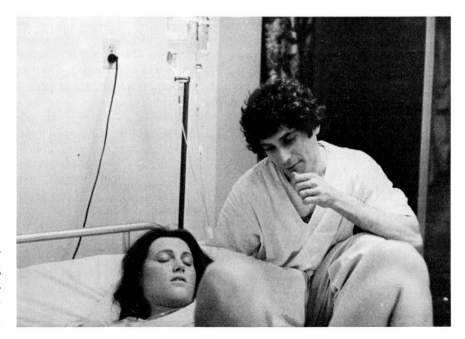

Figure 1-2. Father thoughtfully supports mother during labor and awaits the birth of their child. (Courtesy of Booth Maternity Center, Philadelphia, Pa.)

deliveries, and there is also less danger of mother and newborn acquiring hospital-borne infections. The main disadvantage of home delivery is the lack of emergency services, equipment, techniques, and educated personnel, which are available in the hospital. However, in the minds of some parents this is outweighed by the advantage of home delivery—the ability to be together in familiar surroundings during the birth of their baby.

The current trend toward primary care nursing will undoubtedly encourage a spirit of unity as the parents and their family members relate to the same nurse throughout the childbearing process. The continuum of care begins when the nurse first meets the parents in the clinic or doctor's office, and continues as she follows them through the pregnancy, labor, delivery, and postpartum period, and makes home visits when necessary. This approach is similar to the continuity of care currently provided by the nurse midwife.

NURSE MIDWIFERY

The first nurse midwives in the United States were trained in England and were first employed by the Frontier Nursing Service in 1925. By 1931 the first school for nurse midwifery had opened in New York City, but professional nurse midwives did not enter the organized system of health care until 1955. The United States has been slow to acknowledge the role of nurse midwives and to utilize their services, possibly because the profession has had to outgrow the reputation of the old "Granny midwives," nonprofessionals whose practice was based on experience rather than education.

The last decade has witnessed the growth of a spirit of collaboration and cooperation among health professionals. The nurse midwife is increasingly seen as the teammate of the doctor. In many instances the pregnant woman is seen initially by both the doctor and the nurse midwife. If her condition is not complicated in any way, she may choose to have the nurse midwife follow her throughout her pregnancy and labor. The nurse midwife will deliver her baby and attend to her postpartum and family planning needs, including home visits. The doctor is available for consultation throughout the childbearing process.

The nurse midwife often provides additional services for the parents, such as individual counseling and general health education, arranging for semi-reclining positions during delivery, helping with immediate breast-feeding after birth, and urging the presence of the father or other close relative to support the mother. Parents who have had contact with a nurse midwife usually find the experience beneficial and request the same type of service again. In some groups of pregnant women cared for by nurse midwives, there has been a decrease in the rates of prematurity and neonatal deaths [3].

The American College of Nurse-Midwives is the professional organization that sets the standards for quality care by midwives. It also provides guidelines and accreditation for educational programs and issues a certifying examination. In the 1950s there were five or six such programs; today there are 16 nurse midwifery programs that prepare registered nurses to become certified. Eight of them lead to a master's degree as well. (See the Appendix at the end of the book for a list of these programs.)

The nurse midwife is an outstanding example of the expanded role of the nurse in maternity settings. Clinical nurse specialists with advanced preparation can provide many of the same services (excluding the actual delivery of the baby). These professionals have a broad orientation to health care and relate to families on a very personal level, characteristics increasingly being demanded by the consumer. Because of this, and because fewer physicians are choosing obstetrics as a specialty, the need for prepared nurse practitioners can only be more pressing in the future.

RESEARCH IN NURSING

Every practitioner is responsible for providing quality patient care. Improvements in its delivery can only occur as a result of a strong base of nursing research. Students in nursing, as well as practitioners, have the obligation as professionals to become actively involved in some research activity. A nurse can fulfill this obligation in different ways without actually being involved in designing projects and in collecting data. In fact, it is recognized that true competence in designing research projects is most likely with advanced study.

If nursing is to continue to grow in professional stature, it is essential that it nurture an attitude of curiosity that questions and analyzes the validity of assumptions on which our actions are based. This curiosity moves students or practitioners to question sweeping generalizations found in the professional literature, to wonder why such statements are correct (or incorrect), and to investigate the rationale behind these statements. It stimulates them to question policies that formulate routine aspects of patient care, to evaluate present approaches to it, to wonder about different, more individualized, or better approaches to patient care, and to try some of them to see what results are achieved. This curiosity causes them to want to be knowledgeable about current research in the field, to interpret the findings of such studies critically, and to share this information with their co-workers. It inspires them to be willing to apply the results of clinical research to their own practice and to identify further research problems. Nursing is already characterized by a careful assessment of patients and their environment. An exciting dimension is added when this assessment is used as a basis for developing better methods of patient care.

Many students already use scientific research procedures on a small scale when their curriculum includes independent study. Here they recognize how problems in clinical nursing can be systematically studied, and they have the opportunity to look at those problems creatively, considering a wide variety of approaches for their study and solution. They must identify and critically read relevant research in their subject area, develop a plan for investigating their problem, and implement that plan.

Comprehensive research and critical analysis of the literature naturally precedes application of results of studies to clinical practice. Nurses should not doubt their ability to understand research; there is nothing magical about understanding research that has been carefully documented and clearly presented by the author. Whether it is being read with the purpose of implementing findings in practice or in order to generate new ideas for further research, it is essential for the reader to assess whether the findings are reliable. A methodical, thoughtful, critical analysis of research studies should provide the reader with that assessment.

Castles [2] enumerates certain steps involved in such an approach.

1. Note the credentials of the author. They might bear some relationship to the validity of the research.
2. Look at the title. It should give a clear and comprehensive indication of what the study is about.
3. Look for the definition of the problem and the statement of the purpose. Are they clear?
4. Pay attention to the methodology used. Look at the variables. How were they controlled? Will the findings be valid? Be careful about applying the findings to a general population if the sample was nonrandom, very small, etc. Was the data collection appropriately done?
5. Look at the conclusions of the study. Do they relate to the stated purpose? Are they based on the data? Are they relevant to nursing practice? Were any limitations to the study noted?

Notter [5] and Abdellah and Levine [1] agree that clinical research is a top priority in today's nursing research. Maternity nursing is a "fertile" area for the generation of research ideas; very little has been done in this field. At a time when nursing, particularly obstetrical nursing, is developing in so many new professional directions, we must depend on active and sound nursing research to provide us with the firm foundation for our growing practice.

REFERENCES

1. Abdellah, F., and Levine, E. *Better Patient Care Through Nursing Research.* New York: Macmillan, 1965.
2. Castles, M. R. A practitioner's guide to utilization of research findings. *Journal of Obstetric, Gynecologic and Neonatal Nursing* 4:50, January/February, 1975.
3. Gatewood, T. S., and Stewart, R. Obstetricians and nurse-midwives: The team approach in private practice. *American Journal of Obstetrics and Gynecology* 123:35, 1975.
4. Harrison, L. K. Making a good thing better: The regionalization of neonatal intensive care units. *Journal of Obstetric, Gynecologic and Neonatal Nursing* 4:49, May/June, 1975.
5. Notter, L. The vital significance of clinical nursing research. *Cardio-Vascular Nursing* 8:19, 1972.
6. Schlesinger, E. Neonatal intensive care: Planning for services and outcomes following care. *Journal of Pediatrics* 82:916, 1973.
7. Sklar, J., and Berkov, B. The American birth rate: Evidences of a coming rise. *Science* 189:693, 1975.

FURTHER READING

Birth defect monitoring system. *National Foundation–Maternal Newborn Advocate,* Vol. 2. February 1975.

Chase, H. C., and Nelson, F.   Education of mother, medical care, and condition of infant. *American Journal of Public Health* 63 (Supplement):27, 1973.

Folk superstition and birth rate. (Editorial.) *Science News* 107:104, 1975.

Holden, J., and Holden, L.   Perinatal research laboratories. *Medical Center Quarterly Report of the University of Michigan* 1:7, Winter 1974.

Intensive care for newborns: Are there times to pull the plug? (Editorial.) *Science* 188:133, 1975.

Jones, K., Smith, D., Harvey, M., Hall, B., and Quan, L.   Older paternal age and fresh gene mutation. *Obstetrical and Gynecological Survey* 30:672, 1975.

Lesser, A.   Progress in maternal and child health. *Children Today* 1:7, 1972.

Paul, R., and Hon, E.   Clinical fetal monitoring. *American Journal of Obstetrics and Gynecology* 118:529, 1974.

Quilligan, E.   The obstetric intensive care unit. *Hospital Practice* 7:61, 1972.

Reame, N. E., and Hafez, F. S.   Hereditary defects affecting fertility. *New England Journal of Medicine* 292:675, 1975.

Rising, S.   A consumer-oriented nurse-midwifery service. *Nursing Clinics of North America* 10:251, 1975.

Roberts, D., Farr, L., Guthrie, R., and Nelson, R.   Perinatal care. *Journal of the Kansas Medical Society* 75:259, 1974.

Schlesinger, E., Lowery, W., Glaser, D., Milliones, M., and Mazumdar, S.   A controlled test of the use of registered nurses for prenatal care. *Health Services Reports* 88:400, 1973.

Schneider, J.   Changing concepts in prenatal care. *Postgraduate Medicine* 53:91, 1973.

Terris, M., and Glasser, M.   A life table analysis of the relation of prenatal care to prematurity. *American Journal of Public Health* 64:869, 1974.

U.S. Department of Health, Education, and Welfare, Public Health Service.   Research to improve health services for mothers and children, DHEW Publication (HSA) 74-5121. Washington, D.C., 1974.

U.S. Department of Health, Education and Welfare, Public Health Service.   Promoting community health, DHEW Publication (HSA) 75-5016. Washington, D.C., 1975.

Weigle, J. W.   Teaching child development to teenage mothers. *Children Today* 3:23, 1974.

Westoff, C.   The decline of unplanned births in the United States. *Science* 191:38, 1976.

Chapter 2 Sexuality

SEXUAL DEVELOPMENT

An individual's awareness of his own body is never complete, since his body is constantly changing throughout life. Therefore a person is constantly revising his perception of his body image. His recognition of his body as weak or strong, big or little, sickly or healthy, sexually alive or unresponsive is a significant part of his total sense of identity.

Infancy is filled with experiences that help bring about a sense of the body and its capacities for pleasure and discomfort. Babies are frequently observed exploring their bodies. They learn to be comfortable with their bodies and find them a source of pleasure, especially if their parents are warm and consistent in touching and handling them.

During the preschool years, the child's basic concept of himself as a sexual being is developed. This conception is positively or negatively reinforced by the reactions he receives when he explores or exposes his body. Children at this age begin to question where babies come from, especially if a new baby is expected in the family; however, unless adults bring up the subjects of conception or intercourse, the preschooler is rarely interested in such explicit information.

As Broderick [5] notes, during these years several factors are especially important in the development of the child's sexual identity. One important element is his or her self-image as a boy or a girl, an identification constantly reinforced by adults and other children. In establishing his identity, the preschooler is always absorbing styles, mannerisms, speech patterns, attitudes, and assumptions of people surrounding him. Equally important to his identity are his experiences with adults and children of the opposite sex and his feelings about a lasting relationship with a member of the opposite sex. It is interesting to note that the majority of 5-year-olds are already committed to the idea of eventual marriage for themselves.

Another influential factor on a child's sexual identity is the child's relationship with his parents and the eventual resolution of the conflicts of the oedipal period. If his parents accept his gender at birth and provide a warm, loving, and consistent environment, the child is more likely to incorporate their standards and social values than he would be if discord exists between parents, or between parents and the child. The behavioral patterns established during this period affect the child's future emotional and sexual life.

The experiences of preadolescence are an important shaping force in an individual's sexuality. There is a wide range of knowledge of sexual matters in this age group. Most children have some idea that pregnancy and childbirth are related to sexual intercourse. Girls' questions mainly involve menstruation and pregnancy, while boys ask for definitions of slang terms as well as information about pregnancy and intercourse.

Children of this age tend to group with peers of the same sex, practicing their own sexual roles before interacting comfortably with members of the opposite sex. They may privately choose a special girlfriend or boyfriend, but their choice is usually kept to themselves, giving them an opportunity to fantasize emotional involvement with this special person without fear of rejection or humiliation. While they rehearse this emotional commitment in their own imaginations, they are developing some of the social skills useful in boy-girl relations.

During adolescence there is a shift from questions about menstruation, intercourse, and conception to questions about sexual standards and social relationships between boys and girls. The younger adolescent is concerned with standards and values, whereas the older adolescent is more interested in the psychology of social relationships. Self-understanding and sensitivity to others are the key assets that can be acquired during this period.

For young men ejaculation serves as a symbol of sexual maturity, and for girls menstruation does the same. The frequent erections that a young male adolescent has may be embarrassing at times. Masturbation is his major source of sexual release; although it is a positive and gratifying experience, it also provokes guilt and anxiety. Masturbation rates in females are generally lower. In our society, females are encouraged to be sexually stimulating to men but not to act on their own sexual needs. Girls tend to concentrate on the intense affect-laden portion of relationships and the romance involved.

Later adolescence brings an increase in the opportunity for sociosexual activity. The male who is committed to sex interacts with the female who is committed to romantic love, and in the ensuing courtship, each shares with the other the meaning and content of their respective commitments [5].

Petting is one of the most common forms of sexual behavior during the late teens and early twenties, when the focus is on the strategy of boy-girl relations. This period of life is more supportive to a person's sexual self-image than any other because the process of courtship, which occurs most commonly in this age group, is very flattering. Relationships based on exploitation are usually rejected in favor of those based on mutual concern.

There are a few periods in the life cycle at which there are high rates of sexual activity. These are usually adolescence for the male, the early and romantic years of marriage for men and women, and, for some, later periods of highly charged extramarital affairs. Most of the time sexual activity is less intense.

Cultures that encourage women to respond sexually produce women who generally have a sexual response equal to that of men. If female sexuality is discouraged, female response tends to be inferior. In many Western societies women still have strong negative attitudes about sex and instill these attitudes in their daughters [2]. Masters and Johnson [7] postulate that females have a greater capacity for sexual response than males, and that cultural restraints have been imposed in order to provide a better balance between the sexes.

Middle age can be a difficult period sexually because of decreasing sexual powers, dissatisfaction with some aspects of marriage, and unflattering physical changes.

Sexual difficulties in middle age are closely related to deterioration of self-image and self-confidence.

Advancing age is seen as the end of sexuality by some, and waning sexual prowess is often confronted by ridicule. At age 60, 75 percent of men can achieve intercourse, 30 percent at age 70, and 14–20 percent at 80 [5]. The aging female is capable of orgasmic response indefinitely if regularly exposed to effective sexual stimulation. During menopause many women face an identity crisis as their roles as wives and mothers change when children leave home or husbands die.

RELIGIOUS INFLUENCES

Of all the factors (such as social class, ethnic background, and age) that may influence a person's concept of his sexuality, his religious identity may be one of the most important, since it influences almost every aspect of life.

Jewish history, according to Rabbi Borowitz [3], reflects changes in attitudes toward sexual conduct, varying from restrictive to permissive, depending on the degree of orthodoxy. Jewish tradition has always prized modesty; it has also given full recognition to the sexuality of women, even ascribing to them a greater sex drive than that of men. It praises premarital chastity but imposes no penalty for its violation. Procreation is not considered the sole function of intercourse although contraception other than for medical reasons is regarded as sinful even today by many Orthodox Jews. Abortion is generally considered acceptable when the mother's life or mental health is in jeopardy. Thus, nonpuritanical attitudes accompanied by a self-imposed discipline of sexual restraint appears to be the general trend among present-day Jewish people.

Early Christianity emphasized the monogamous family and the moral upbringing of children. Sex was often confused with sin. Women's sexuality and pleasure in sex was denied, while men were inhibited in their sexual attitudes. For both men and women, sex was associated with guilt. Sexual intercourse was considered acceptable only in marriage and only for the purpose of procreation, and many prohibitions were placed on the manner in which intercourse could take place. Even today in certain states, married couples can be convicted as criminals for using certain positions of intercourse or forms of caresses, such as oral-genital contact.

Generally, attitudes of Protestants toward sexuality [10, 14] rely less upon religious authority than those of Catholics or Jews, but this does not imply greater sexual freedom. Early Protestant church leaders saw sexual drives as basic needs and wished to create a more accepting atmosphere; however, prudery and shame became the prevailing attitudes. Luther doubted that any man or woman could be free from lust since the libido was overwhelmingly strong. Marriage then became a remedy for concupiscence. Calvin saw sex in marriage as proper and decent, not lustful. Contemporary Protestantism includes attitudes ranging from acceptance of premarital expressions of affection to disapproval of dancing and movies. Supporters of a traditional morality are in the majority and disapprove of sex outside of marriage. Divorce is permitted, however, and contraception is acceptable.

Catholicism, more than the other major religions, has definite rules regarding the sexual behavior of its followers [12]. While it does not deny the pleasures associated with sexual intercourse, it sees procreation as its main purpose. Premarital and extramarital sex are not allowed. The fundamental premise is based on a relationship between sex and marriage which involves two basic concerns: the protection of human life in every form and respect for the meaning or significance of an act as revealed in its objective "natural" structure. Any deliberate attempt to inhibit the normal structure and progress of the physiological process initiated when a couple has intercourse constitutes an objective immoral act. Thus the rhythm method of contraception is the only acceptable one, since it involves cooperation with "nature" through periodic abstinence. Pope Paul VI reiterated this position in the encyclical, *Humanae Vitae,* emphasizing that the marital act must always be open to procreation.

During the past 20 years, a number of Catholic scholars have seriously questioned the adequacy of the Church's sexual ethics. The Council Fathers of Vatican II took these criticisms under consideration. They recognized the implications of the current population growth trend, acknowledging the need for some form of family regulation. They displayed a mature understanding of the sexual dimensions of conjugal love. This may have marked the beginning of a careful reformulation of the specifically Catholic approach to human sexuality in the light of contemporary cultural and theological developments.

The underlying philosophy remains the same, however. Since sexual relations are designed both to unite the partners as persons and to provide for the continuity of the human race through parenthood, responsible sex can be engaged in only by married couples. Their commitment to a community of life and love within which they can strive for mutual fulfillment and happiness helps them create the human environment in which children can be fittingly raised.

SOCIOECONOMIC INFLUENCES

While religion may have significant influences on sexuality, so too may cultural and socioeconomic background. In today's middle class there is certainly much less role segregation than existed in the past. More women now maintain jobs outside the home and share childrearing with their mates. Today's ideal of marriage is a relationship between husband and wife built on happiness, communication, and mutual gratification. This is also true in the sexual sphere, where there is emphasis on the partners' recognizing each other's needs and working toward satisfaction for both.

Brenton [4] sees this shift as a challenge for today's men. He notes that the contemporary male faces sexual responsibilities far exceeding those of men in the past. Today a man must gratify both himself and his sexual partner. He must make sure he is a good lover. In addition, he must cope with the sexually liberated woman, something that can require a considerable amount of adjustment.

Many contemporary women suffer from sexual inhibition caused by their socialization, by feelings of guilt, and by overemphasis on the importance of sex in addition to the new expectations of mutuality. All of these factors may serve to intensify the problem of sexual adjustment for couples today.

In the lower socioeconomic groups role segregation is still predominant, clearly defining what role is appropriately male or female. In general the male is still viewed as the head of the household and expects to offer little help in the household tasks and childrearing. The double standard is still more firmly entrenched in the lower class than in the middle class. Further, in families of lower socioeconomic status there is a tendency for men and women to enjoy the company of and rely heavily on a close-knit group of friends and relatives of the same sex.

In general, a larger percentage of the youth in the lower socioeconomic class have intercourse at a younger age than those in the middle class. Boys are expected to engage in sex with girls whenever the opportunity arises. A reputation for "making out" is very valuable within peer groups. Thus, boys must learn patterns of seduction and their ability is then judged by their peers.

Girls, on the other hand, operate under different rules. In some subcultures girls are rated according to their degree of promiscuity. Virgins are highly valued and often protected, especially in Italian, Greek, Spanish, and Portugese societies [11]. Girls who have sex with only one boy may have status, especially if they later marry him. More promiscuous girls are regarded as "easy lays." Overall within these subcultural groups, girls are protected from sexual stimulation, and efforts are made to conceal from them basic facts about sex and their future sexual roles.

According to research done by Rainwater [8, 9], many young black girls in the ghettos are not expected to be virginal unless they are not mature enough or unless they lack the opportunity. The fear of being taken advantage of or getting into trouble, however, may leave them with an ambivalence toward having intercourse. Having sex may also be looked on as a test or symbol of maturity. Pregnancy, however, is seen as the real measure of maturity for the young woman, just as fathering a child confers maturity on boys and young men. If the girl does become pregnant, value is placed on establishing the identity of the father since this confers a form of legitimacy on the birth. Within the black ghetto family many parents feel helpless about adolescent sexual behavior, and, while they do not necessarily have an attitude of acceptance toward illegitimate birth, they are more tolerant of it as a reality of life.

SEXUAL OUTLETS

In all classes, sexual relations within marriage are considered preferable. While masturbation, oral-genital lovemaking, and erotic dreams may release sexual tension, intercourse provides the major sexual outlet for most men and women. As with any facet of a relationship, sexual intercourse becomes entwined in a complex of emotions—love, affection, and companionship, as well as physical attraction.

Historically, in some groups intercourse has been viewed as a husband's pleasure and a wife's duty. Today it is generally recognized that it should be mutually satisfying, thus enhancing intimacy and nurturing a growth of trust between partners. This approach is important, for as Kinsey and associates [6] note, many partners report pain and nervousness following intense arousal that is not followed by orgasm. Two main deterrents to reaching orgasm may be fatigue and preoccupation;

therefore, an awareness of the feelings and responses of the partner is essential in lovemaking.

While biological mechanisms are involved, learning is also required to find optimal patterns of sexual gratification for both partners. It should be kept in mind that everyone at times may experience difficulties of shyness, aversion, or unresponsiveness. During pregnancy when a couple's usual technique becomes uncomfortable for either partner or is no longer satisfying, experimentation may become necessary. Preferable positions may involve them lying on their sides either face to face or with the man entering the woman from the rear.

In addition to varying positions, other techniques may be employed during pregnancy. Oral-genital contact may be used, perhaps for the first time. In talking with an expectant couple, nurses might mention that many couples rely on this technique more frequently during pregnancy, when their usual method is no longer satisfying. Oral-genital contact may be used to achieve orgasm, or it may be used in foreplay to arouse either partner and to maintain or effect an erection in the male.

Masturbation is another technique that is often used during pregnancy, particularly by the male partner. While its use normally begins in childhood and peaks during adolescence, masturbation is very common in the middle and later years. Better educated men, both single and married, tend to masturbate more often than those in the lower socioeconomic class. Women who have difficulty achieving orgasm are advised to try masturbation so that they may learn about their body's responses in a private and relaxed way.

Most authorities now agree that masturbation should be viewed as a normal sexual outlet. This has hardly been the view throughout history, however. To our grandparents it was a sinful perversion that caused warts, impotence, blindness, or even madness. To carry on the battle against masturbation, a public figure named Henry Varlie delivered a lecture in 1833 to an attentive audience. The 3000 men listened as he dealt with onanism, or self-abuse, a practice as common as it was hateful and injurious. He pointed out the results—a low stature, contracted chest, weak lungs, liability to a sore throat, a tendency to cold, indigestion, depression, drowsiness, and idleness. In addition, he declared that disease, decay, and death among young men were chiefly caused by this terrible practice. Needless to say the lecture was a success and was subsequently published in book form. Respected physicians then advocated a treatment—cold showers and exercise in the open air. While all of this hardly changed the public's masturbating practices, it did have an effect on attitudes toward them. Some people still attribute premature ejaculation, impotence, or lassitude to masturbation, but there is no proven direct relationship [1, 13].

While masturbation is considered a normal practice, it can be considered excessive if it becomes the exclusive form of sexual expression when other alternatives are available. It may be used as a conscious substitute for interpersonal love and, in this way, may signify withdrawal, reinforcing timidity about forming social and sexual relationships. When used excessively it may also signify a deeper underlying problem in a relationship, perhaps a breakdown in communication or perhaps the inability of a couple to come to sexual terms with each other. During adolescence excessive masturbation may be a symptom of conflicts such as boredom, frustration, loneliness, poor self-image, school pressures, or conflicts with parents. The adolescent uses masturbation to relieve tension, but the conflicts themselves must be resolved, usually through counseling.

Before nurses can help others cope with their sexual needs, they must be aware of their own sexual values. They must recognize the influences their life experiences have had on their feelings about their own sexuality. Nurses must also be sensitive to others' views on sex and sexuality that may be quite different from their own, and they must respect others' rights to those views. Perhaps most of all, nurses must recognize that people's sexual needs are as important as the more obvious physical needs that are traditionally identified.

REFERENCES

1. Alexander, J. Masturbation as a substitute. *Man and Woman* (Part 27) 2:729, 1972.
2. Auerback, A. The Psychology of Human Sexual Development. In J. G. Howells (Ed.), *Modern Perspectives in Psycho-Obstetrics.* New York: Brunner/Mazel, 1972.
3. Borowitz, E. *Choosing a Sex Ethic (A Jewish Inquiry).* New York: Schocken, 1969.
4. Brenton, M. *The American Male.* New York: Coward-McCann, 1966.
5. Broderick, C. Normal Sociosexual Development. In C. Broderick and J. Bernard (Eds.), *The Individual, Sex, and Society.* Baltimore: Johns Hopkins Press, 1969.
6. Kinsey, A., Pomeroy, W. B., Martin, C. E., and Gebhard, P. H. *Sexual Behavior in the Human Female.* New York: Pocket Books, 1965.
7. Masters, W. H., and Johnson, V. E. *Human Sexual Inadequacy.* Boston: Little, Brown, 1970.
8. Rainwater, L. Crucible of identity: The Negro lower-class family. *Daedalus* 95:172, 1966.
9. Rainwater, L. Sex in the Culture of Poverty. In C. Broderick and J. Bernard (Eds.), *The Individual, Sex, and Society.* Baltimore: Johns Hopkins Press, 1969.
10. Seymour, J. The Importance of Ethics—Moralistic Consideration in Counseling upon Sexual Matters. In H. L. Silverman (Ed.), *Marital Therapy.* Springfield, Ill.: Thomas, 1972.
11. Sjovall, T. The Development of Contraception: Psychodynamic Considerations. In K. Elliott (Ed.), *The Family and Its Future.* London: Churchill, 1970.
12. Thomas, J. L. The Catholic Tradition for Responsibility in Sexual Ethics. In J. C. Wynn (Ed.), *Sexual Ethics and Christian Responsibility.* New York: Association Press, 1970.
13. Toner B. Masturbation—the realities. *Man and Woman* 1:204 (Part 8), 1972.
14. Wynn, J. C. (Ed.). *Sexual Ethics and Christian Responsibility.* New York: Association Press, 1970.

FURTHER READING

Adams, B. *The American Family.* Chicago: Markham, 1971.
Church, J. *Understanding Your Child from Birth to Three.* New York: Random House, 1973.
Comfort, A. (Ed.). *The Joy of Sex.* New York: Crown, 1972.
Goode, W. J. (Ed.). *The Contemporary American Family.* Chicago: Quandrangle, 1971.
Grummon, D., and Barclay, A. (Eds.). *Sexuality: A Search for Perspective.* New York: Van Nostrand Reinhold, 1971.
McCary, J. *Human Sexuality.* Princeton: Van Nostrand, 1967.
Rayner, E. *Human Development.* London: Allen & Unwin, 1971.
Reiss, I. L. *Readings on the Family System.* New York: Holt, Rinehart, & Winston, 1972.
Reiss, I. L. *The Family System in America.* New York: Holt, Rinehart, & Winston, 1971.
Sherman, J. *On the Psychology of Women.* Springfield, Ill.: Thomas, 1971.

Chapter 3 Structure and Function of the Reproductive Organs

STRUCTURE OF FEMALE REPRODUCTIVE ORGANS

The female reproductive organs consist of the external genitalia and internal organs.

External Organs

The female external genital structures are collectively called the *pudenda* or *vulva* and include the mons pubis, labia majora, labia minora, clitoris, and vestibule or pudendal cleft (Figure 3-1).

The most anterior is the *mons pubis* or *mons veneris,* an adipose cushion shaped as an inverted triangle, lying over the anterior surface of the symphysis pubis and covered with pubic hair. Continuous with the mons, two folds of adipose tissue, the *labia majora,* extend downward and merge, forming the *posterior commissure.* The outer surface of the labia majora is covered with hair, while the inner surface appears moist and more delicate. In addition to adipose tissue, the labia majora contain connective tissue rich in elastic fibers, sebaceous glands, and many veins. These veins may become varicosed, which is an important point for the nurse to remember if shaving this area is part of preparation for delivery. In addition, hematomas may develop in the labia following the trauma of delivery. In nulliparous women the labia majora meet at the midline and thus provide some protection for underlying structures. After childbearing, they tend to gape. The labia majora correspond to the scrotum in the male.

The *labia minora* are two thin folds of connective tissue lying beneath the labia majora. Similar in appearance to mucous membrane, they contain sebaceous follicles, occasional sweat glands, a few nonstriated muscle fibers, a rich variety of nerve endings, and many blood vessels that dilate during sexual excitement. Anteriorly, the labia minora are divided into two portions: the upper, which forms the prepuce, or clitoral covering, and the lower, which joins the ventral surface of the clitoris to form the *frenulum clitoridis.* Posteriorly, the labia minora merge at the *fourchette,* located behind the posterior commissure.

The *clitoris* is a projection of erectile tissue, nerves, and blood vessels situated where the labia minora divide anteriorly. Its physiological function is to initiate or intensify levels of sexual tension. It consists of the erectile body, which contains two corpora cavernosa, and the glans, made up of a small mass of erectile tissue fitted over the pointed end of the body and covered with very sensitive epithelium. The clitoris is the equivalent of the male penis.

*Figure 3-1. External
female genitalia.*

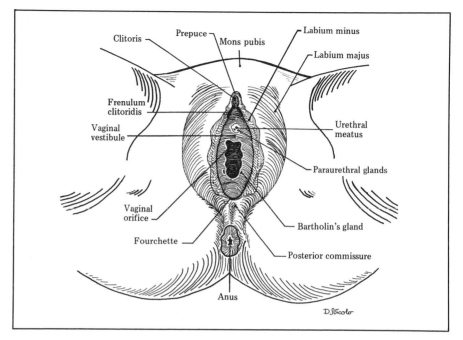

The *vaginal vestibule,* or *pudendal cleft,* is that area bounded by the labia minora and extending from the clitoris to the fourchette. It is perforated by the openings of the urethra, paraurethral glands, vagina, and ducts of Bartholin's glands.

The *urethra* is situated between the clitoris and vagina. Its orifice has the appearance of a vertical slit or of an inverted V with its margins in contact with each other. The openings of the two ducts of the *paraurethral* glands (Skene's glands) are located on each side of the orifice. They are homologous to the male prostate and are particularly susceptible to gonococcal infection.

Two bean-shaped *Bartholin's glands,* similar to the bulbourethral glands in the male, open on either side of the vagina. They produce a mucoid material in response to sexual stimulation, but this is a negligible factor in *primary* vaginal lubrication. They are subject to various infections, including gonorrhea.

Bounded anteriorly by the pubis and posteriorly by the coccyx, the *perineum* has a diamond shape. It can be divided into anterior and posterior regions by a line drawn between the ischial tuberosities. The anterior section is called the urogenital diaphragm, with deep transverse perineal muscles and the urethral sphincter. The posterior portion, referred to as the pelvic diaphragm, forms a sling for the urethra, vagina, and rectum, and provides constrictor action for the vagina and rectum. It contains two main muscle groups: the coccygeal and the levator ani. The levator ani is composed of the iliococcygeal, the pubococcygeal, and puborectal muscles (Figure 3-2).

Another structure found in the posterior portion between the vagina and anus is the *perineal body,* which provides the main support to the pelvic floor. It consists of the levator ani and a number of other muscles, the bulbocavernous, the superficial transverse perineal muscles, and the external sphincter ani, all of which meet mid-

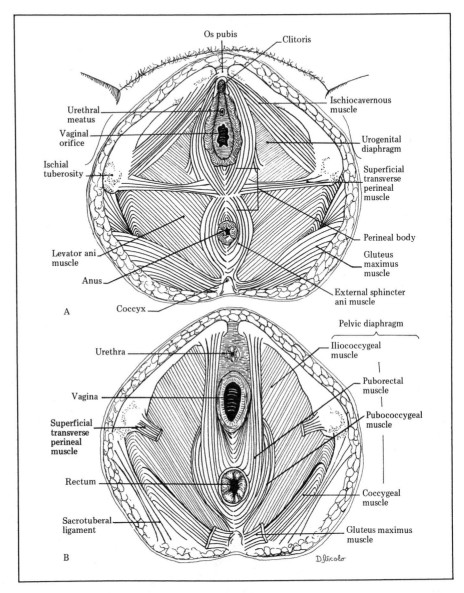

way at the central tendon of the perineum. This is the area most likely to be lacerated while being stretched by the descending fetal head during childbirth. (When the term perineum is used, it commonly refers to the region between the vagina and rectum, even though that region is only a small part of the entire perineal structure.)

The *hymen,* a thin fold of vascularized mucous membrane at the vaginal orifice, separates the internal from the external genital organs. Occasionally it is completely absent or it completely closes the lower end of the vagina, but most often it is centrally perforated. Anatomically, neither its absence nor its presence can be considered a criterion for virginity, although the intact hymen usually ruptures with the first intercourse. After childbearing, the remnants of the hymen form scarlike nodules.

The *vagina* is a relatively insensitive, well-vascularized musculomembranous tube that extends from the vulva to the uterus and lies between the bladder and the rectum. It functions as the excretory duct of the uterus, the female organ of copulation, and part of the birth canal during labor.

The vaginal wall has an outer fibrous coat, a middle muscular layer, and an inner mucous lining corrugated by thick transverse ridges or *rugae*. These are found in the lower part of the vagina, especially in young women, and tend to become obliterated with repeated childbirth. The mucous layer contains considerable glycogen that, when broken down into lactic acid by the action of Döderlein's bacillus, contributes to the acidity of the vagina, particularly in pregnancy (Figure 3-3).

The vagina is directed upward and backward from the vulva, but in the supine position it is directed almost precisely posteriorly. It is approximately 9 centimeters (3½ inches) long, with the posterior wall being longer than the anterior. The upper

Figure 3-3. Side view of female genitourinary anatomy.

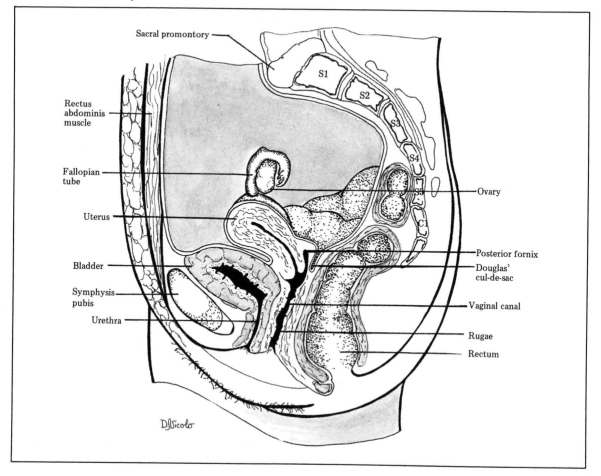

Sacral promontory
S1
S2
S3
S4
Rectus abdominis muscle
Fallopian tube
Uterus
Bladder
Symphysis pubis
Urethra
Ovary
Posterior fornix
Douglas' cul-de-sac
Vaginal canal
Rugae
Rectum

DJNicolo

portion of the posterior wall is separated from the rectum by a deep fold of peritoneum, which forms the *Douglas' cul-de-sac* (or pouch of Douglas).

The upper part of the vagina surrounding the cervix ends in a blind vault which is divided into anterior, posterior, and two lateral *fornices.* Their thin walls allow internal pelvic organs to be easily palpated. The posterior fornix is the deepest and provides surgical access to the peritoneal cavity.

Normally the walls of the vagina lie in contact with each other. The upper portion is easily distended, but the lower vagina, surrounded by the musculature of the pelvic and urogenital diaphragms, offers more resistance.

Glands are normally absent from the vagina, and secretions from the uterus keep the canal moist. The character of the secretions varies with the phase of the menstrual cycle. Before puberty, vaginal pH ranges between 6.8 and 7.2. After puberty, the pH is lowest in midcycle and highest premenstrually, ranging between 3.5 and 4.0. Three to four days before and one day after ovulation, cervical mucus increases in quantity and becomes less viscous; this causes it to be less resistant to penetration by spermatozoa.

The character of vaginal secretions also changes under sexual stimulation. After one-half hour of sexual stimulation without intercourse, the vaginal secretions increase and reach a pH of 4.25 to 4.5 [4]. Droplets of vaginal lubricating material can then be seen throughout the rugal folds of the vagina.

Internal Organs

The female internal reproductive organs include the uterus, fallopian tubes, and ovaries (Figure 3-4).

UTERUS

The uterus, a hollow, thick-walled, muscular organ weighing approximately 60 grams (2 ounces), is located in the pelvic cavity between the bladder and the rectum. Its position is slightly anteflexed over the bladder. It serves for the reception, retention, and nutrition of the fetus.

The pear-shaped upper two-thirds of the uterus is known as the *corpus* (or *body*). The uppermost portion between the insertion of the fallopian tubes is called the *fundus.* At both lateral edges, near the insertion of the fallopian tubes, are two sections called the *cornua.* Pacemakers that initiate uterine contractions and control their rhythm are most often found in these areas. (The cervix, discussed later, forms the lower one-third of the uterus.)

The wall of the corpus is composed of three layers: serous, muscular, and mucous. The serous coat, or *perimetrium,* is a peritoneal covering that is firmly adherent to the outside of the uterus and covers the fundus and most of the body.

The muscular coat, or *myometrium,* is composed of bundles of smooth muscle united by connective tissue containing many elastic fibers. The muscle fibers progressively decrease and the fibrous tissue increases toward the lower uterus. The cervix contains mainly fibrous tissue with a small amount of muscular and elastic tissue; thus, it is firmer and more rigid. The fundus is the most muscular part of the

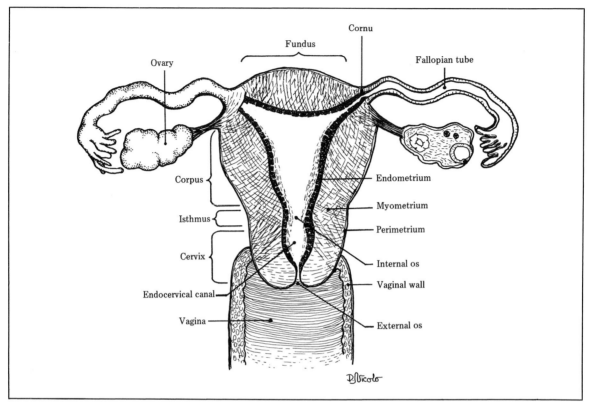

Figure 3-4. Internal female reproductive organs.

uterus. During pregnancy the muscle content of the upper portion of the uterus increases without a similar increase in the cervix.

The myometrium is arranged in three layers, which become more distinct in pregnancy. They include an outer hoodlike layer that covers the fundus and extends to various ligaments, and a thin internal layer consisting of sphincterlike fibers around the openings of the tubes and the internal os of the cervix. Between these two lies a dense network of muscle fibers perforated in all directions by blood vessels. The main portion of the uterine wall is formed by this layer; each of its cells interlaces with the next. After delivery, these cells have the ability to contract and, as a result, constrict blood vessels.

The mucous coat, or *endometrium,* which lines the slitlike uterine cavity, is covered with columnar, partially ciliated epithelium. It is perforated by a large number of minute openings, the mouths of the uterine glands. These glands secrete a thin alkaline fluid that keeps the uterine cavity moist. The endometrium normally varies in thickness, being quite thin after menstruation. It then increases rapidly in thickness and before the next menstrual period contains many convoluted glands and numerous blood vessels.

Knowledge of the arrangement of the blood vessels in the endometrium is of value in understanding certain aspects of female physiology. The uterine and ovarian arteries and their branches carry blood to the uterus. The arterial branches enter the uterine wall at a slant, become parallel to the surface, and are called *arcuate arteries*. From these, *radial arteries* branch out toward the endometrium at sharp angles. Smaller *basal arteries* branch from the radial arteries. The endometrial portions of the radial arteries have a corkscrew appearance and are called *coiled* arteries. The walls of these arteries are very sensitive to hormonal influences, especially those causing vasoconstriction. The coiled arteries are thought to play a part in menstrual bleeding (Figure 3-5).

The position of the uterine artery is of significance, since the uterine artery and the ureter are in close proximity at the level of the internal os. It is at this point that the ureter may be accidentally ligated, injured, or cut during pelvic surgery.

The *isthmus* is the lowermost portion of the uterine body and connects with the supravaginal portion of the cervix. The mucous layer of the isthmus is less complex and less affected by periodic changes of the menstrual cycle. In the last months of pregnancy, the isthmus, normally indicated by a slight uterine constriction, becomes more distinct. During labor it becomes part of the lower uterine segment.

The lower one-third of the uterus, cylindrical in shape and projecting into the upper portion of the vagina, is called the *cervix*. It contains a central spindle-shaped canal, the *endocervical canal,* which communicates with the uterus above and the vagina below. The supravaginal portion contains a small opening, the *internal os;* its lower portion, or vaginal part, contains the *external os*. This lower part is described as having anterior and posterior lips, both of which are usually in contact with the posterior wall of the vagina. If the lips project toward the anterior vaginal wall, the uterus may be retroverted (tipped posteriorly).

The external os varies in appearance from a small oval opening in a nulligravida to a transverse slit following childbirth. The cervix of the nulligravida feels like the tip of the nose, whereas in the gravid woman, it feels softer, like the ear lobe or lips.

The cervix is basically composed of connective tissue, some smooth muscle fibers, elastic tissue, and many blood vessels. Peripherally, the cervix contains circular muscle fibers that connect with the uterine myometrium above. The mucosa of the endocervical canal is composed of columnar epithelium. Mucous cells of this epithelium furnish the thick tenacious secretions of the cervical canal. Occasionally the endocervical glands become occluded and result in the so-called nabothian cysts.

Ligaments.   Ligaments extend from the sides of the uterus and give it support. The principal ligaments around the uterus are the broad, round, and uterosacral ligaments (Figure 3-6).

The *broad ligaments* are two winglike structures that extend from the lateral margins of the uterus to the pelvic walls and divide the pelvic cavity into anterior and posterior sections. Each broad ligament consists of a fold of peritoneum containing several structures. The inner two-thirds serves as an attachment for the fallopian tubes, while the outer one-third forms the *suspensory ligament* of the ovary and contains the ovarian blood vessels. The broad ligament allows anterior-posterior movement of the uterus but opposes lateral motion. The lower portion of this ligament is thickened; it is continuous with the connective tissue of the pelvic floor. The most dense portion, the *cardinal ligament,* is firmly united to the upper

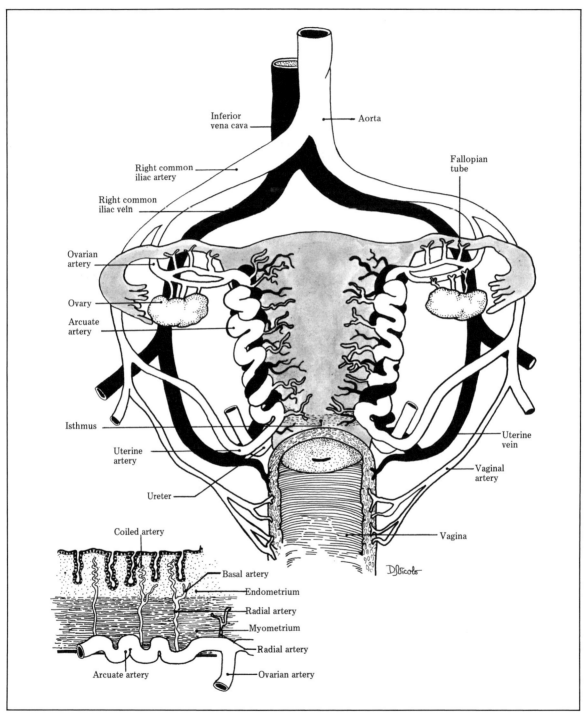

Figure 3-5. Blood supply to the vagina, uterus, fallopian tubes, and ovaries.

Figure 3-6. Ligaments supporting the uterus in the pelvic cavity.

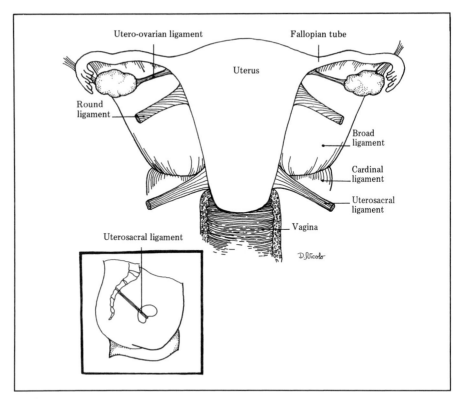

portion of the cervix and lateral margins of the uterus. It encloses the uterine vessels and ureters and offers base support to the uterus.

The *round ligaments* are fibromuscular cords which arise from the lateral surface of the uterus below the insertion of the fallopian tubes. Each runs outward and upward in a fold of peritoneum continuous with the broad ligament. They pass through the inguinal canal and terminate in the labia majora. Their function is to help maintain the uterus in its anteflexed position.

The *uterosacral ligaments* originate from the upper posterior portion of the cervix and insert into the fascia over the second and third sacral vertebrae. They aid in keeping the uterus in its normal position, exerting traction on the cervix and pulling it into the posterior fornix.

Ligament support causes the usual position of the uterus to be slightly anteflexed. In a standing woman, the uterus is almost horizontal, with the fundus resting on the bladder. Distention of the bladder and/or rectum can influence uterine position. While the body of the uterus is free to move anteriorly and posteriorly, the cervix is anchored by the cardinal and uterosacral ligaments.

Nerve Supply.   The uterus is innervated principally from the sympathetic nervous system and also from the parasympathetic and central nervous systems. The sympathetic fibers maintain uterine tone by stimulating muscle contraction and promoting vasoconstriction. Stimulation from the parasympathetics has an opposing effect by inhibiting uterine muscle contraction and promoting vasodilatation. Action of the parasympathetics allows for intermittent uterine contractions.

The eleventh and twelfth thoracic nerve roots carry sensory fibers from the uterus, transmitting the pain of uterine contractions to the central nervous system. Motor fibers going to the uterus leave the spinal cord at the seventh and eighth thoracic vertebrae. The separation of the motor and sensory levels permits the use of epidural and spinal anesthesia in labor.

FALLOPIAN TUBES

The fallopian tubes are a pair of ducts, richly supplied with elastic tissue, which convey oocytes to the cavity of the uterus. Except for a distal portion, they are enclosed in a fold of peritoneum known as the *mesosalpinx*. The tubes, approximately 11 centimeters ($4\frac{1}{2}$ inches) long, are divided into four sections: the interstitial portion, isthmus, ampulla, and infundibulum.

The *interstitial portion* is found within the anterolateral wall of the uterus and is the most muscular section of the tube. Immediately adjacent to the interstitial segment is the straight, narrow *isthmus.* The *ampulla,* continuous with the isthmus, is the longest and widest portion of the tube; it is there that fertilization takes place. The ampulla ends in the *infundibulum,* or *fimbriated end,* the funnel-shaped outer portion of the tube that extends into the abdominal cavity. The lining of the infundibulum contains folds continuous with those of the ampulla, and it is these folds that give the end of the tube its fimbriated appearance. The longest fold reaches toward the tubal pole of the ovary. It is believed to aid in conducting the ovum from the ruptured follicle into the lumen of the tube.

The tubal structure is composed of several layers of tissue. The outside covering is peritoneum, beneath which is a tissue coat containing nerves and many blood vessels. Next, the muscle layer is divided into outer longitudinal and deeper, thicker circular fibers. These undergo constant rhythmic contractions, which are weakest during pregnancy and strongest during the transport of ova. The mucous lining of the tube contains ciliated and nonciliated epithelium. The current created by the cilia in both the fallopian tubes and the uterus flows from the fimbriated ends, where the cilia are most abundant, to the external os of the uterus. During the menstrual cycle the mucosal lining undergoes growth associated with increased secretory activity. Occasionally diverticula extend through the mucosal lining into the muscular wall; these diverticula may possibly contribute to the development of ectopic or extrauterine pregnancies.

OVARIES

The ovaries are two small, almond-shaped organs having the dual function of ovum development and hormone production. In the adult, the organs are connected with the broad ligament of the uterus by a peritoneal fold called the *mesovarium.* The ovaries are supported by two additional ligaments running within the broad ligament. The ovarian ligament connects one pole of the ovary to the uterus, while the suspensory ligament, containing the ovarian vessels and nerves, connects the opposite pole of the ovary to the lateral pelvic wall. The ovaries receive their blood supply from the ovarian arteries, which branch off the aorta below the renal arteries.

The exterior of the ovaries varies in appearance with age. In young women it is smooth with small clear follicles; in the mature woman, more corrugated; in the elderly woman, markedly convoluted.

The ovary is composed of an outer zone, the cortex, and an inner zone, the medulla. The *cortex* varies in thickness with age, becoming thin with advancing years. It contains connective tissue cells and fibers, among which are scattered ovarian follicles in various stages of development. Of the 300,000 primary oocytes present at birth, the majority degenerate without reaching maturity. The outermost portion of the cortex, the *tunica albuginea,* appears dull and white. The ovarian *medulla,* or central portion, is composed of loose connective tissue and contains a large number of arteries and veins, nerve fibers, and a small number of smooth muscle fibers.

Breasts

The breasts are generally considered accessory glands of reproduction. Their growth and function involves the coordinated functioning of the nervous system, reproductive system, and hormones. The breasts are composed of a mass of glandular tissue and are supported by fibrous tissue; they contain a thick layer of fat and many blood vessels (Figure 3-7).

The *nipple,* located near the center of the breast, contains a considerable number of muscle fibers and a rich nerve supply. The nipple is an erectile organ by virtue of muscle contraction and vascular engorgement; it becomes firmer and more prominent as a result of stimulation. Surrounding the nipple is a thin, pigmented, circular area of skin, the *areola,* which contains roughened elevations that represent sebaceous glands (Montgomery's tubercles or Montgomery's glands).

Each breast contains a network of ducts, which branch into a network of alveolar units. The *alveoli* are sacs made up of a layer of secretory cells (*acini cells*) surrounded by a covering of myoepithelial cells that contract to force milk into the duct system in response to stimulation. A group of alveoli makes up a *lobule,* and a group of lobules makes up each of the 15–20 *lobes* of the breast. Intralobular ducts from the alveoli lead to lactiferous ducts and then widen to form *lactiferous sinuses* or milk reservoirs behind the areola. Then, becoming constricted once more, some 8–15 of the ducts open on the surface of the nipple. Lymph vessels in the breast are numerous and, for the most part, join the lymph nodes of the axilla. The majority of lymph vessels follow the lactiferous ducts and converge toward the nipple, joining a plexus under the areola.

Breast size depends largely on the amount of superficial fat, but also on the amount of glandular tissue present. The amount of glandular tissue is very small in women who are not lactating. Therefore, breast size alone is not a good predictor of a woman's future ability to produce an adequate milk supply. Developments at

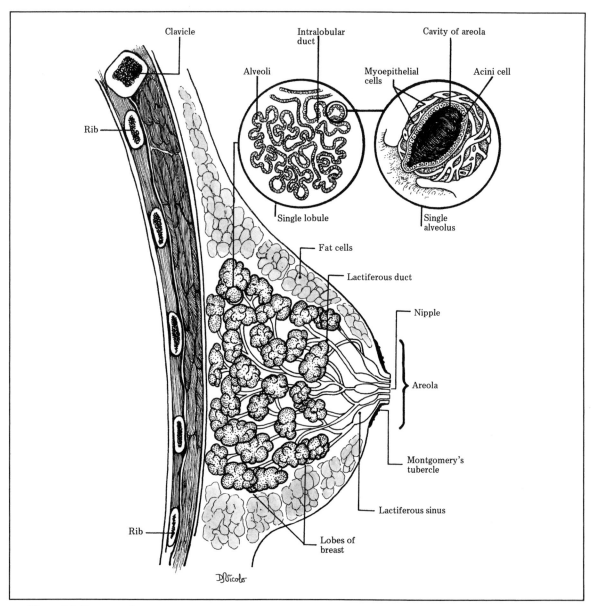

*Figure 3-7. Breast and
    ductal system.*

puberty include increasing amounts of ovarian hormones, a conspicuous growth and branching of the ductal system, and extensive depositing of fat in the breasts. A characteristic differentiation of glands occurs in pregnancy. Breast tissue atrophies at the time of menopause.

FUNCTION OF THE FEMALE REPRODUCTIVE ORGANS

A woman's reproductive function has a specific beginning and end. *Puberty* represents the beginning of reproductive life, and the climacteric, or *menopause,* represents its ending. Puberty covers a time span during which many maturational changes are taking place, including a rapid change in size and shape of the body, maturation of the gonads and the reproductive tract, and the development of secondary sexual characteristics.

While a growth spurt begins at approximately 8 years of age, most growth occurs between the ages of 10 and 15, when fatty deposits develop on the hips and shoulders. The breasts and pubic hair begin to develop at about the same time, between the ages of 8 and 13, and axillary hair will develop about two years later. Menarche (the beginning of menstruation) usually occurs between the ages of 10 and 14, although a wider age range (9–17 years) would be considered normal. The average age of menarche in the United States is now $12\frac{1}{2}$ years [6]. Over the past 100 years, the onset of menstruation in this country has been occuring at a progressively earlier age, as a result, according to some, of the better nutrition of American youth. More recent findings indicate that the decline in the age of menarche has ended [5]. There are variations in the timing of all the above processes, but the sequence remains the same. It is not known what changes initiate puberty, but current theory suggests that hypothalamic maturation is necessary. Following this, the pituitary is stimulated to release follicle-stimulating hormone (FSH) and luteinizing hormone (LH). The gonads and adrenals respond by producing steroid hormones, which influence the growth and development at puberty. A knowledge of the functioning of these steroid and pituitary hormones is essential to an understanding of their roles in the menstrual cycle and in reproduction.

Pituitary Hormones

The pituitary hormones include FSH, LH, and prolactin. *FSH,* a glycoprotein, is produced and secreted by the anterior pituitary in response to a releasing factor from the hypothalamus. This substance travels to the pituitary via the hypophyseal-portal system.

FSH release is influenced by the level of estrogen or by neurological impulses from higher brain centers. In the absence of estrogen, FSH-releasing factor is uncontrolled, and FSH is secreted in larger amounts. This situation occurs after surgical removal of the ovaries or after menopause. Levels of FSH can be reduced by administration of exogenous estrogens.

Functions of FSH include stimulation of ovarian follicle growth and ovarian estrogen production. However, hormone production and ovulation will not occur unless LH is also present. The FSH level fluctuates throughout the menstrual cycle, with its peak in the middle of the cycle. The level remains low throughout pregnancy, reflecting pituitary inactivity.

LH, also a glycoprotein, is produced and secreted by the anterior pituitary by the same mechanism as that of FSH. Release of LH is regulated by feedback effects of steroid hormones (estrogen or progesterone) on the hypothalamus. Neural impulses may also affect FSH and LH gonadotropin levels by being channeled into the hypothalamus from other areas of the brain as a result of changes in the internal or external environment. Therefore, such factors as light or emotional state can influence reproductive function.

Levels of LH are low in childhood and gradually rise to a plateau at puberty. In the mature female there is a midcycle surge just before ovulation. The administration of estrogen and/or progesterone can inhibit the midcycle surges of LH and FSH; this forms the basis of action of oral contraceptives.

Early in the menstrual cycle LH, in association with FSH, causes changes in the ovarian theca and granulosa cells; these changes result in estrogen production. LH is instrumental in causing the fully developed follicle to rupture when the proper ratio of LH to FSH develops. It initiates the formation of the corpus luteum, which responds to LH by increased hormone secretion. LH is responsible for the accumulation in granulosa cells of cholesterol or cholesterol-like substances, which are apparently the precursors of progesterone.

Prolactin is a pituitary protein also known as mammotropin, luteotropin, or lactogenic hormone. While prolactin has not been isolated in pure form in humans, its activity stimulates milk formation in mammalian species when the breasts have been primed by prior quantities of estrogen, progesterone, and adrenal steroids. High doses of estrogen and/or progesterone will prevent the release of prolactin, whereas suckling and estrogen in low doses stimulate its release. In addition to stimulating the production of milk, prolactin facilitates breast growth through development of the lobulo-alveolar structures.

Ovarian Hormones

The ovarian hormones are estrogen and progesterone. *Estrogens,* the hormones of femininity, are responsible for the development and maintenance of female secondary sexual characteristics. Both men and women have circulating estrogens and androgens. The relative amount of androgens determines body type, breast development, hair growth, and reproductive activity. An imbalance of androgens in women can interfere with estrogen production and the response of the target organ to the hormone.

Estrogens are steroid growth hormones that have a specific effect on tissues derived from the müllerian ducts: the fallopian tubes, endometrium, the musculature of the uterine body, and the cervix. Estradiol, the most active estrogenic substance, is the principal ovarian secretory product and precursor of many urinary estrogen metabolites. In the ovary it is produced by the thecal cells of the follicle and the luteinized granulosal cells of the corpus luteum. During pregnancy estradiol is also produced by the placenta. In addition to estradiol, there are other natural estrogens, estrone and estriol, as well as a number of synthetic estrogens.

In the mature female, blood levels of estradiol and excretion of urinary metabolites have two peaks during the menstrual cycle: at ovulation (approximately day 14) and at the height of the luteal phase (approximately day 21). During the four to five days prior to the next menstrual period, estrogen secretion decreases rapidly. The estrogen levels rise progressively in pregnancy. The majority of urinary estrogen in pregnancy is estriol. Estrogens are found in the amniotic fluid and in the fetal circulation in higher concentrations than those found in the maternal circulation.

Estrogens affect a number of tissues in specific ways.

1. *Vagina:* The vaginal epithelium changes from a thin, columnar layer to a multi-layered structure.
2. *Cervix:* Under the influence of estrogen, the cervix increases in size and vascularity and develops mucous glands. The cervical mucus increases in quantity, increases in pH, becomes less viscous, and is more readily penetrated by spermatozoa. Microscopically, the dried mucus assumes the pattern of a fern (Figure 3-8).
3. *Uterus:* Estrogens cause proliferation of endometrial glands and blood vessels, hypertrophy of the myometrium, and an increase in electrical and contractile activities.
4. *Fallopian tubes:* The fallopian tubes are dependent on estrogen for their contractility, secretion, and function, since estrogens cause the mucosal lining and musculature to develop.
5. *Ovary:* Estradiol exerts a local effect, stimulating growth of the ovarian follicle even in the absence of FSH. It potentiates ovarian response to pituitary gonadotropins.
6. *Breasts:* Growth and development of the nipple, areola, and breast ducts occur under the influence of estrogens.
7. *Endocrine glands*
   a. Pituitary: Effects of estrogen on the pituitary have already been discussed (see p. 33).
   b. Thyroid: Serum thyroid-binding globulin is increased, resulting in an increased protein-bound iodine level.
   c. Adrenal: Estrogens cause a decrease in adrenal hormone metabolism but lengthen the half-life of the adrenal steroids in the blood.

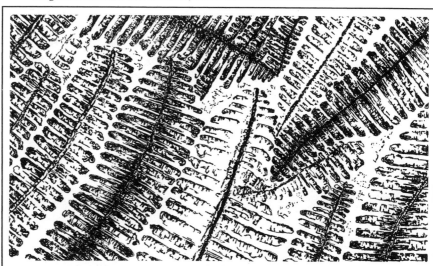

Figure 3-8. Diagram of fern pattern seen on microscopic examination of cervical mucus at midcycle in normal menstruating women.

8. *Skeletal system:* Increased estrogen levels in young girls lead to premature epiphyseal closure, and estrogens can have a positive influence on the calcium balance, upon which bone integrity depends.
9. *Skin:* The estrogens are responsible for an increase in skin pigmentation, particularly in the breast areola.

Progesterone has been described as the hormone of pregnancy. Unlike estrogen, it has no primary growth-initiating effect but rather affects tissues already under the influence of estrogen. Progesterone is responsible for the uterine endometrial and myometrial changes that permit and maintain implantation, and it contributes to decreased uterine contractility.

The major sources of progesterone are the corpus luteum and, in pregnancy, the placenta, and it can also be produced in the adrenal gland and the ovarian follicle. The main metabolite of progesterone is pregnanediol. Its presence varies with the phase of the menstrual cycle. During the follicular phase, the urinary pregnanediol levels and blood progesterone levels are barely detectable. Progesterone blood levels peak approximately one week after ovulation and formation of the corpus luteum. Progestins (synthetic forms of progesterone) act synergistically with estrogen to inhibit hypothalamic stimulation of pituitary gonadotropin production and release.

Progesterone affects a number of tissues in specific ways.

1. *Vagina:* Under the influence of progesterone, the vaginal lining decreases in thickness.
2. *Cervix:* Progesterone causes the secretions of the cervix to become scanty, more viscous, and impermeable to spermatozoa. The ferning pattern is absent when the dried mucus is viewed microscopically.
3. *Uterus:* The *endometrium* changes from a proliferative to a secretory type. Changes in the uterine glands reflect increased tortuosity, glycogen deposits, and evidence of secretion. Likewise, blood vessels proliferate, becoming more tortuous and coiled. The above changes are conducive to proper nutrition for the implantation and retention of the ovum.

   The *myometrial* and *smooth muscle* contractions are milder and less frequent. This action is partially responsible for the uterine ability to retain the growing fetus without expulsion prior to term.
4. *Breasts:* Progesterone causes growth of the acini cells and lobules, preparing them for lactation.
5. *Central nervous system:* Through action at the level of the hypothalamus, progesterone causes the increase in body temperature that occurs after ovulation.
6. *Renal:* Research suggests that progesterone causes an increase in aldosterone secretion with a resulting retention of water and electrolytes. The mechanisms of action remain unclear [3].

Reproductive Cycle

The reproductive cycle is dependent on constant harmonious interactions among the central nervous system, the pituitary gland, and the reproductive tract. In the mature woman, the reproductive structures undergo a series of changes that is repeated approximately every 28 days. This 28-day cycle has three phases. The first, or *menstrual* phase, is the period of active bleeding. It is followed by the *proliferative* phase (or *follicular* phase), during which the ovarian primordial follicles, which contain the oocytes, mature. This is also known as the estrogenic phase because estrogen is the primary female steroid produced during this period. The third, or *secretory,* phase includes the formation of the corpus luteum and its secretion of estrogen and progesterone. This is also referred to as the *luteal* or *progestational* phase. The menstrual and proliferative phases of the cycle precede ovulation.

MENSTRUAL PHASE

The onset of vaginal bleeding designates the first day of the menstrual phase and also the first day of the 28-day menstrual cycle. During the preceding secretory phase, the endometrium has developed into three distinct layers: the zona basalis (next to the myometrium), the zona spongiosa, and the zona compacta (the outermost layer). Menstrual bleeding follows the degeneration of the spongiosa and compacta endometrial layers resulting from the congestion of blood vessels and formation of small hematomas. Approximately 4–24 hours before the onset of bleeding, the coiled arteries become constricted, which causes these two layers to receive an inadequate supply of blood. Following the period of vasoconstriction, the coiled arteries relax, hemorrhage ensues, and the degenerated compacta and spongiosa layers slough off. Menstrual bleeding, which is mostly arterial, lasts for three to five days. A wide variation exists in duration and amount of bleeding, although the average amount is 50–150 milliliters.

PROLIFERATIVE PHASE

The nine-day proliferative phase follows the period of menstrual bleeding. During this portion of the cycle, ovarian primordial follicles, which contain the oocytes, are stimulated by pituitary FSH and LH and ovulation occurs. During each cycle one mature follicle (graafian follicle) makes its way to the surface of the ovary. The follicle consists of an ovum surrounded by a layer of granulosa cells. The granulosa cells are enveloped by circles of specialized stromal cells, the *theca interna,* and a layer of less differentiated cells, the *theca externa*. It is believed that the granulosa supply the ova with nutritional stores and developmental information. The theca interna is the site of estrogen formation.

The increase in follicle size is accomplished by development of a fluid-filled cavity, the *antrum,* as well as by granulosa cell proliferation. As the fluid cavity enlarges, the ovum is pushed to one side, surrounded by a mass of granulosa cells, the *cumulus oophorous,* with which it is discharged at the time of rupture. While the follicle is still very small, a clear elastic membrane, the *zona pellucida,* envelops the ovum. It probably persists until after the ovum has reached the uterus. Attached to the zona pellucida is a single layer of granulosa cells, called the *corona radiata*. The corona radiata remains with the ovum after ovulation but must be separated before fertilization can take place (Figure 3-9).

At maturity the follicle protrudes above the surface of the ovary. The point of rupture and subsequent discharge of the ovum becomes very thin and is known as the *stigma*. Actual rupture occurs gradually and is probably caused by increased

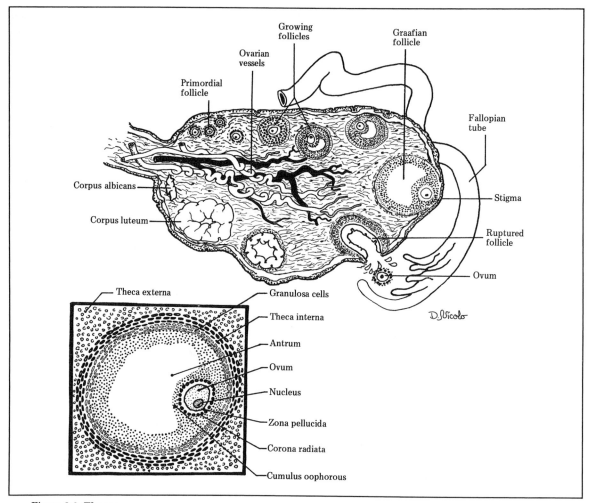

Figure 3-9. The ovary, showing maturation and release of ovum. Inset (in box) shows a developing graafian follicle.

distensibility and local enzymatic destruction of the follicular wall. Usually only one follicle ruptures each month. Many, however, reach the halfway point and then regress.

Estrogen secretion begins on day one of the menstrual cycle and reaches a peak just before the preovulatory surge of FSH and LH, which presumably triggers ovulation. The estrogen levels decline just prior to or with ovulation, but increase again in the next half of the cycle. Progesterone is present at low levels prior to ovulation and is secreted by both the ovary and adrenal gland. During the proliferative phase, the endometrium responds to increased estrogen levels by general thickening of the endometrial layers and elongation and coiling of the glands.

OVULATION

There is marked variability in the length of menstrual cycles. Researchers report that 95 percent of all cycles are between 15 and 45 days long, with an average of 28 days [1]. Ovulation marks the midpoint of a 28-day cycle. Since in any cycle ovulation occurs approximately 14 days before the first day of the next menses, the secretory phase is relatively constant in length.

Ovulation can be detected in a number of ways. Approximately 25 percent of all women experience *mittelschmerz,* or pain in the lower abdomen on or about the day of ovulation. It is thought to result from peritoneal irritation by fluid or blood escaping from the ruptured follicle. During or just after ovulation, increased levels of progesterone cause a rise in body temperature. (This temperature pattern forms the basis for the rhythm method of contraception.) Cervical mucus increases in amount and changes from an opaque to a clear substance, with decreased viscosity. Due to the high estrogen levels at the time of ovulation, cervical mucus forms a ferning pattern microscopically. The demonstration by biopsy of a secretory endometrium is a strong indication that ovulation has occurred. Another means of determining that ovulation has occurred is the demonstration of an increase in serum progesterone.

Detection of ovulation is important in order to facilitate or avoid conception. Since the life spans of the sperm and ovum are limited, fertilization must take place within about 24 hours after ovulation if conception is to occur.

SECRETORY PHASE

The secretory phase begins around the time of ovulation. It is characterized by increased progesterone secretion, corpus luteum formation, and further endometrial development. About the middle of the secretory phase, estrogen reaches a second peak in the menstrual cycle.

The *corpus luteum,* or yellow body, is formed by the collapsed follicle. The follicle initially fills with blood that is replaced by lipid-rich luteal cells. The theca and granulosa cells left behind in the ovary proliferate and, together with the luteal cells, form the corpus luteum. The corpus luteum produces large quantities of progesterone and some estrogen. The unique feature of the corpus luteum is its limited life span, thereby limiting the secretory phase of the menstrual cycle to a more constant period. After an average life of 10–14 days, the luteal cells degenerate, causing a withdrawal of estrogen and progesterone. These cells are replaced by connective tissue, forming the *corpus albicans.* If, however, fertilization occurs, the corpus luteum remains active during the first trimester of pregnancy.

During this phase the endometrium becomes markedly increased in thickness and extremely vascular, succulent, and rich in glycogen. The endometrial arteries are more coiled and closer to the endometrial surface, making an ideal site for implantation and growth of the fertilized ovum.

Other signs of increased serum progesterone and corpus luteum formation include breast tenderness, fluid retention, and the symptoms of premenstrual tension.

OOGENESIS

Gametogenesis is the term applied to the process by which primordial or primitive germ cells are transformed to mature germ cells, or *gametes.* In females, primitive germ cells, called oogonia, are transformed through reduction division into the mature oocyte. The essential biological feature of gametogenesis is this reduction division or meiotic cellular division. *Meiosis,* characterized by a long and unusual prophase, results in the reduction of the diploid number of chromosomes, 46 in humans, to the haploid number of 23. Each mature oocyte contains the haploid number of chromosomes, with 22 autosomes and one sex chromosome (the X chromosome) (Figure 3-10).

In the first of the two maturation divisions, the *primary oocyte* undergoes an early meiotic or reduction division. In the process of division, one daughter cell receives the majority of the cytoplasm plus 23 chromosomes and is called the *secondary*

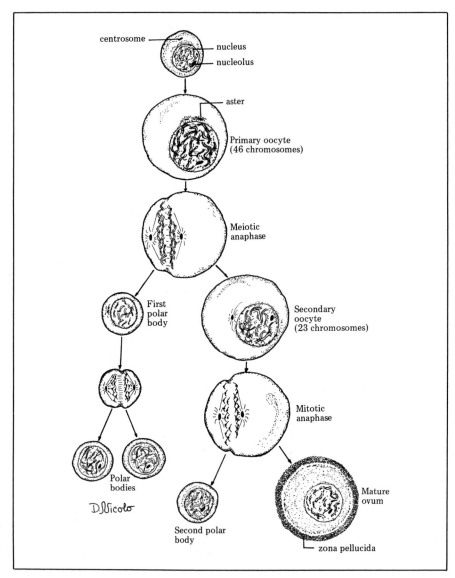

Figure 3-10. Maturation of female reproductive cells, resulting in formation of one mature ovum.

oocyte. The other daughter cell receives 23 chromosomes but little cytoplasm, and is referred to as the *first polar body.* This reduction division is thought to occur immediately prior to ovulation.

If fertilization occurs, the secondary occyte is capable of completing a second maturation division, this one mitotic in nature. Again, both daughter cells contain 23 chromosomes. One daughter cell receives the majority of the cytoplasm and is called the *mature ovum.* The other daughter cell, which receives little cytoplasm, is called the *second polar body.*

The mature ovum differs from typical cells because of its large size and protective envelope, the zona pellucida. Another important difference is that, under ordinary circumstances, the mature ovum is incapable of further cell division because it possesses no centrosome—a deficiency that is corrected by the spermatozoon if fertilization occurs. If the secondary oocyte does not meet with a spermatozoon, it degenerates or passes through the genital passages and is cast off and lost.

STRUCTURE OF THE MALE REPRODUCTIVE ORGANS

The male reproductive organs include external and internal structures (Figure 3-11).

External Organs

The external organs of the male consist of the penis and the scrotum. The *penis* is the male organ of copulation; it is attached to the anterior and lateral walls of the pubic arch and lies in front of the scrotum. The skin of the penis is thin, highly pigmented, and freely moveable. It is covered with hair only at the base.

Structurally, the penis is composed chiefly of cavernous (erectile) tissue, and it contains the urethra. The engorgement of cavernous tissue with blood produces a considerable enlargement of the penis and its erection. Two longitudinal columns of erectile tissue, the *corpora cavernosa,* are located laterally. They are spongelike, contain large venous sinuses, and form the chief bulk of the organ. The *corpus spongiosum* (or *corpus cavernosum urethrae*) is the smaller third longitudinal column, which is also composed of erectile tissue. It is centrally located beneath the corpora cavernosa and contains the urethra. Toward the distal end of the penis, the corpus spongiosum expands, and, spreading toward the dorsal surface, forms a cap, the *glans penis.* This covers the conical end of the united corpora cavernosa and contains the urethral orifice. Overhanging the glans is the *prepuce,* a fold of loose skin. (This foreskin is removed in circumcision.) The penis receives its blood supply from the internal pudendal arteries and its nerve supply from the pudendal nerve and pelvic sympathetic plexus.

The *scrotum* is a pouchlike continuation of the abdominal wall located behind the penis. It is divided by a septum into two sacs, each containing and supporting one of the testes and its epididymis. The scrotum is more pigmented than the rest of the body and is covered with sparse hair. In the subcutaneous tissue of the scrotum are small muscle fibers, the *tunica dartos,* which contract with decreased temperature

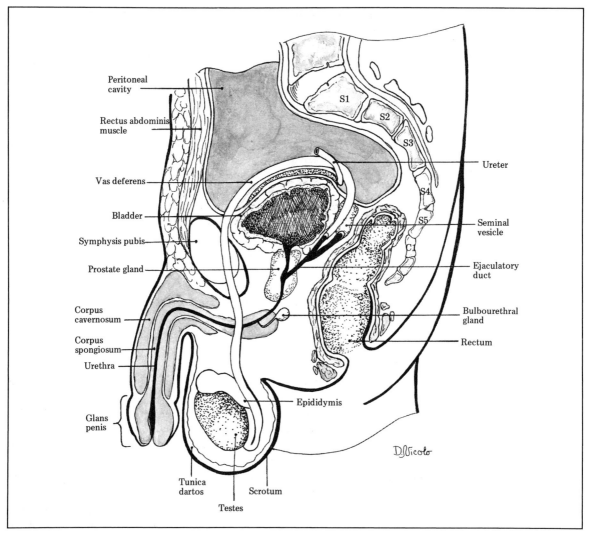

Figure 3-11. Side view of male genitourinary anatomy.

and give a more wrinkled appearance to the scrotum. This response causes the testes to assume a position closer to the perineum, where they absorb body heat and maintain a temperature compatible with the viability of spermatozoa. Under normal temperature conditions, the fibers are relaxed and the scrotum is pendulous and free from wrinkles. In the adult, the temperature in the scrotal sac is about 2° C (5° F) lower than that in the abdomen. This lower temperature is essential for the production of sperm. If the testes are kept at an elevated temperature for long periods of time (as with prolonged high fever or undescended testes), sterility may result.

A serous membrane, the *tunica vaginalis,* lines the walls of the scrotal sac. It resembles the peritoneum in structure and appearance. The scrotum, like the penis, receives its blood supply from the internal pudendal arteries.

Internal Organs

The internal male reproductive organs are the gonads or testes, a series of ducts (the epididymis, the vas deferens, and the urethra), and accessory glands (the seminal vesicles, the prostate, and the bulbourethral or Cowper's glands). The spermatic cords are internal supporting structures.

The *testes,* a pair of nearly symmetrical oval bodies situated in the scrotum, are the reproductive glands of the male that correspond to the ovaries in the female. They are covered by a dense, white, inelastic fibrous tissue called the *tunica albuginea.* Inside, fibrous septa extend into the testis and divide it into about 250 wedge-shaped lobes. Each lobe contains one to four narrow coiled tubes, the *seminiferous tubules,* which, if uncoiled, would measure about 60 centimeters (24 inches) in length. Male reproductive cells (spermatogonia) at different stages of development are found within these tubules. Smooth musclelike cells in the walls of the tubules cause tubular contraction. This contraction is thought to promote transport of spermatozoa and fluid within the tubules toward the *rete testis,* a network of larger straight ducts. About 20 small coiled ductules leave the upper end of the rete testis, perforate the tunica albuginea, and enter the head of the epididymis (Figure 3-12).

In addition to reproductive cells, rather large *Sertoli's cells* are found within the testis. Spermatids (developing reproductive cells) attach themselves to the Sertoli's cells, which may provide the spermatids with nutrient material, hormones, or enzymes necessary for their maturation into spermatozoa. The *interstitial cells of Leydig* are also scattered among the tubules and are responsible for the production of male hormones.

The ductules leaving the testis open into the *epididymis,* a single convoluted duct that ends in the vas deferens. The epididymis is a tube nearly 5 meters (16 feet) long that is coiled into a space of about 4 centimeters (1½ inches) on the posterior aspect of the testis.

The *vas deferens* (*ductus deferens*), the excretory duct of the testis, is a direct continuation of the duct of the epididymis. It ends, after a course of about 46 centimeters (18 inches), by joining with the duct of the seminal vesicle to form the ejaculatory duct. The peristaltic activity of its middle muscular layer is responsible for the passage of sperm along the duct. The vas deferens, together with nerves, lymphatics, and blood vessels, form the *spermatic cord.*

The *ejaculatory duct* is approximately 2.5 centimeters (1 inch) long, penetrates the base of the prostate gland, and opens into the prostatic portion of the urethra. It ejects sperm and seminal vesicle fluid into the urethra.

The *urethra* is the last connecting link from the testis to the exterior. It is supplied with mucus derived from a large number of small glands located along its entire length, and also from the large bilateral bulbourethral glands, or Cowper's glands, located near its origin.

Accessory Glands of Reproduction

The *seminal vesicles* are two membranous pouchlike tubes lying behind the base of the bladder. The tube of each vesicle ends in a straight narrow duct, joining the vas deferens to form the ejaculatory duct.

Figure 3-12. Male ductal system and developing reproductive cells. Enlargement on right shows cross section of seminiferous tubule and spermatogenesis.

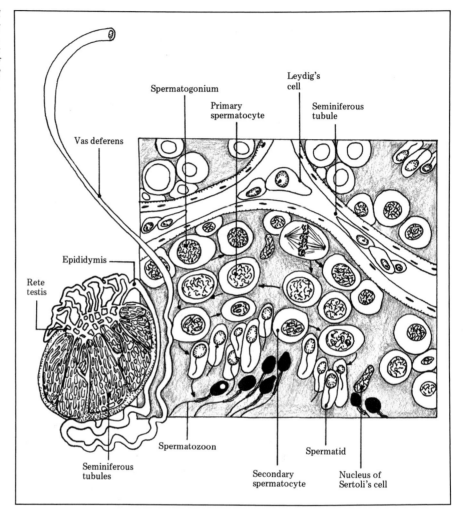

The seminal vesicles are lined with secretory epithelium. The mucoid secretion contains much fructose, small amounts of ascorbic acid, inositol, ergothioneine, five of the amino acids, phosphoryl choline, and prostaglandins. During ejaculation, the seminal vesicle empties its contents into the ejaculatory duct while the vas deferens empties sperm. The seminal vesicle secretion adds bulk to the ejaculated semen. The fructose and other substances in the fluid probably provide nutrients and protection for the ejaculated sperm. Research suggests that prostaglandins may promote uterine contractions that help propel sperm toward the fallopian tubes [2].

The *prostate gland* is a chestnut-sized conical structure that surrounds the first several centimeters of the urethra. During ejaculation, the capsule of the prostate contracts simultaneously with contractions of the vas deferens and seminal vesicles, adding its thin, milky, alkaline fluid to the bulk of the semen. The alkalinity is important in fertilization, since the relatively acid fluid of the vas deferens may inhibit sperm fertility. It also helps to neutralize the acid vaginal secretions and enhance sperm motility.

The *bulbourethral glands* (*Cowper's glands*) are pea-sized structures found beneath the prostate on either side of the urethra. They contribute alkaline fluid to the semen.

FUNCTION OF THE MALE REPRODUCTIVE ORGANS

As in the female, puberty evokes a rapid growth spurt and many maturational changes in the male. At about age 10 a young man's testes, prostate, seminal vesicles, and penis begin to enlarge. By age 11, axillary sweating and odor appear, followed by pubic hair at 13, and enlarged larynx, axillary hair, and hair on the upper lip by 14. The average age at which boys acquire the ability to produce and ejaculate spermatozoa is 15, but it is not abnormal to find a range of 9 to 17 years. By age 18 the shoulders have broadened and the muscles have hypertrophied. At age 21 practically all skeletal growth has stopped.

During puberty the pituitary gland is stimulated to release FSH and LH (interstitial cell stimulating hormone). FSH facilitates the production of spermatozoa, while LH acts on the Leydig cells of the testis to release androgens. The level of these androgens serves as a feedback mechanism to regulate the amount of LH secreted from the pituitary.

Of these androgens, *testosterone* is the most significant male hormone. It is formed by the interstitial cells of Leydig, which lie in spaces between the seminiferous tubules. These cells are active in the fetus and the newborn, possibly due to stimulation by a placental hormone, chorionic gonadotropin. They become active again after puberty, and at both of these times secrete large quantities of testosterone. After the age of 40, the testosterone level decreases rapidly.

After secretion by the testes, testosterone circulates in the blood. Either it becomes fixed to tissues where it performs intracellular functions, or it is degraded into inactive products that are secreted in the urine as 17-ketosteroids.

The functions of testosterone are many. During fetal development it is responsible for the development of the penis, scrotum, prostate gland, seminal vesicles, and genital ducts. It provides the stimulus for descent of the testes. Given exogenously in the case of undescended testes in a child, it can cause descent if the inguinal canal is large enough.

Testosterone is essential for the development of primary and secondary sex characteristics in the male. After puberty, it stimulates enlargement of the penis, scrotum, and testes until about the age of 20. Testosterone influences the distribution of body hair and makes it more prolific, but it decreases the growth of hair on the top of the head. Therefore, baldness results from large amounts of androgenic hormones as well as from genetic background.

The effects of testosterone on the skin include an increase in thickness, increased ruggedness of subcutaneous tissues, and increased pigmentation due to elevated melanin production. Testosterone increases the rate of secretion of sebaceous glands and is therefore believed to contribute to acne.

Under the influence of testosterone, the total quantity of bone matrix increases. The bones become thicker and longer and the muscles increase in mass as a result of the hormone's general protein anabolic function. This function is also thought to be the cause of the increased number of red blood cells produced in the male.

Testosterone may increase the basal metabolic rate. It also causes hypertrophy of the laryngeal mucosa and enlargement of the larynx, which results in the characteristically lower male voice.

Other androgens are produced by the male, but their masculinizing effects are slight. Estrogen is also produced in small amounts, perhaps by the seminiferous tubules or by the interstitial cells of the testes. Its function in the male is unknown.

Spermatogenesis

Spermatogenesis occurs in the seminiferous tubules during active sexual life beginning at puberty and continuing throughout the remainder of life. It is stimulated by FSH in the presence of adequate testosterone. The tubules contain two or three layers of *spermatogonia* (primitive germ cells) along the outer border of the tubular epithelium. From puberty on, these cells continually proliferate and differentiate to form mature spermatozoa. Each cell is capable of producing four descendant cells (Figure 3-13).

At the time of sexual maturity, the spermatogonia become active and mature to form *primary spermatocytes*. Each primary spermatocyte undergoes an initial meiotic maturation division. The two resulting descendant cells, or *secondary spermatocytes,* contain the haploid number of chromosomes (23 chromosomes). These two cells divide mitotically during the second maturation division to form a total of four *spermatids*. Without further division the four spermatids, containing equal amounts of cytoplasm, are gradually transformed into four mature spermatozoa over a period of about two weeks. Each spermatozoon contains 22 autosomes and one sex chromosome, either an X or a Y.

During transformation each spermatid loses most of its cytoplasm and elongates into a spermatozoon with a head, neck, body, and tail. The head contains the nuclear material in a compact mass, and it is this part that fertilizes the egg. At the front of the head is a small structure called the *acrosome,* which is believed to play a role in the entry of the sperm into the ovum (Figure 3-14).

The *centrioles* are found in the neck of the sperm and the *mitochondria* are found in the body. Attached to the body of the sperm is a long tail, which has a structure similar to that of cilia; it contains large amounts of adenosine triphosphate, which energizes its movement. When deposited in the vagina the tail begins to move back and forth, driving the sperm forward at a maximum speed of 30 centimeters (12 inches) per hour.

Sperm mature in the epididymis; they develop their power of motility and become capable of fertilization within one to 14 days. Sperm are relatively dormant as long as they are stored (some are stored in the epididymis but most are stored in the vas deferens). As a result of their own metabolism, sperm secrete considerable CO_2 into the surrounding fluid, and the resulting acidity inhibits their activity. They are immotile at a pH greater than 12 or below 3. Sperm die rapidly in a strongly acidic

Figure 3-13. Maturation of male reproductive cells, resulting in formation of four mature sperm.

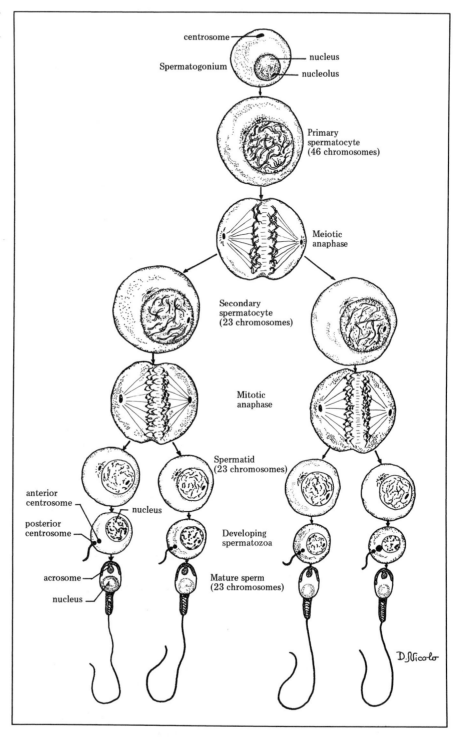

Figure 3-14. Mature sperm.

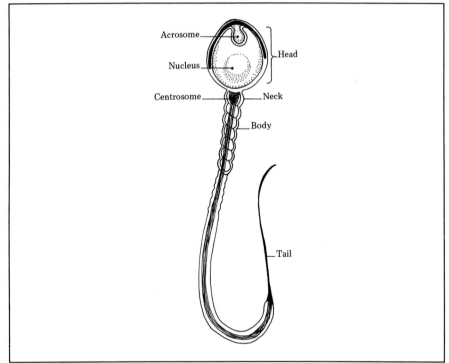

environment, while a neutral or slightly alkaline medium greatly enhances their activity. Their activity is also increased with an increase in temperature, but this also causes an increase in their rate of metabolism and thus shortens their life span. The average life of sperm in ejaculated semen at normal body temperature is 24–72 hours [2].

Hyaluronidase, an enzyme found in the acrosomes of the sperm heads, has the ability to break down intercellular cementing substances. When the ovum is expelled from the follicle, it is surrounded by the corona radiata, which must be removed before fertilization can occur. Hyaluronidase is thought to cause these cells to disperse, allowing the sperm to reach the ovum.

Seminal fluid consists of the ejaculum minus the sperm. Sixty percent of the seminal fluid comes from the prostate, 30 percent from the seminal vesicles, and the remainder from the epididymis and bulbourethral glands. It functions as a suspending medium, provides fructose and buffers, and contains substances that transform sperm into highly mobile cells.

Semen, a white viscous liquid with a pH of 7.35–7.50, consists of the seminal fluid plus the sperm. It normally forms a gel after leaving the male urethra, but becomes more liquid within 10–15 minutes. The amount of semen per ejaculation is about 3 milliliters, with about 120 million sperm per milliliter. A man is likely to be infertile when the number of sperm falls below 20 million per milliliter. It is possible that semen contains a mucolytic enzyme, similar to hyaluronidase, which can dissolve the mucous plug that frequently forms in the uterine cervix.

REFERENCES

1. Chiazze, L., Jr., et al.   The length and variability of the human menstrual cycle. *Journal of the American Medical Association* 203:377, 1968.
2. Guyton, A. C.   *Textbook of Medical Physiology* (4th ed.). Philadelphia: Saunders, 1971.
3. Reid, D. E., Ryan, K. J., and Benirschke, K.   *Principles and Management of Human Reproduction*. Philadelphia: Saunders, 1972.
4. Shepard, R. S.   *Human Physiology*. Philadelphia: Lippincott, 1971.
5. Sullivan, W.   Boys and girls are now maturing earlier. *New York Times,* January 24, 1971.
6. Zacharias, L., Wurtman, R. J., and Schatzoff, M.   Sexual maturation in contemporary American girls. *American Journal of Obstetrics and Gynecology* 108:833, 1970.

FURTHER READING

Greenhill, J. P., and Friedman, E. A.   *Biological Principles and Modern Practice of Obstetrics.* Philadelphia: Saunders, 1974.

Hellman, L. M., and Pritchard, J. A.   *Williams Obstetrics* (14th ed.). New York: Appleton-Century-Crofts, 1971.

Jacob, S. W.   *Structure and Function in Man.* Philadelphia: Saunders, 1970.

Masters, W. H., and Johnson, V. E.   *Human Sexual Response.* Boston: Little, Brown, 1966.

Romanes, G. J. (Ed.).   *Cunningham's Textbook of Anatomy.* London: Oxford University Press, 1972.

Chapter 4   Contraception, Infertility, and Therapeutic Abortion

THE BIRTH RATE in the United States has been declining steadily during the past several years. One underlying factor has been the development of the nuclear family constellation, which promotes a couple's independence; it no longer seems desirable or valuable to many people to have a large number of children, which may have been an asset in the extended family group. What used to be sole functions of the family (i.e., socialization, education, food production) have been taken over by larger specialized institutions. The large middle class of today's society sees upward mobility as a goal within reach, so that a large number of children becomes a liability rather than an asset. In addition, the changing status of women, which involves the recognition of their individual goals and aspirations beyond that of motherhood, has been influential in decreasing family size. Although Catholicism discourages artificial methods of contraception, the majority of Catholic women report that they have used or will use them. Most other religious affiliations encourage parents to have only the number of children for whom they can adequately provide.

Because of these factors and because of the increased availability of contraceptive information and methods, it seems obvious that couples are planning their families; they are making choices about whether to have children, how many children to have, and when to have them. Contraception is the means by which family planning becomes a reality. It should be noted here that family planning, in its broad application, is also concerned with assisting infertile couples to become pregnant.

Most couples face decisions about contraception and often therapeutic abortion or infertility prior to coping with a pregnancy that proceeds to term. The traditional approach of nurses in counseling only the woman, and mainly after a pregnancy, is outmoded. Health education that includes sexuality, family planning, and preparation for parenthood should be imparted to both the woman and the man before choices actually have to be made.

CONTRACEPTION

Contraception is hardly a new practice but rather one that has been used through the ages. Wives of North African desert tribesmen mixed gunpowder solution to prevent pregnancy. Egyptian women inserted pessaries made from crocodile dung into their vaginas or used tampons made from lint soaked in citrus juice. They also partially hollowed out lemon halves and fitted them over the cervix. The Chinese swallowed 14 live tadpoles three days after menstruation.

During the second century, Greek women made vaginal plugs of wool soaked in sour oil, honey, cedar gum, and fig pulp, while others ate the uterus of a female mule.

During the sixth century, Byzantine women attached a tube containing cat liver to their left foot. In the Middle Ages potions were prepared from willow leaves, iron rust or slag, clay, and the kidney of a mule. European brides in the seventeenth century were taught to sit on their fingers while riding in their coaches, or in a figure-flattering move, to place roasted walnuts in the bosom, one for every barren year desired [7].

In the early 1900s, Margaret Sanger, a nurse in New York City's Lower East Side, became incensed at the high incidence of criminal abortions and the high maternal death rate that followed. Accordingly, in 1916 in New York, she organized the first birth control clinic in the United States, only to be sent to jail as a result. Because of her initial persistence, birth control programs eventually became internationally funded by the Planned Parenthood Federation. Today the nurse in the hospital or community has broad opportunities to introduce the topic of family planning. This may be done initially during routine examinations, at the time of premarital examination, or in the prenatal period, as a part of the many kinds of planning being done at this time. The mother is usually very receptive immediately post partum in the hospital, as well as when she is seen in the pediatrician's office during the period when coping with the baby occupies much of her energy and she is highly motivated to allow sufficient time before having to cope with another baby.

One of the most important factors in a nurse's ability to discuss family planning is her* understanding and acceptance of her own attitudes and feelings regarding sex, sexuality, and the role of women in society. She is then more likely to be able to accept, without being judgmental, a variety of standards and modes of sexual behavior (e.g., an unmarried woman's need for contraception).

Since sharing contraceptive information involves very intimate areas of an individual's life, it is necessary that first contacts with couples be warm and meaningful. When a nurse enjoys the couple's respect and confidence, it is easier for her to perceive the couple's needs and to facilitate their choice, understanding, and use of a particular method. Because the nurse is in a key position, it is imperative that she know the facts about the various contraceptives; she should also know about the couple's attitudes, customs, mores, and vocabulary. She should be aware of the contraceptive methods used most frequently in the local community; this knowledge may be influential in helping couples make their choices. In many health centers, workers from the community are being trained and supervised by nurses to disseminate information about available services and to participate in activities within the center. These paraprofessionals can speak very effectively to couples as peers and as personal users of various contraceptive methods.

Follow-up appointments or perhaps a home visit by the family planning nurse should be scheduled to give the couple a chance to have their additional questions answered. In their expanded roles, nurses are doing counseling as well as performing routine vaginal examinations, taking Papanicolaou (Pap) smears, and fitting contraceptive devices. Although maternal-child health services are the traditional vehicles for sharing contraceptive information, nurses need to remember that patients

*She and her are used throughout this book in reference to the nurse to avoid repetition of "he and she" and "him and her." This usage is not in any way intended to exclude the many male nurses nor does the information in this book apply only to female nurses.

in other health situations might like these resources to be made available to them. Postponement of pregnancy can be as important as medical treatment for a woman who has heart disease, cancer, tuberculosis, venereal disease, mental illness, or another disabling condition.

While some of the older methods of contraception were fairly successful, obviously today's methods enjoy far greater success rates. However, even today, methods that should be technically very reliable can have high failure rates. This may be due to misinformation regarding the method or may be caused by ambivalence or a negative attitude toward the method on the part of either the user or health personnel. Some methods require more motivation on the part of the user than others, which can contribute to increased failure rates. People also may be inadequately informed about the variety of methods available. In addition, people may not have adequate access to facilities where they may obtain today's methods of contraception. They may be unaware the service exists, or there may be a problem of distance to a health facility, inconvenient hours for service, or inordinate expense.

Condoms

Although condoms are a very old method of contraception, they were originally developed to protect against venereal disease during the Renaissance. During the eighteenth century their value as a contraceptive was recognized and their use for this purpose became widespread during the nineteenth century after the discovery of vulcanization. Because of their long history, condoms have accumulated a number of synonyms, such as rubbers, skins, coats, softies, covers, protectors, shoes, bags, and prophylactics.

The earliest condoms were made from fabric impregnated with drugs, or from the intestinal membranes of animals, usually sheep. Today there are approximately 60 brands on the market, some without a lubricant, some lubricated with a "dry" lubricant such as a silicone compound, and others packaged with a wet lubricant, either a water gelatin colloid or a solution of glycerine in water. The lubricants often contain a preservative that acts as an antibacterial agent and also enables these condoms to be stored intact in a foil or plastic package at normal temperatures for approximately five years [6]. The two most common condom shapes are those with a dome-shaped end, and those with a nipple or reservoir end.

When used consistently, condoms are a highly effective method of contraception. Breaks or tears have been cited as causes of failure, but the most common cause of failure is irregular use. It has been estimated that over 99 percent of the condoms sold in the United States are free of defects. Pregnancy rates when using condoms have been reported as low as 2.6 per 100 women using the method for a year, and as high as 18 percent [6]. Since the method requires motivation and some technical skill on the user's part, as well as the expense of purchasing the condoms, the failure rates vary according to a group's education and socioeconomic level.

Condoms are unrolled onto the erect penis before any leakage of semen has occurred. In uncircumcised males, the foreskin is retracted prior to application. When the condoms with dome-shaped ends are used, approximately 1 centimeter ($\frac{1}{2}$ inch) of the condom should be allowed to protrude beyond the end of the penis. This acts as a reservoir and decreases the pressure of the semen against the tip of the condom during ejaculation. Air should be expelled from this reservoir before the condom is completely unrolled onto the penis. (This should also be done with the condom with the nipple end.) If this step is omitted, the trapped air may be released during the thrusting motions, escaping through the open end of the condom and carrying drops of semen with it.

After ejaculation the penis should be withdrawn from the vagina, with the condom held firmly at the base of the penis. If this is not done, the condom may slip off easily as detumescence occurs.

Overall, this method has many advantages. The condom has proven reliability, is inexpensive, requires no physician visit or prescription, has a long storage life, is portable, and can be purchased in relative secrecy from vending machines. It may also help protect against venereal disease and *Candida* and *Trichomonas* infections (this protection also depends on other health measures such as a good handwashing and proper condom disposal).

Although the condom has been used for many years, its use has decreased as other methods have become available. This is probably due to such disadvantages as fear of breakage, difficulty or discomfort encountered when insertion is attempted (with nonlubricated types of condoms), and the need to interrupt lovemaking to apply the condom. This may only add to the anxiety of a man who is already uncertain about his ability to maintain an erection.

Men often complain of impaired sensation during intercourse, but this may be an advantage in men who ejaculate prematurely. Women also occasionally complain of being unable to feel the ejaculation. Some women who value "cleanliness" prefer their partners to use condoms, since then the semen does not touch them.

Diaphragms

A diaphragm resembles a cup, with a circular rim and a dome made of thin rubber; its size ranges from 45 to 105 millimeters (1.8 to 4.1 inches) in diameter. The purpose of the diaphragm is to block access to the cervical canal by covering the external os and thus act as a barrier between sperm and egg.

For the diaphragm to be effective, however, it is essential that it be used with a vaginal spermicidal cream or jelly. About a teaspoon of cream or jelly is placed inside the dome of the diaphragm, and more is spread around the rim. Some women find it facilitates insertion if they spread some jelly or cream on the other side of the dome also.

For insertion, the diaphragm is squeezed together so that the rim sides touch, with the dome side down. When the diaphragm is properly inserted, the dome covers the cervix and the woman then tucks the anterior rim under her pubic bone. She must check to see that the dome has covered her cervix by feeling for the cervix with her index finger.

A woman may squat to insert her diaphragm, or she may stand placing her foot on a chair or the toilet, or lie on her back with her knees bent. The diaphragm and spermicide may be inserted 1 hour prior to intercourse and should not be removed for a minimum of 6 hours following intercourse. Should intercourse take place a second time within the 6-hour period, an applicator of spermicide should be injected into the vagina (without removing the diaphragm) prior to lovemaking.

The diaphragm is removed by hooking an index finger under the front rim and pulling downward and outward. Removal may be facilitated by bearing down as though having a bowel movement. An introducer (or inserter or director) may also be used to insert or remove the diaphragm. For insertion, the diaphragm is stretched over the introducer, spermicide is applied as already described, and the diaphragm is directed into the vagina, with the front end placed in the posterior fornix. When it is in place, the diaphragm can be unhooked with sideward motion of the introducer. The woman then tucks the anterior rim under her pelvic bone. By using the hook end of the introducer the diaphragm may be removed (Figure 4-1).

After use, the diaphragm should be washed with warm soapy water, dried, and dusted with cornstarch or talcum. Cared for in this way it should last between two and four years; however, it must be inspected for holes or thinning prior to each insertion.

Diaphragms must be fitted to the individual by a physician, nurse, or health care worker prepared in this area, since a good fit is essential for its success. A virgin may be fitted with the diaphragm; however, after several months of sexual activity she should have the size rechecked, since she may now require a larger one. Diaphragm fit should also be checked following pregnancy or abortion, pelvic surgery, or a loss or gain of 10 or more pounds.

There are no side effects associated with the use of a diaphragm except in those rare people who are allergic to spermicides or rubber. However, the method does require high motivation, planning, patience, intelligence, some degree of mechanical aptitude, visits to a physician for fitting, and a prescription. There may also be associated psychological problems for the woman who is uncomfortable touching her genitalia. The overall failure rates vary from 3 to 12 percent, depending on the group studied.

Cervical Caps

The function of a cervical cap is much like that of a diaphragm; it fits over the cervix and imposes a barrier between the sperm and egg. It is an old method that is com-

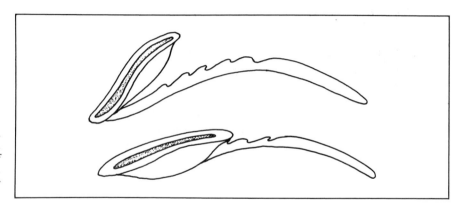

Figure 4-1. Diaphragm and inserter. Diaphragm attached to hooked end of inserter (top). *Diaphragm hooked and ready for insertion* (bottom).

mon in Europe. Cervical caps are made of rubber or plastic and are smaller, thicker, and less flexible than diaphragms. Rubber caps may be left in place for 24 hours at a time, while plastic ones may be left in place between menstrual periods, which separates their insertion from the sex act. There are no side effects attributed to caps; their failure rate is 7–8 percent. Spermicide may be inserted with rubber caps, but it is not necessary.

Vaginal Creams, Jellies, and Foams

Vaginal creams contain a spermicide and a base, which is usually a soft soap or an oil in water emulsion. The cream may be used alone or in conjunction with a diaphragm or condom. When not used with a diaphragm, the cream is inserted by means of a vaginal applicator. Many people feel that vaginal creams are the best substances to be used when a condom or diaphragm will not be used, since the creams adhere well to tissue surfaces. This is viewed by some as a disadvantage, since the creams coat the penis during intercourse and tend to cling to the labia and vulva as the penis is withdrawn.

Contraceptive vaginal jellies contain a spermicide and a translucent gelatin base. They can be used alone or with a diaphragm or condom. When not used with a diaphragm, the jelly is introduced into the vagina by using an applicator. However, many investigators feel that when used alone the jellies are inferior to vaginal creams since they do not disperse and adhere as well to tissue surfaces. Both creams and jellies are less effective when used alone than when used with a condom or diaphragm. Their failure rate averages 30 percent.

Some lubricating jellies that are often sold alongside contraceptive jellies in stores are intended for vaginal lubrication rather than for contraceptive purposes. When purchasing a jelly for contraceptive purposes one should check to see that it states on the label either that it contains a spermicide or that it is for contraceptive purposes.

Foams are sold in aerosal containers. The foam is sprayed into an applicator and then inserted into the vagina, where it expands immediately, giving nearly instant protection. When used alone the foams are not as effective as when used with a condom, but they are considered by many to be more effective than creams or jellies.

Foaming tablets are also available. The foam-producing ingredients, tartaric acid and sodium bicarbonate, are mixed with other substances, including a spermicide. The mixture is pressed into a tablet and wrapped in foil. When the tablet is moistened (either by the secretions in the vagina or by wetting with saliva or water prior to insertion), the result is a foam plug that acts as a barrier and also as a releasing agent for the spermicide.

It takes approximately 5 minutes for the tablet to react completely. The failure rate is high, and a common side effect is an unpleasant burning sensation within the vagina. The tablets also need to be placed as far into the vagina as possible. As with the diaphragm, when foams, creams, or jellies are used, douching should not take place for at least 6 hours after intercourse (douching is not really necessary at all).

Chemical methods cannot be separated from the sex act and must be used shortly before intercourse begins. The chemical agent must be added again if intercourse is to be repeated. With chemical methods it is also necessary to understand the method and the mechanics involved. Some women are repelled by the manipulation involved, while others incorporate it into their foreplay.

Rhythm

The rhythm method of contraception is based on the facts that the egg is fertilizable for about 12 hours (not more than 24 hours) and that sperm usually maintain their total ability to fertilize for not more than 48 hours after ejaculation (although some have been found to survive in the female reproductive tract for as long as seven days). Thus, theoretically a woman is potentially fertile for two days before ovulation and one day after—a total of four "unsafe" days per cycle. Even though it is known that ovulation occurs 14 ± 2 days before the onset of the next menstrual period, unfortunately it is impossible to make an accurate prediction of when ovulation will occur in each cycle, particularly if the cycles vary in length. There are two methods of rhythm birth control, which may be used singly or in combination to determine when ovulation occurs and to compute the number of infertile and fertile days per cycle.

With the *calendar method,* the accuracy of determining infertile days is greatly improved if the dates of the twelve previous cycles are known. If all the cycles were 28 days long, for example, the fertile phase would begin on day 10: 28 days minus 16 (14 plus 2 days for a long progestational phase or early ovulation) minus 2 more days for sperm life span. The fertile phase would end on day 17: 28 days minus 12 (14 minus 2 days for a short progestational phase or late ovulation) plus 1 day for ovum life span.

Since most cycles vary in length, the shortest cycle as well as the longest must be considered. The day on which menstruation begins is considered to be *day 1* of the cycle. In the general formula for the calendar method, the fertile phase extends from and includes the 18th day before the end of the shortest cycle through the 11th day before the end of the longest cycle. If, for example, a record of menstrual dates during the preceding twelve cycles shows that a woman has cycles as short as 23 days and as long as 33 days, her projected fertile phase for the current month would begin on day 5 (23 minus 18) and end on day 22 (33 minus 11).

It is fortunate that not very many women in their prime childbearing years (age 20–30) have such a wide range of cycle lengths, since if the woman in the example has an active flow of 4 days and her next menstrual period on day 24, she would have only two "safe" days. This would hardly be acceptable to most sexually active couples; this emphasizes the extremely strong motivation a couple must have if rhythm is to be successful. With *conscientious* use of this calendar rhythm method, the pregnancy rate is in the vicinity of 15 percent.

A woman may actually fail to ovulate once or twice a year. In these cases her menstrual flow, if there is any, will be slightly different in quality, amount, and duration, and it may occur earlier in the cycle. To safely use the rhythm method, she must not have intercourse until she has had at least two periods of normal flow, since ovulation may recur at any time after failure to ovulate.

It is possible to shorten the "unsafe" phase (as determined by the calendar method) with the use of the *basal body temperature method.* The basal body temperature is taken with a special thermometer that records 35.5°–37.8° C in 0.05° rather than 0.1° units (96°–100° F in 0.1° rather than 0.2° units), so that minute temperature shifts may be read easily. The temperature is taken for 5 minutes, preferably rectally, at the same time each morning immediately upon wakening after at least 5–6 hours sleep. It is important that the temperature be taken before any kind of physical or emotional activity (e.g., eating, drinking, smoking, getting out of bed) and recorded at the time so that it is not forgotten.

The daily charting of the basal body temperature will reveal a characteristic pattern or curve, so that it is possible to determine the time of ovulation when there is a sudden and maintained shift of at least 0.3° C (0.5° F) (Figure 4-2). This temperature shift reflects the thermogenic action of progesterone produced by the corpus luteum following ovulation, although the time relationship between the temperature rise and ovulation is still controversial. At the time of ovulation there may be a slight transient drop in temperature but this is not a constant finding [12].

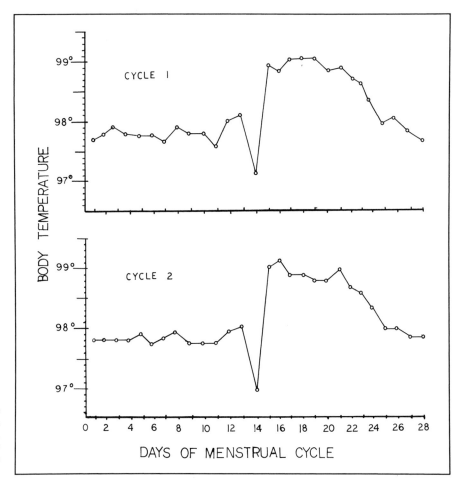

Figure 4-2. Basal body temperature during two menstrual cycles. Ovulation probably occurred on day 14 of each of these cycles.

Pinpointing ovulation is important for infertile couples as well as those hoping to avoid pregnancy, since infertile couples will want to take maximum advantage of their opportunities for fertilization. For the couple seeking contraception, the woman's "safe" period has begun when her temperature has been elevated by at least 0.3° C (0.5° F) for three consecutive days. This method is successful when intercourse is limited to the postovulatory period.

The basal body temperature method can be combined with the calendar method to determine a primary safe phase prior to ovulation, since the temperature rise only determines the *end* of the abstinence period. Failures are more probable in this primary phase, however.

Although rhythm is effective when used correctly, necessity of a prolonged period of abstinence makes the method unacceptable to many couples. According to the National Fertility Survey, the use of all types of rhythm contraception fell significantly in the United States between 1965 and 1970. In 1965, 15 percent of couples using contraception used the rhythm method; in 1970 only 7 percent used it. Since the woman bears the responsibility of determining safe periods, she must be capable of accurate perception, faithful adherence to schedule, and simple calculations. In addition, her partner must be content to let her determine when intercourse is permissable; if he fears being dominated, he will not be able to tolerate this. By dictating periods of abstinence, the rhythm method makes the need for spontaneous sex impossible to meet. For those women in whom the sex drive is highest at ovulation, rhythm is extremely difficult to practice at the time when it is most necessary.

SALIVA TEST

The accuracy of the rhythm method may be increased through the use of a new test using paper that is treated chemically to react with alkaline phosphatase in the saliva. The amount of alkaline phosphatase rises just before ovulation and turns the test paper blue at that time.

Coitus Interruptus

Coitus interruptus (withdrawal) requires the man to withdraw his penis immediately before he begins to ejaculate, a moment when the closest possible physical union is desired. It is also a time when the typical male impulse is to penetrate the vagina as deeply as possible. Consequently many couples find the use of coitus interruptus very frustrating, although some have relied on it for years with both success and satisfaction. Coitus interruptus is the oldest known form of contraception and, in some parts of the world, is still used more often than the condom and the pill. Depending on the care and timing of the man, the pregnancy rate is 8–40 percent.

Since even one drop of semen may contain 10,000 to 100,000 sperm, the effectiveness of coitus interruptus depends largely on psychological factors. Withdrawal is best practiced by a conscientious man with a thorough knowledge of his own body, extremely good self-control, and a very strong desire to protect his partner. The woman has to be content to restrain her activity during intercourse so that she does not threaten her partner's control over his own sexual excitement.

The technique may be ineffective because of premature ejaculation and because sperm may still enter the vagina even when coitus is interrupted. This can occur if a drop of semen escapes before ejaculation, or if the ejaculation occurs in stages, or if intercourse is interrupted after some portion of semen is already in the vagina. Some men are unable to withdraw in time, or they may ejaculate at or near the woman's moist external genitalia, in which case sperm are able to travel into the vagina.

Some men refuse to accept this method of birth control because they are unwilling to forego the pleasures associated with completing intercourse in the usual manner. They may also fear that it may eventually damage their health, causing prostatitis, impotence, or premature ejaculation—fears that are not supported by evidence. The woman's sexual responsiveness may be lessened by psychological stress, such as anxiety over whether her partner will withdraw in time. Interruption of intercourse may also mean that her orgasm may not be as strong on these occasions or that it may not be reached at all.

Postcoital Douche

The theory behind douching as a contraceptive measure is that semen can be flushed from the vagina before sperm have had a chance to enter the cervix. However, it is known that immediately after the ejaculation of semen into the vagina, the sperm penetrate the cervical mucus; some are passively carried to the place of fertilization in as short a time as 2–10 minutes; and some reach the internal os in 1.5–3 minutes. Since the woman must have extraordinary speed if her postcoital douche is to reach the sperm, its efficacy as a contraceptive measure is extremely doubtful. The pregnancy rate associated with it is at least 36 percent.

Intrauterine Device

Medical literature during the 1880s reported the use of intrauterine devices (IUDs) or intracervical devices for both contraception and treatment of gynecological disorders. These devices were unpopular because it was believed that they initiated abortions and that they were associated with pelvic inflammations. In the early 1900s, opposition again developed shortly after two new models, silkworm gut rolled into rings and a coil of silver wire (Gräfenberg ring), were introduced. The IUD as a contraceptive was revived in 1959 by two physicians (one in Israel and one in Japan), with resulting low pregnancy rates and no serious side effects.

Since the early 1960s several types of polyethylene IUDs have become available, including the spiral, loop, and bow (Figure 4-3). Their flexibility allows them to be inserted rather simply: The IUD is straightened full length in a narrow plastic tube and is inserted under sterile conditions into the uterus through the cervix; it then resumes its original shape as it is pushed from the inserter into the uterine cavity. The plastic devices are kept completely in the inserter for no more than 1 or 2 minutes to keep them from losing their shape "memory." Those with strings that project from the cervix can usually be removed by gentle traction. Pregnancy rates with IUDs in place are 2–3 percent, depending on the device used.

In recent years IUDs have become increasingly popular contraceptives as more

Figure 4-3. Types of IUDs. 1. Double coil. 2. Lippes loop. 3. Bow. 4. Copper 7. 5. Spiral. 6. Copper T.

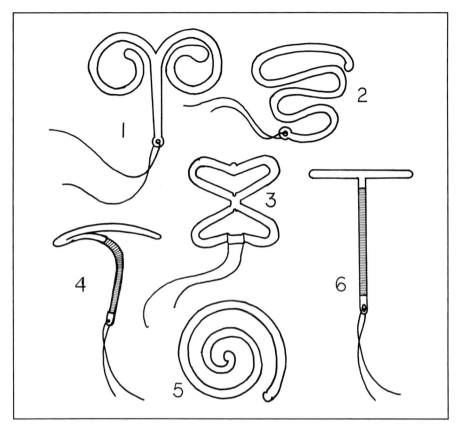

highly qualified scientists and physicians participate in contraceptive research. Rapid population growth, especially in underdeveloped countries, has created a need for more methods of population control. New inert materials have made it possible for IUDs to remain in the uterus for indefinite periods, and new treatments for pelvic inflammatory disease have made that a less serious complication.

With more research into IUD development, new and improved models continually appear for clinical use, some with only small changes and others based on entirely new principles. One of these is an IUD made of plastic and containing metallic copper—the copper T. The T shape was designed to avoid distortion of the uterine cavity and thereby reduce the incidence of endometrial bleeding and of painful contractions and expulsion of the device.

Unfortunately the T device, while well tolerated, was ineffective in preventing conception; a copper wire around the stem improved its effectiveness. It is thought that as the copper diffuses into tissue fluids it reduces the viscosity of uterine secretions and lyses cervical mucoid substances. In this manner it may prevent implantation as well as significantly change cervical mucus and the transport of sperm [10]. A modification of this copper T is the copper 7, which, because of its unique size, shape, and flexibility, may be inserted easily without dilatation of the cervix, even into the uterus of a normal nulliparous woman.

Another modification incorporates progestogens into devices, which apparently enhances their effectiveness, decreases their expulsion rate by diminishing uterine contractility, and reduces vaginal bleeding and spotting.

EFFECTIVENESS AND RETENTION

Pregnancy rates and expulsion rates vary with the type and size of the IUD, the duration of its use, and the age and parity of the woman. The larger sizes are associated with higher pregnancy rates; the smaller sizes are associated with lower rates. Highest pregnancy rates exist for bows, then loops, then spirals. With a large loop, the pregnancy rates are highest for the first year and get lower with each subsequent year.

The actual effectiveness of the IUD approaches the theoretical effectiveness since it does not depend on daily or periodic medication or on insertion before, during, or after intercourse. To lessen the chance of unnoticed explusion, the woman should be taught to examine herself about once a week for the presence of the strings protruding from her cervix. Since a large proportion of expulsions occur at the time of the menstrual flow, especially during the first few periods following insertion, she should examine tampons or perineal pads to see if the device has been expelled. She should report expulsions immediately so that a new device can be inserted; she should be reminded to use other contraceptive measures in the interim.

IUDs of smaller sizes are associated with higher expulsion rates. The highest expulsion rates occur with spirals, then loops, then bows. Expulsion rates decrease with the age of the woman and, in most age groups, with parity.

INDICATIONS AND CONTRAINDICATIONS

The IUD is most appropriate for women who prefer a method that requires no precoital preparation, who wish to dissociate intercourse from contraceptive measures, who are not successful in the use of other birth control methods, or who have contraindications to the use of other methods. The IUD should not be used by women who have pelvic inflammatory disease, known or suspected pregnancy, cervical or uterine cancer, uterine malformations or fibroids, or a history of abnormal uterine bleeding.

TIME OF INSERTION

A convenient time for insertion is during the woman's postabortion or postpartum check-up, which is a time when the cervix is still somewhat dilated, the risk of pregnancy is low, and her motivation for a method of contraception is high. Another time of choice is during the menstrual flow, when the cervix is again somewhat relaxed, the chance of pregnancy is minimal, and any bleeding after insertion (which could alarm the woman) is hidden in the menstrual flow.

If she has no difficulties, the woman can wear the plastic or stainless steel IUD indefinitely until menopause, although she is instructed to have an annual check-up. Copper-bearing IUDs are replaced from time to time, usually at two-year intervals.

In clinics in the United States the IUD is the method of second choice, behind the pill and only slightly ahead of the diaphragm. In some of the developing countries, however, it forms the backbone of national family planning programs. IUDs are still most suitable for populations not accustomed to continued use of any form of preventive medicine.

MODE OF ACTION

The mechanism of IUD action is not yet fully understood. Major theories suggest that it acts as an abortifacient, mechanically traumatizing the endometrium and implanted embryo, or that it stimulates increased peristalsis of tubal and uterine musculature, propelling the fertilized and unfertilized ova into the uterus prematurely. Some researchers postulate that the IUD alters corpus luteum function and life span. Others point to an increase in the quantity of inflammatory cells in the uterine cavity, which may be toxic to the embryo. Still another theory suggests that the IUD stimulates phagocytosis, with a resulting decrease in sperm number. The foreign-body reaction appears to be the unifying principle for contraceptive action, either through local tissue reaction or through hormonal changes in the woman [10].

SIDE EFFECTS AND COMPLICATIONS

The most common side effect (along with pain and discomfort) is bleeding, i.e., menorrhagia, metrorrhagia, or both. Women should be informed that they may normally expect some bleeding and some cramping after IUD insertion. The first few menstrual periods after insertion tend to be heavier and last longer than previously, and they are sometimes followed by postmenstrual staining or spotting. These symptoms tend to disappear within three months, but sometimes they are severe enough to cause the woman to have the IUD removed. (About 20–30 percent of women either have the device removed for these reasons or expel it involuntarily.) Associated cramping is usually eased by application of heat and by analgesics.

Infrequently some men have complained of pain during intercourse. This complaint was particularly associated with the Margulies spiral, which had a stiff, beaded projection from the cervix into the vagina. A few men complain about the nylon strings that protrude from the cervix; in these cases the strings are usually clipped shorter. Ordinarily the IUD does not interfere with intercourse, douching, or use of tampons.

The most important complication associated with IUDs is that of pelvic infection which occurs in 2–3 percent of women, usually during the first year following insertion. Most of the pelvic inflammatory disease associated with IUDs is diagnosed as preexisting chronic or subchronic infection, exacerbated by the insertion procedure rather than a new infection. It is doubtful that IUD insertion can cause infection, since the bacteria in the cervical mucus carried along on the device are generally of low virulence. The host defenses of the endometrium are usually adequate to combat these organisms within a very short period of time. Most of these cases are mild and are treated with antibiotics, with or without removal of the device.

Perforation of the uterus is another infrequent complication of IUD insertion and is usually asymptomatic. There is no evidence at this time that the IUD has any carcinogenic effect.

EFFECTS ON FERTILITY AND REPRODUCTION

Fertility after removal of an IUD appears to be unimpaired. Although there is no evidence that the presence of an IUD can cause an ovum to implant ectopically, ectopic pregnancies seem to be somewhat more frequent among women who conceive with IUDs in place than among women in general. The incidence of spontaneous abortion also appears to be somewhat increased if pregnancy occurs with the device in place. It is usually possible to remove the device without disturbing the pregnancy; however, in most cases the IUD is left in place and is found on the membranes or in the placenta at the time of delivery. Its presence has not been correlated with fetal malformation or injury [17].

PSYCHOLOGICAL IMPLICATIONS

Peaceful, secure, trusting women adapt well to the IUD. They do not have to be highly motivated or well organized. Some women may feel uncomfortable with the idea of a foreign body inside them or may fear that it will cause cancer. With support and reassurance they are usually able to react more positively.

The use of the IUD is contraindicated in women who have an unusually strong need to feel control over themselves. Sometimes such women become anxious when they are not permitted spur of the moment changes of mind regarding their fertility. However, since this method of contraception is dissociated from intercourse, women with guilt feelings about birth control may have fewer conflicts about using the IUD rather than the pill. On the other hand, the IUD is not usually an acceptable contraceptive measure for women who have strong feelings against abortion.

Oral Contraceptives

MODE OF ACTION

Oral contraceptives work by inhibiting the release of follicle-stimulating hormone (FSH) and luteinizing hormone (LH) from the pituitary. Normally, as the pituitary releases FSH, follicular growth occurs in the ovary and estrogen production increases. Estrogen levels peak just before the preovulatory surge of FSH and LH, which presumably triggers ovulation.

Following ovulation, the corpus luteum produces progesterone. The oral contraceptives decrease the level of FSH in the blood by providing estrogen and inhibit LH release by supplying progesterone. The estrogen and progesterone provided by the pill inhibit ovulation but do cause endometrial changes and menstruation. The changes caused by the pill make the endometrium unfavorable for implantation and the cervical mucus more viscid and hostile to sperm.

There are two main types of oral contraceptives marketed in the United States, the sequential and the combination pills. Sequential pills contain synthetic estrogen for the first 15–16 pills and synthetic progesterone and estrogen for the next five pills. This type mimics nature since it patterns itself after the normal release of these hormones. However, sequential pills have a higher failure rate than the combined pills because the former are less likely to inhibit the LH surge. The combination pill contains estrogen and progesterone in each pill.

The pills are supplied in a number of ways. Some preparations have 28 pills per packet, the last seven being placebos. In the first month that a woman takes these, she takes the first pill on the fifth day of her period, and then takes a pill each day until the packet is empty. When this happens she simply begins another packet.

A woman taking 21-day pills begins her first packet on the fifth day of her period. One pill is taken daily for 21 days, then the pills are discontinued for 7 days; a new packet of pills is begun on the eighth day. The menstrual period will occur during the 7 days without the pill.

Combination oral contraceptives are sold under the names Enovid, Norinyl, Norlestrin, Ortho-novum, Ovral, and Ovulen, among others. Since synthetic estrogens and progesterones are much more potent than natural forms, they are given in much smaller doses than the amounts of estrogen and progesterone produced by the body. Oral contraceptives are sold in varying hormone doses, since the correct dose depends on individual body chemistry: A particular woman may have undesirable side effects from one preparation and none from another.

If a woman forgets a pill, she should take it as soon as she remembers it and take her next one when it would normally be due. If she misses two pills, she should take the normal one for that day plus one of the missed pills and take two pills the next day to prevent breakthrough bleeding. She should also use another method of contraception, such as a cream, jelly, or foam, during the remainder of that menstrual cycle while she finishes the packet of pills. Some physicians may also advise a woman to use a cream, jelly, or foam during her first packet of pills, since new pill users make more mistakes at this time than later. Fewer mistakes are made if a woman establishes a schedule and takes the pill at approximately the same time every day. Many physicians also caution women to use another contraceptive during the first week of her initial package of pills, since it will take this long for her to be protected.

SIDE EFFECTS AND COMPLICATIONS

A number of side effects have been attributed to oral contraceptives. There had been some concern that they increased the incidence of cervical cancer, but no causative relationship was proved to the satisfaction of the Food and Drug Administration. In cases of preexisting breast cancer, however, the pill would be contraindicated, since it would cause exacerbation of the disease. Recent findings indicate an increase of endometrial carcinoma in young women taking sequential oral contraceptives and an increase of liver tumors in women of any age taking any of a variety of oral contraceptives [9, 11, 14].

A causative relationship has been established between thromboembolic disorders and the use of oral contraceptives. Deaths related to use of the pill have been attributed to blood clots in the vessels of the lungs and brain, although most often thrombus formation in pill users originates in the deep leg veins. While the death rate from blood clots caused by the pill has been reported to be 1.5 per 100,000 users per year in 20- to 34-year-old women, the risk of a woman's dying as a consequence of pregnancy and giving birth in a developed country in the same age group is 23 per 100,000 live births. In women between 35 and 44 years of age, the death rate from blood clots attributed to the pill is 3.9 per 100,000 users versus 57 maternal deaths per 100,000 live births. It has also been reported that death rates attributed to the pill may be substantially reduced by using only the pills with the lower estrogen content. There does not appear to be a higher failure rate associated with these lowered estrogen doses.

Because of the risk of thromboembolic disease, the American Medical Association advises that any woman using the pill who has severe leg or chest pains, coughs up blood, has difficulty breathing, or has sudden severe headache or vomiting, dizziness or fainting, disturbances in vision or speech, or weakness or numbness of an arm or leg should discontinue the pill and contact her doctor immediately.

In addition to thromboembolic disease, the oral contraceptives can produce temporary symptoms that are common during actual pregnancy. A woman may experience nausea, breast tenderness, weight gain or occasionally weight loss, and chloasma. The nausea, breast tenderness, and weight gain usually clear up during the first to third cycles as the woman's body adjusts to the synthetic hormone levels. The chloasma may remain even after the woman is no longer taking the pill.

Other side effects that have been attributed to oral contraceptive use include amenorrhea, lighter periods, headache, hair thinning, regression of gum tissue, eye complaints (such as blurred vision and eyes tiring more easily), and changes in sex drive and appetite. Some women who have borderline hypertension develop definite hypertension while on the pill. The elevated blood pressure returns to normal following discontinuance of the pill. Occasionally women develop corneal edema and are unable to wear their contact lenses. Women who are long-term users of oral contraceptives may also have changes in their vaginal pH from acidic to alkaline and thus an increased incidence of vaginal infections.

Breakthrough bleeding is an annoying side effect for many women. Often the estrogen dose is inadequate to maintain the integrity of the endometrium and it begins to slough. Some physicians will advise a woman to take two pills daily rather than one for the remainder of that packet, thus shortening that cycle; she then resumes taking the normal one pill per day starting on day 5 of the following cycle. A woman may also be asked to stop taking her pills at the first sign of breakthrough bleeding. This allows menstruation to begin; pill taking is then resumed on day 5 following the beginning of the menstrual flow. If a definite flow does not begin, pill taking resumes seven days after the last pill was taken.

Oral contraceptives are contraindicated in women with abnormal liver function, since some progestins can cause retention of bile or decrease its rate of flow and in turn cause jaundice. The pill is likewise contraindicated in women with diabetes, since it interferes with glucose utilization. It is usually also contraindicated in women with a history of thromboembolic disease, hypertension, heart and kidney disease, uterine fibroids, migraine, and mental depression.

Some have also expressed concern that the ability to become pregnant will be decreased after using oral contraceptives for a few years. However, clinical studies indicate that this is not the case and that in fact 90 percent of the women attempting to become pregnant after discontinuing the pill do become pregnant within a year. There is also no evidence to indicate that pill use causes any abnormalities in the offspring of former pill users.

Clinical studies have reported a deficiency of vitamin C, vitamin B_6, and folic acid in women who use the pill. Some researchers now question whether some of the pill's side effects are due to deficiencies of these vitamins. Many physicians advise women using the pill to take vitamin supplements to eliminate this problem if the vitamins have not been incorporated into their brand of pill.

Oral contraceptives are generally avoided for nursing mothers. The pill may cause a decrease in the mother's milk supply, and the hormones do pass through the milk. The long-range effects of these hormones on the infant are not known at this time.

Experimental Methods

There is now in use an experimental pill consisting of long-acting estrogen and progestin given only once during a cycle. A long-acting progestin may also be given as an injection. Some of these preparations provide protection up to 84 days. The main side effect is menstrual irregularity, with irregular bleeding and occasionally heavy bleeding and periods of amenorrhea. Other side effects include headache, dizziness, nervousness, and nausea.

Another experimental method consists of placing a plastic ring containing a progestin in the vagina. The hormone diffuses through the ring slowly; the ring is left there during the cycle and removed during the menstrual flow. Progesterone has also been incorporated into a capsule and implanted in the skin for diffusion over a number of months.

Diethylstilbestrol is used as a postcoital contraceptive given within 72 hours after intercourse; it has been shown to be a highly effective contraceptive method, with relatively few side effects other than nausea. However, the use of diethylstilbestrol in the maintenance of pregnancy has been discontinued, since there have been a number of reports of vaginal cancer in female offspring of mothers treated with that drug during their pregnancy [5]. Postcoital progesterone preparations are now being tested and show satisfactory initial findings. Their main side effects appear to be menstrual irregularities.

Also under investigation is a mini-pill, which consists of small doses of progestin (0.35 milligrams). While large doses of progestin will inhibit ovulation, these smaller doses usually do not but appear to have an antifertility effect by acting on the cervical glands to increase the antisperm properties of cervical mucus or by interfering with the endometrial secretory phase; occasionally, in an extremely sensitive individual, ovulation is inhibited. Side effects of this method include occasional headaches, digestive disorders, and menstrual irregularities, including amenorrhea and spotting. The failure rate is higher than that of the combination pill but comparable to that of the IUD and diaphragm.

Sterilization

FEMALE STERILIZATION

History has always recorded a much greater interest in the sterilization of women rather than men—from the use of chastity belts to various experimental surgical procedures. In ancient times closure of the vaginal entrance was achieved by sewing up the vulva and passing a ring through the labia majora, with the aim of preserving the purity of women by preventing adultery and illegitimate pregnancy. Sterilization itself was first proposed by Hippocrates as a means of reducing hereditary insanity. Oophorectomies were performed by the ancient Egyptians; the first tubal sterilizations were done in 1880.

By 1921, 42 different procedures had been proposed, and at the present time there are over 100 surgical techniques for sterilizing women. Generally these are variations on the following approaches: simple tubal ligation, tubal ligation with partial resection, cornual resection, bilateral salpingectomy, burial of tubal stump in the broad ligament or in the uterus, transuterine cauterization of cornu, injection of sclerosing solutions into tubes, burying the ovary in the broad ligament, fimbriectomy, hysterectomy, and, more recently, electrocoagulation and transection via celioscopy or laparoscopy.

The choice of the specific procedure depends on many factors, among which are the patient's age, weight, history of previous pelvic surgery, presence of systemic or pelvic disease, risk of future pregnancies, failure rate and complexity of procedure, and the timing of the operation (whether or not post partum). Other factors to be considered include the safer alternative of vasectomy in the partner, psychological factors, type of anesthesia, and availability of hospital or outpatient facilities.

Because of the expense and lack of trained personnel, surgical sterilization has not had much effect on the world population. Costs of sterilization should decrease as outpatient procedures are developed and refined, older techniques and their failures are evaluated, and culdoscopic and laparoscopic techniques are introduced. Elective voluntary sterilization is being increasingly used as a legitimate method of birth control, and it may yet prove to be a significant factor in population control. However, sterilization is still difficult for many patients as well as physicians to accept and is a step that should not be taken without serious consideration of its permanence.

Current Methods. In 1919 Madlener developed a more or less dependable method for female tubal ligation (at about the same time satisfactory techniques for vasectomy were developed). Today the tubal ligation techniques of Pomeroy (1930) and Irving (1950) are still widely used. (Figure 4-4).

Following the introduction of fiberoptics in 1964, endoscopic techniques began to be developed; laparoscopic sterilization, (first developed in 1966), has become increasingly popular. During this procedure, which requires a very small abdominal incision, a pneumoperitoneum is produced with carbon dioxide, and the tubes are visualized, grasped with forceps, and electrocoagulated, excising a portion of each. This may be done on an outpatient basis.

Figure 4-4. A. Pomeroy tubal sterilization. Tubes are tied with plain catgut and a portion is resected. B. Irving tubal sterilization. Portions of the tubes are resected and the uterine stumps are buried in the uterine musculature. 1. Ligation and resection of the tube. 2. Securing opening in uterine musculature. 3. Tube being buried in the uterine musculature.

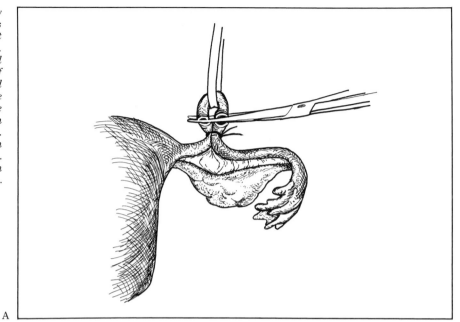

A

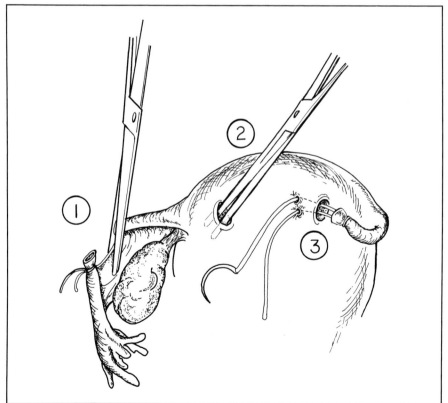

B

Hysterectomy, of course, is another method of sterilization, one which is sometimes more easily accepted by Roman Catholics than procedures specifically designed to prevent conception. However, hysterectomy has a higher mortality associated with it.

On an experimental basis, intrauterine instillations of chemical cytotoxic agents for sterilization have been suggested, e.g., ethanol (100%) or ethanol and formalin (2 or 5%), which results in tubal obstruction. The endometrium does not seem to be affected. Studies are being made of tissue glues, for injection directly into either the fallopian tubes or the vas deferens, possibly producing closure of the tubal passageway.

Time of Procedure.   Although tubal ligations are performed at varying times, the first 48 hours post partum is a convenient period, since the patient is already in the hospital and her tubes are readily accessible. After 48 hours, tubal edema may make surgery more difficult, increase the risk of hemorrhage and infection, and contribute to a higher failure rate. Some increase of gynecological disorders is associated with tubal ligations, but this is attributed to preexisting disease rather than to any interference with ovarian or uterine function.

MALE STERILIZATION

Vasectomy, the leading surgical procedure used for male sterilization, is also the leading method of contraceptive sterilization requested today. Compared to female sterilization, it is less expensive, less time-consuming, easier to perfom, and more widely available and involves no risk to life. It does not affect sex drive, ability to enjoy intercourse, amount of ejaculate, or the quality, duration, or frequency of erection. The procedure is being performed in public health departments, hospital clinics, and doctors' offices.

The purpose of vasectomy is to sever the vas deferens in each testicle, thus making it impossible for sperm to pass from the testes into the urethra. The vas is severed and ligated in the straight portion, which is relatively close to the ejaculatory duct (Figure 4-5). This portion of the vas is contained in the spermatic cord, along with blood vessels, lymph vessels, and nerves. The parts of the spermatic cord that lie within the scrotum can be located by feeling the posterior portion of the sac on either side. Once located, the spermatic cord is injected with a local anesthetic, a small incision is made, and the vas deferens is isolated. The vas is then ligated and resected, or the ends may be electrocoagulated; then they are buried in surrounding structures, and the skin is closed. The procedure is then repeated on the other testis. The skin incisions in each testicle are covered with sterile gauze pads, which are held in place by some type of scrotal supporter. Both the pads and supporter may be removed after a day.

Following the procedure the man is asked to go home, rest, and apply an ice bag to the incisional area. Two aspirin tablets every 4 hours are recommended if he has pain. He is asked to keep the incisions dry and, while he may shower after a day, he should avoid swimming and baths. For two to three days following the procedure, he should avoid heavy physical activity, and some physicians recommend abstinence

Figure 4-5. Vasectomy. Vas deferens has been ligated and cut. Sperm are now blocked from entering ejaculatory fluid.

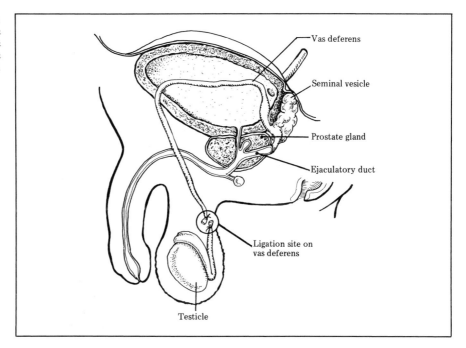

from intercourse. Vasectomies usually are performed Friday afternoon or evening, so that a minimum of time is lost from work. A man whose work does not require heavy physical activity may return to work when he feels comfortable.

Men must be told that they may not be sterile for two months or more following the procedure; therefore, they should bring a semen specimen less than 5 hours old to the clinic or doctor's office two to three months following surgery. Many physicians request two samples several weeks apart. The semen is examined for sperm content; a man is considered sterile when two samples of semen have been aspermatic.

Reported failure rates vary, but in general the method is more reliable than oral contraceptives. Failure may result from recanulization of the vas, ligation of a structure other than the vas, or failure to use another method of contraception during the unsafe period immediately following the procedure.

The most common side effects are bleeding (hematomas) and infection; the formation of spermatic granulomas may also occur. Spermatic granulomas are small tumorous masses formed in response to sperm that has escaped in the testes, either from the ligated ends of the vas or through a ruptured epididymis. The granulomas are usually very small and present no problems; however, they are excised if they do cause pain.

The severed vas can be rejoined through an operation called vasovasotomy. However, fertility rates following the procedure remain low, even though sperm are present in the ejaculate. It has been speculated that the low fertility rates may be due to antibody formation in the man from his unejaculated sperm that are phagocytized as they age and deteriorate. This antibody reaction causes inactivation of sperm and may account for decreased fertility following reanastomosis of the vas deferens.

Some men have been encouraged to have vasectomies by the existence of banks to store frozen sperm. It has been reported that sperm may be preserved $2\frac{1}{2}$–10 years or more in cold storage, used for artificial insemination, and result in normal offspring [3, 18]; however, these reports are controversial. The first individual born through the use of frozen sperm was 21 years old in 1974. As of mid-1972 a reported 300–400 healthy newborns conceived through the use of frozen sperm had been reported, and this group had a lower incidence of birth defects than that usually quoted for the normal population. The sperm banks have also been used to store semen of infertile men. The stored semen can be spun down and concentrated prior to artificial insemination.

PSYCHOLOGICAL IMPLICATIONS OF STERILIZATION

Since many couples in the United States have their desired families at an early age, sterilization has become an inviting alternative to long-term use of temporary contraceptive measures for both men and women. The choice of this option should be made only after very serious consideration, since the reversal of male and female sterilizing procedures has not yet had a high rate of success. This leaves little room for a change of mind following circumstances such as death of existing children or remarriage. Nurses play a vital role as listeners and as counselors when patients are contemplating such a step, helping them to make their decision based on knowledge of all the implications of the procedure.

As a rule, fewer than 5 percent of those men and women who are sterilized express regret over the decision. On the contrary, most report unchanged or improved health. When the fear of pregnancy has been removed, the couple's sex drive increases, as does the frequency of intercourse; many marriage bonds have become stronger. However, if the sterilization has been performed against the wishes of one partner, the result can be devastating to the relationship.

The emotional and psychological impact of the loss of reproductive capacity can be very great, although more men than women tend to equate sterilization with castration. Roman Catholics may have more conflicts to resolve and may express guilt following the procedure. An individual who has had previous psychiatric problems is likely to be more disturbed while coping with the ramifications of being sterilized.

LEGAL ASPECTS

Accepted legal opinion supports the position that purely voluntary sterilization is permissable provided that both partners have been informed of the implications of the procedure, including the chance of failure, and that permission in writing has been given. In most states the consent of the patient alone is all that is needed, provided that he or she is legally competent, although it is highly desirable that both partners sign the permit. Lawfully married minors or "emancipated" minors (15 years or older and living apart from parent or guardian) may legally give consent; otherwise they need the consent of a parent or guardian.

INFERTILITY

Fertility is greatest in men and women around the age of 24. A woman's fertility gradually diminishes around the age of 30 and declines rapidly thereafter. Without using a method of contraception, 25 percent of all sexually active women will become pregnant in the first month, 63 percent in six months, 75 percent in nine months, 80 percent in a year, and 90 percent in 18 months. According to the American Fertility Society, a couple who has had unprotected intercourse for a period of a year and who have not conceived may be considered infertile and are entitled to an infertility examination [8]. The infertility can be said to be primary if the couple has produced no children; it is secondary when a viable offspring has been born previously.

Prior to more elaborate testing procedures, the couple should have thorough histories taken and thorough physical examinations performed. The woman's history would include her age at puberty, her menstrual, gynecological, and obstetrical history, and past and present illnesses. The couple should be interviewed separately and together regarding frequency of coitus and sexual technique. Attitudes toward intercourse may also be determined in these interviews.

Laboratory tests should be performed for urinary sugar and protein, complete blood count, serology, and semen analysis. Chest x-rays and thyroid function should be evaluated. The woman's pelvic examination could show an unduly tight hymenal ring, cervical or vaginal abnormalities, or deviations in the position and outline of the uterus, tubes, or ovaries. When nothing can be found to demonstrate infertility by means of these procedures, other factors must be investigated more thoroughly.

Infertility is reportedly due to cervical problems in 20 percent of the couples, tubal problems in 30 percent, hormonal problems in 15 percent, and sperm deficiencies in 30 percent; these percentages vary according to the population studied. Low socioeconomic groups are reported to have higher tubal factors, often as a result of gonococcal or enterococcal pelvic inflammatory disease or postabortion sepsis. Despite all the progress in fertility management, there are 5–10 percent of all couples who are medically healthy and in whom no cause for infertility can be established.

Female Infertility

CERVICAL AND UTERINE FACTORS

An incompetent cervix can be a factor in infertility if the woman's history indicates two or more second-trimester abortions. The pregnancies usually terminate suddenly and painlessly after spontaneous rupture of the membranes, usually with no primary bleeding. Treatment can be performed surgically by placing plastic tubules or dacron mesh around the circumference of the internal os.

The quality of cervical mucus can be a problem; it may be improved by low doses of estrogen, making it more favorable to penetration by sperm. The estrogen may also enhance ovarian response to pituitary gonadotropins. Progesterone and estrogen given during the luteal phase may also enhance endometrial quality, which aids in implantation.

Submucous uterine fibroids may disturb endometrial function or be large or numerous enough to prevent or interfere with implantation or fetal growth. These fibroids are diagnosed by palpation, curettage, or hysterography and are treated by surgical removal (Table 4-1). Third-degree retroversion of the uterus has also been considered to be a predisposing factor in infertility and may be treated with an intravaginal pessary.

Congenital anomalies, including bicornuate, septate, and double uteri, may also be contributing factors. Diagnosis of these anomalies is made by curettage or hysterography. Surgical treatment consists of removing the septum, joining the cornua, or uniting the horns of a double uterus (after the medial halves have been excised). Surgery should be delayed, however, until it has been established that a pregnancy cannot be maintained without intervention. If surgery is necessary, the woman should be advised to wait from eight to 12 months after the operation before attempting to become pregnant. Delivery is usually by cesarean section in order to minimize possibilities of uterine rupture and fetal loss.

TUBAL FACTORS

Occluded tubes may be opened by time, a period of sexual abstinence, antispasmodics, and weight loss. Some investigators believe that repeated tubal insufflations with carbon dioxide at pressures as high as 300 milligrams of mercury, along with pelvic heat and sexual abstinence, are superior to tubal surgery.

Surgical treatment (tuboplasty) for a closed oviduct is advisable when the male partner is normal and female reproductive function seems otherwise normal. The tuboplasty may take the form of a salpingolysis (separation of peritubal adhesions) or a salpingoplasty (opening of the totally occluded distal end of the tube). Reconstruction of the midsegment, cornual segment, or interstitial segment may also be performed.

Following surgery there is an increased incidence of tubal pregnancies. Smoldering pelvic inflammatory disease may also be reactivated at the time of tuboplasty. Formation or reformation of adhesions following tubal surgery is a major reason for failure to become pregnant. To reduce the incidence of adhesions, anti-inflamma-

Table 4-1. Diagnostic Tests Used for Infertility

Test	Procedure	Finding
Hysterosalpingogram	Cervix is injected with radiopaque dye, which flows into the uterus and fallopian tubes; radiological examination follows	Determination of malformations, patency, or tumors
Laparoscopy	Small abdominal incision is made; laparoscope is passed into pelvic cavity	Visualization of ovaries, fallopian tubes, and uterus
Tubal insufflation (Rubin's test)	Carbon dioxide is introduced through the cervix into the uterus and fallopian tubes	Normally, pressure readings show a rise and fall. Shoulder pain signifies tubal patency

tory agents such as dexamethasone sodium phosphate (Decadron) and antihistamines such as promethazine hydrochloride (Phenergan) may be given preoperatively, intraperitoneally during surgery, and postoperatively for two days. Hydrocortisone may also be injected into the uterus and lavaged through the tubes postoperatively four to five times during the first two weeks after surgery to decrease the incidence of postoperative tubal adhesions [8].

OVARIAN FACTORS

The major ovarian abnormalities involved in infertility are irregular ovulation or anovulation and the anatomical and functional changes caused by endometriosis. It is essential in treating infertile couples to determine whether or not ovulation occurs; the methods most commonly used are endometrial biopsy, records of basal body temperature, and examination of vaginal cells and cervical mucus. The anovulation or oligo-ovulation may be due to pituitary, thyroid, adrenal, or ovarian dysfunction.

The ovarian cortex in Stein-Leventhal syndrome shows fibrosis and follicular cysts and is associated with anovulation. Following treatment with ovarian wedge resection, menstrual irregularity is corrected in many women, and ovulation and pregnancy following the procedure have been reported to occur in 13–89 percent of the women (depending on the population studied). Young women with irregular bleeding or endometrial hyperplasia are also believed to benefit from wedge resection, but it is recommended that they first be treated with administration of estrogen-progestin combinations.

Treatment.   Two pharmacological agents commonly used in treating anovulation are clomiphene citrate and human menopausal gonadotropins (HMG). Clomiphene is used in anovulatory women who have follicular function and adequate endogenous estrogen but lack adequate and cyclic stimulation by pituitary gonadotropic function. These women usually have normal or slightly decreased total pituitary gonadotropins but lack the midcycle burst of LH which causes release of the mature follicle. Clomiphene is believed to have an antiestrogenic effect that promotes a midcycle burst of LH.

Ovulation may be expected to occur in approximately 70 percent of women with secondary amenorrhea following clomiphene therapy; of this group, 40 percent will become pregnant. If pregnancy does not occur, it may be due to accelerated tubal transport or inadequate treatment time with the drug. Some resulting pregnancies are aborted before the fourth week. Women are advised not to attempt to become pregnant during the first treatment cycle, since the incidence of abortion is increased at this time, particularly if prolonged amenorrhea existed previously. Spontaneous abortion is not increased in pregnancies occurring after the first treatment cycle.

The incidence of multiple pregnancy in women who conceive following clomiphene therapy is increased to approximately 1 in every 16 pregnancies. The increase is undoubtedly due to fraternal twinning and superovulation after taking the drug.

The most striking side effect during therapy is ovarian enlargement due to the enlargement of cystic follicles, cystic corpora lutea, or other physiological cystic structures. These physiological cysts regress spontaneously within seven to 28 days following cessation of therapy, and the drug is administered again only after the ovaries have returned to pretreatment size. The drug should never be given to a woman who has an ovarian cyst.

Ovulation may also be induced by administration of the gonadotropic substances FSH and LH extracted from the urine of postmenopausal women, followed by doses of human chorionic gonadotropin (HCG). One preparation of menopausal gonadotropin, Pergonal, is in general use. In the course of the development of the drug, its FSH conent has varied; currently each ampule contains 75 IU of FSH, 75 IU of LH, and 10 milligrams of lactose. Women with persistently low or absent gonadotropins may be treated with Pergonal if pituitary or hypothalamic tumors and cysts have been ruled out. Women with primary gonadotropin insufficiency and hypothalamic amenorrhea usually respond promptly to HMG and HCG therapy.

Women with normal gonadotropin levels are usually given at least six courses of clomiphene therapy before resorting to gonadotropin administration. Women who fail to ovulate with clomiphene alone may ovulate after clomiphene and HCG sequential therapy, e.g., 10 days of clomiphene followed four days later by a dose of HCG. Women who fail to respond to this therapy will usually respond to HMG if the ovaries have not been depleted of follicles.

Pergonal does not appear to influence the incidence of abortion in subfertile women the way clomiphene does. Following treatment with Pergonal, multiple births occur in approximately 20 percent of pregnancies, the majority of which are twin births. If no other cause for infertility exists, the pregnancy rate within the first two treatment cycles is 50 percent.

The recommended initial dose of Pergonal is one ampule given intramuscularly for nine to 12 days followed by 10,000 IU of HCG given one day after the last dose of Pergonal. If the woman's ovaries become unusually enlarged, the dose of HCG may be omitted for that treatment cycle. Daily intercourse is encouraged, beginning on the day prior to administration of HCG and continuing until ovulation becomes apparent by the various indicators.

Couples attempting to conceive without the aid of drugs but by following the woman's basal body temperature are advised to have intercourse during days 11, 13, and 15, or 12, 14, and 16, of a 28-day cycle. It is not necessary to abstain before these days to increase sperm count, since evidence indicates that the motility decreases even though the count may increase. Men who have intercourse four or more times weekly have lower counts, but their partners have a higher rate of conception. Following intercourse the woman should remain supine for approximately an hour to facilitate upward sperm migration.

Much experimentation is now occurring with hypothalamic-releasing factors. Currently a luteinizing hormone/releasing hormone (LH-RH) and a follicle-stimulating hormone/releasing hormone (FSH-RH) are under investigation. They offer the advantages of being inexpensive and safer than gonadotropins and clomiphene [15].

OTHER FACTORS

Endometriosis has also been identified as a factor in infertility. In women with endometriosis the expectation of pregnancy is about one-half that of the general population; the incidence of sterility in these women approaches 30–40 percent.

Endometriosis may be treated with analgesics and patience, surgery, or hormones, or a combination of the above. Pregnancy is considered the best treatment by some; they administer increasing doses of estrogen and progestins for six to nine months to initiate a pseudopregnancy. This produces a decidual reaction in the areas of the endometriosis, and these areas undergo degeneration and necrosis and hopefully are absorbed, thus improving fertility. This treatment is successful 50 percent of the time if there is no other cause of infertility, and if the endometriosis involves only the ovaries.

Male Infertility

A man's fertility depends on his production of an adequate number of normal mature sperm (at least 20 million to 40 million per milliliter of semen, with 80 percent normal forms). His fertility also depends on his being able to ejaculate and on his ability to produce an ejaculum which undergoes spontaneous enzymatic liquification within 30 minutes.

As the sperm move through the epididymis, they mature and become increasingly capable of motility and fertility. Mature sperm are stored in the end of the epididymis and the vas deferens, where they can survive for a much longer time than in the female reproductive tract. Their survival in the epididymis depends upon the endocrine activity of the testicular Leydig cells; this endocrine activity is responsible for the condition of the epididymal and ductal epithelium. Leydig cell failure leads to poor sperm motility, as a result of the absence of the hormonal support necessary for sperm maturation as well as their passage through the duct system.

Sperm are inactive in the epididymis and are transported through the duct via peristalsis and the spastic contractions at ejaculation. Sperm take about three weeks to pass through the duct system, a time which is influenced by the frequency of ejaculation. After a prolonged period of abstinence from ejaculation, there are often a high proportion of dead and aging sperm in the semen. After ejaculation the average man requires 30–40 hours to regain his normal sperm count. A man with a sperm count per ejaculation (2–4 cubic milliliters) of below 100–200 million is probably infertile. Specimens for semen analysis are obtained by masturbation or coitus interruptus, collected in a clean, dry glass jar, and transported to the doctor's office no later than 2–3 hours after collection.

Normally during ejaculation a sympathetic reflex action causes the sphincter of the urethra to close, while a parasympathetic reflex causes the external sphincter to open and the ejaculate is forced out through the urethral meatus. The contraction of the internal sphincter prevents retrograde passage of the semen into the bladder (retrograde ejaculation), which would result in a lack of seminal fluid upon ejaculation. This lack may occur following disruption of the internal sphincter as a result of surgery, the use of some antihypertensive blocking agents, or diabetic neuropathy.

At ejaculation, sperm respond to their changed environment by an increase in motility and metabolic activity; they rapidly become exhausted and die, probably as a result of the increased availability of oxygen. The life span of sperm at room and body temperature is relatively short, but their life may be prolonged by refrigeration, in some cases by increasing carbon dioxide tension and by freezing after treatment with a protective substance such as glycerol. Since sperm lose some motility in the process of freezing and thawing, sperm which already have poor motility are not the best specimens to be frozen.

Stored semen is used to artificially inseminate the woman, a procedure timed to coincide with her ovulation, at which time the semen will be introduced into the vagina near the cervix with a syringe. Artificial insemination may be accomplished with the husband's sperm (AIH), or if he is azoospermic, with a donor's sperm (AID). AID, while medically sound, may have legal, religious, and social implications that should be discussed with the couple.

FACTORS AFFECTING MALE FERTILITY

A common cause of male infertility is a *varicocele,* which consists of dilated left scrotal veins due to incompetent valves in the left internal spermatic venous system with retrograde flow of blood from the renal vein into the scrotal circulation. In addition to increasing heat in the area, this blood from the renal vein may also carry a relatively high concentration of toxic metabolic substances such as steroids, which are potential inhibitors of spermatogenesis. This condition is surgically corrected, not with removal of the dilated veins but with the interruption of the left internal spermatic vein to prevent the retrograde flow of blood. This procedure usually results in an increase in sperm motility and a decrease in immature sperm forms [1].

If the *semen volume* is less than 1 milliliter but is otherwise of normal quality, infertility may result from failure of the seminal fluid to make contact with the cervix. Artificial insemination is sometimes used in this case. Semen volume is occasionally increased by the administration of gonadotropins in high doses [1].

In most men the greatest concentration of motile normal sperm is in the first portion of the ejaculate. Insemination with this portion of the ejaculate often solves fertility problems, particularly when the man has a semen volume of 3 milliliters or more, with low sperm density or increased semen viscosity. Pregnancy also sometimes occurs in this case if the male withdraws his penis after the release of the first portion of the ejaculate [1].

Endocrine imbalances (i.e., decreased levels of pituitary gonadotropin, Leydig cell failure, thyroid dysfunction) may have a devastating effect on male fertility.

Impotence, a factor in about 5 percent of male infertility problems, may have many causes, including diabetes, anticholinergic drugs, tranquilizers, certain antihypertensives, and surgery [1].

Sexual frequency may be related to infertility. If intercourse is too infrequent, not enough sperm will be deposited during the fertile period; however, if intercourse is too frequent, the semen may be of poor quality. Intercourse every other day during the fertile period is sometimes recommended. The woman should avoid immediate ambulation and/or douching. Sometimes couples have reported the use of spermicidal jellies as lubricants—an easily remedied cause of infertility [1].

Epididymal obstruction (congenital or secondary to infection from gonorrhea or tuberculosis), *testicular failure* (due to mumps, trauma, or tumor), or *cryptorchidism* may result in azoospermia. It is now thought that if the testes have not descended by the time a child is 5 years old, irreversible changes begin to occur. If the testes remain outside the scrotum until puberty, the male will be unable to produce sperm, since the testes have been subjected to the higher intra-abdominal temperature. Since Leydig cells are heat resistant, androgen function and secretion will continue. However, if the testes remain undescended by 30–35 years of age, hormone secretion will decrease as well. Active therapy with gonadotropins, followed by orchiopexy, is indicated between 5 and 9 years of age [1].

Sometimes, in association with epididymitis, the sperm penetrate the walls of the epididymis and invade surrounding tissue. In some infertile men this may result in the phenomenon of autoimmunization against their own sperm; the sperm appear to be ejaculated in an *agglutinated* condition. Other cases of sperm agglutination are sometimes remedied by ascorbic acid therapy, which increases the activity of antiagglutinin in the semen [1].

It is also possible that vaginally deposited sperm can provide an antigenic stimulus in susceptible women, who respond by developing antispermatozoal antibodies. These may be individual specific (only one partner's sperm) or species specific (any human sperm). It has been reported that if a condom is used during intercourse or if a couple abstains for periods ranging from two to six months, antibody titers will decrease, and pregnancy is likely to follow unprotected intercourse [1].

While *age* is not an important factor in sperm production, fertility is reduced with aging. *Allergic reactions* or *anxiety* or *emotional tension* can also have temporary adverse effects on sperm production [1].

Of the systemic diseases *diabetes* has a specific effect on fertility, since the accompanying vascular changes may accelerate aging. Diabetes may result in calcification of the vas deferens along with impotence and retrograde ejaculation [1].

With *chronic renal failure* there is often endocrine dysfunction, low levels of testosterone, oligospermia with poor motility, and germinal cell arrest. Although libido sometimes improves with continued dialysis, spermotogenesis often does not. Libido, potency, and ability to ejaculate may greatly improve after kidney transplant, but most of the patients on immunosuppressive therapy remain oligospermic. Return of ovulation and subsequent pregnancy have been reported in female patients. In most cases of *paraplegia* and *quadriplegia,* testicular atrophy is slow and progressive [1].

Infertility may also result from nutritional deficiencies in vitamin A (which causes germinal cell hypoplasia), vitamin B complex (which affects pituitary function), vitamin C (which affects sperm antiagglutinin), or certain trace elements such as zinc (which affects spermatogenic epithelium) [1].

Acute febrile or viral illnesses may result in temporary depression of sperm production and poor semen specimens. To much *heat* affects the seminiferous tubules, arresting spermatogenic maturation. Frequent hot baths or close fitting or thermal underwear may be contributing factors. Usually the semen returns to normal within three months after the extra heat is removed. Although no firm conclusions have been reached, it has been shown that *heavy smokers* have severe disturbances of sperm motility and decreased testosterone levels [1].

Damaged chromatin in *irradiated spermatozoa* may be incapable of fertilizing or of contributing to the normal development of the fertilized ovum. If a man receives 225 rads to his testes prior to puberty, it is predicted that three of every five of his children will have detrimental mutations. Therefore diagnostic x-rays and therapeutic radiation in boys should not be done without truly valid indications. Recovery of fertility in the adult male after accidental sterilization by nuclear radiation has been reported within 41 months [1].

Certain *drugs* adversely affect spermatogenesis. Colchicine arrests cell division at metaphase. Methotrexate interferes with folic acid metabolism in nucleic acid synthesis. Testosterone inhibits spermatogenesis by inhibiting pituitary FSH secretion. Nitrofurantoin (Furadantin) depresses spermatogenesis by interfering with carbohydrate metabolism in the germinal epithelium, producing primary spermatocyte arrest. Monoamine oxidase inhibitors are reported to produce an increase in the sperm count followed by a profound drop. Medroxyprogesterone (Depo-Provera) causes depression of sperm count and motility after a single injection; the use of such injections to induce periods of male sterility is currently under investigation [1].

MEDICAL THERAPY

Androgens may be used if there is a normal sperm count but decreased motility; they help to create an environment in the epididymis conducive to the development of motility. Clomiphene has been used to stimulate endogenous gonadotropin production in males with low sperm counts and normal or low FSH and interstitial cell–stimulating hormone levels. Semen responses have generally been unpredictable. Exogenous gonadotropins have been used in the past to stimulate testicular, germinal, and hormonal activity. Large doses of chorionic gonadotropin have shown good results.

Psychological Implications

Infertility causes feelings of frustration, guilt, and depression; tests and treatment for it often bring about anxiety and fear [19]. A third party inquiring into private sexual activity is not without serious implication. The resulting tensions add their inhibiting effect to whatever organic factors are present via the hypothalamic pituitary pathways, via autonomic smooth muscle systems, or by pathways not fully delineated.

Adoption has been recommended as a treatment in psychological infertility for those couples in whom no physical reason for infertility can be found, as has a Hawaiian vacation precisely timed with the fertile phase.

The tension involved in attempting to overcome infertility can cause a man to become emotionally impotent. It can also cause uterine or possibly tubal spasm, decreasing the chances of rapid passage of sperm.

THERAPEUTIC ABORTION

Historical and Legal Aspects

Laws and attitudes toward abortion have vacillated throughout history and may continue to do so. Catholic doctrine for 300 years, from 1450 to 1750, made specific distinctions about the status of the fetus in the mother's womb. The distinction, based on the concepts of "ensoulment" and "unensoulment," permitted abortion in the period up to 40 days of gestation. For the last century the Catholic Church has been opposed to any form of abortion; however, recent opinion polls carried out in the United States show that the majority of Catholics polled believe that the decision about abortion should be made by a woman and her doctor [4].

Orthodox Jews have been opposed to abortion in the past and remain so, while those less orthodox are not. Likewise some Protestant denominations have opposed abortion in the past and remain opposed today, while many no longer take an antiabortion stand.

There was a time in the early history of the United States when there was no legal prohibition against termination of pregnancy before quickening. Abortion reform began in the 1820s, as a response to the high mortality of surgical procedures in general, particularly of those carried out by back alley abortionists, and as a result of a movement by some to impose an ascetic morality on all. Laws passed by the states during this period outlawed abortion except when necessary to preserve the life of the woman.

On January 22, 1973, the United States Supreme Court, recognizing a woman's right to privacy and the current adequacy of medical practice, ruled in effect that in the first trimester of pregnancy the abortion decision is to be left to the woman and her doctor. The state of residence may not prohibit abortion in the second trimester but may regulate its procedures in the interest of protecting the woman's health; these regulations could include where abortions can be performed and who can perform them. During the final weeks of pregnancy the state may choose to protect the potential life of the fetus by prohibiting abortion except where necessary to preserve the life or health of the woman.

Since the Supreme Court decision, follow-up studies in the states that liberalized their abortion laws show a decrease in maternal mortality, a decrease in hospital admissions for women with complications of illegal abortion, a decrease in spontaneous abortion, and a decrease in out-of-wedlock births. Maternal mortality in New York City during the period October 1969 to March 1970 was 5.63 deaths per 10,000 live births, while during the comparable period of October 1970 to March 1971 (after a law had been passed permitting abortion on request) maternal mortality dropped to 2.6 deaths per 10,000 live births [6].

Statistics from San Francisco General Hospital reflect the California experience. In 1967 the hospital's rate of septic abortion was 68 women per 1000 live births; after California's liberalized abortion law took effect, the rate of septic abortion dropped to 36 per 1000 live births in 1968 and to 22 per 1000 live births in 1969. The spontaneous abortion rate also dropped since, as one report notes, many abortions listed as spontaneous were not spontaneous but induced. The rate in 1967 was 125 per 1000 live births and dropped to 49 per 1000 live births in 1969. Maternal deaths from abortion fell in California from 8 per 100,000 live births in 1967 to 3 per 100,000 in 1969 [13]. Comparable changes can now be seen in many states with new, more liberal abortion laws.

Whether or not a state has a restrictive or liberalized law on abortion probably will not significantly change the number of abortions performed; abortions have been with us throughout history. In the past, abortion has been attempted by taking various drugs, starving, placing hot coals on the abdomen, jumping from high places, lifting heavy objects, diving into the sea from cliffs, sitting on a bucket of hot ammonia water, or inserting bent twigs or wires into the uterus as curettes. Substances such as lye, pine oil, alcohol, lysol, or other liquids were (and sometimes still are) also used to perform abortions. The complications from these various methods include hypotension and renal failure, infection, liver abnormalities, infarction, and necrosis of portions of the uterus.

The horrors of these methods and their subsequent complications dramatically underline the fact that decisions on abortion are made individually in response to social, economic, moral, religious, and psychological factors, regardless of the status of the law. Liberalized laws should place more of the actual procedures under medical supervision.

Psychological Aspects

Many nurses, especially those who have worked in maternity for some years, have difficulty caring for women who choose to terminate their pregnancies. Their orientation toward preserving life, as well as their own religious and moral philosophy, runs counter to abortion. Groups of nurses who work with women choosing abortions find it helpful to have counseling sessions among themselves, in which they can explore their own thoughts and feelings about the procedure. In no instance should nurses be forced to care for patients having abortions when they themselves are opposed to the procedure. The experience is detrimental both to the nurses and to the women seeking abortions, who are already under stress and in need of care. Inevitably there is a decrease in the quality of care the nurses are able to provide, and their feelings about abortion are communicated to the woman, often leaving her with residual feelings of guilt.

A woman under the stress of carrying an unwanted pregnancy is in need of help. She has a right to expect counseling from nurses or other health professionals that will enable her to mobilize her inner strengths and outer resources. She needs an environment where she can openly examine her thoughts, wishes, and uncertainties without fear of judgment or coercion. The experience should help her toward a greater self-understanding and a feeling that she has some control over her life.

Counseling sessions should explore past psychological and medical history, including past pregnancies, abortions, and living children, and the woman's experiences during pregnancy, labor, and delivery. It is important to know if the present pregnancy was planned or the result of contraceptive failure or failure to use a contraceptive. It is also vital to ask how she feels about this pregnancy, if she has made any decision about what to do, if she has felt life, and if she is now thinking in terms of a baby as opposed to an abstract pregnancy. All alternatives must be explored: having the baby and keeping it, adoption, foster care, or termination of the pregnancy.

Her religious feelings and convictions are important. Her current life situation should be explored, including her economic resources, current stresses, and availability of emotional support. What is the relationship with the man involved? How will other significant people in her life react? Will she receive any support from them whatever her decision? How does she see this pregnancy affecting her future career or marriage goals? How does she feel about herself, about men, and about her own sexuality?

The nurse in counseling should help her focus on these important factors; she should also correct misinformation and supply any information the woman might wish. Throughout the sessions the nurse must be objective, refraining from judgment and intense emotional involvement. The woman must make her own decision; when she has made that decision the nurse should assist her in getting care through referral services.

If the woman chooses an abortion, the nurse should refer her to an appropriate agency as soon as possible, because the complications of therapeutic abortion are lowest during the first trimester. The risk of complications is three to five times greater when the abortion is performed in the second trimester. Recent reports indicate that the majority of therapeutic abortions are now being performed during the first trimester, and the trend is toward a greater percentage being done during this period. Late abortions have been reported as being most frequent in young women under 18, black women, nonprivate patients, and women with six or more children [16].

Methods of Therapeutic Abortion: First Trimester

The methods of abortion used during the first trimester (sometimes up to as late as fourteen weeks) are dilatation and curettage (D&C) or uterine aspiration (vacuum aspiration). These procedures are usually performed in an outpatient facility.

DILATATION AND CURETTAGE

A woman about to have a D&C performed is asked to avoid eating 3–4 hours prior to the procedure, to avoid vomiting and aspiration (even though the anesthesia is usually a paracervical block—only rarely is general anesthesia used). A bimanual examination is performed to check the angle of the uterus, following which the depth of the uterine cavity is measured with a uterine sound. This latter measure also assures the physician that the cervical canal is open. The canal is then dilated and the endometrium is scraped with a curette. The entire procedure takes approximately 20 minutes. Although the rate of complications is low, uterine perforation, cervical lacerations, infection, and hemorrhage can occur.

VACUUM ASPIRATION

Vacuum aspiration was developed in China in 1958 and has since become popular in the United States, where it was introduced in 1966. Preparation for the procedure is the same as for D&C. A bimanual examination checks uterine position, paracervical block is usually given, the uterus is measured, the cervix is dilated, and the endometrial lining and products of conception are aspirated by a hollow tube called a vacurette.

Some physicians may scrape the endometrium with a curette afterward to ensure the removal of all placental tissue. The procedure is faster than D&C, produces less blood loss and less chance of uterine perforation, and requires less anesthetic. Some reports show a lower rate of complications with vacuum aspiration than with D&C.

Methods of Therapeutic Abortion: Second Trimester

Methods of abortion used during the second trimester include hysterotomy and intrauterine injection of saline or prostaglandins; hospitalization is required for each of these procedures. Because of the duration of the pregnancy, actual labor is involved in second-trimester abortions induced by saline or prostaglandins. Unlike most women in labor (who are about to have full-term infants that have been expected for some time), most women undergoing abortions have had the additional stress of deciding to terminate an unwanted pregnancy, finding health personnel and a facility to have the abortion performed, and having a procedure done to initiate labor prematurely. These women can use all the support the nurse can provide—remaining with the woman during the procedure, helping her breathe and push properly, encouraging her by telling her that she is doing well and that labor is progressing, giving frequent back rubs in the lumbar area, and administering properly timed analgesics.

HYSTEROTOMY

Hysterotomy consists of incising the uterine wall, removing the products of conception, curetting the endometrium, and closing the incision. General or spinal anesthesia is used for the abdominal surgery. The method is not used often.

SALINE INJECTION

After the fourteenth to sixteenth week of pregnancy, the amniotic sac is large enough and contains enough fluid for the saline injection procedure to be possible. A solution of 20–50% sodium is exchanged for an equal amount of amniotic fluid via amniocentesis (passing a catheter through the abdominal wall and into the amniotic cavity). A total of 50–200 milliliters of sodium solution is exchanged for amniotic fluid. It is believed that fetal destruction is caused by the increased osmotic pressure of the amniotic fluid.

Labor begins in 24 to 72 hours; the products of conception are usually completely expelled, making curettage unnecessary. The most serious complication of saline induction is intravascular absorption of the injected saline, leading to hypernatremia. The saline may be absorbed through torn blood vessels, through injection into myometrial or placental vessels, or by abnormally rapid transfer to the maternal circulation from fetal membranes. If this occurs the woman will experience severe headache and thirst; if not treated, she will show signs of hypotension, bradycardia, apnea, and alterations in consciousness. Women who have kidney or cardiac problems should not have saline abortions.

PROSTAGLANDINS

Prostaglandins act as abortifacients by producing strong uterine contractions; they have been found to be relatively ineffective when used orally. Both intravenous and oral administration of prostaglandins have produced severe nausea, vomiting, and diarrhea as side effects. However, when prostaglandins are injected into the uterus, the required dose and the side effects are both decreased. After 14–16 weeks, prostaglandins are injected into the amniotic sac via amniocentesis. Prostaglandins have also been injected into the uterus through the cervix, but this method is used less frequently. Uterine contractions usually begin within a few hours following the injection; the majority of pregnancies are aborted within approximately 24 hours.

Proponents of prostaglandin abortions note that the induction time is shorter than that of saline injection when used in the second trimester. They note that uterine stimulation with oxytocin is often needed with saline abortion and is not required with the prostaglandin method. They also report that some degree of disseminated intravascular coagulation occurs in all patients undergoing saline abortions [2].

LAMINARIA

Recently an old technique for dilating the cervix is regaining popularity. A laminaria tent (a cylinder made of the stem of a seaweed or other suitable material) is inserted into the cervix; as the material absorbs water and expands it dilates the cervix, thus aiding the abortion procedure.

Follow-up Care

Following an abortion a woman should avoid douching and using vaginal sprays and tampons and should avoid intercourse, according to some physicians, for two weeks to prevent infection. If she has heavy bleeding (approximately twice that of her normal period), a temperature over 38° C (100.5° F), foul-smelling discharge, nausea and vomiting, or pain, she should see her physician at once. She can expect to have a menstrual period again in four to eight weeks following the procedure.

All women should be seen for follow-up care after a therapeutic abortion to check for complications, including psychological problems. Reports show, however, that severe psychological aftereffects are uncommon and that the predominant reaction appears to be relief. Many women report moderate depression several days after the procedure. During the counseling session after the abortion or on follow-up visits, contraceptive information should be offered; the woman should be provided with a method of her choice.

REFERENCES

1. Amelar, R. D., and Dubin, L. Stimulation of Fertility in Men. In E. S. E. Hafez and T. N. Evans, (Eds.), *Human Reproduction.* New York: Harper & Row, 1973.
2. Anderson, G. Prostaglandin versus saline for midtrimester abortion. *Contemporary Ob/Gyn* 4:91, 1974.

3. Ersek, R. A.   Frozen sperm banks. *Journal of the American Medical Association* 220:1365, 1972.
4. Gallup, G. H.   Abortion? Let doctor and patient decide, majority says. *Philadelphia Inquirer,* August 25, 1972.
5. Herbst, A. L., Robboy, S. J., and Scully, R. E.   Clear cell adenocarcinoma of the vagina and cervix in girls: An analysis of 170 registry cases. *American Journal of Obstetrics and Gynecology* 119:713, 1974.
6. Hubbard, C. W.   *Family Planning Education.* St. Louis: Mosby, 1973.
7. Kistner, R. W.   *The Pill.* New York: Delacorte, 1968.
8. Kistner, R. W.   The infertile woman. *American Journal of Nursing* 73:1937, 1973.
9. Lyon, F.   The development of adenocarcinoma of the endometrium in young women receiving long-term sequential oral contraception. *American Journal of Obstetrics and Gynecology* 123:299, 1975.
10. Moyer, D. L., and Shaw, S. T.   Intrauterine Devices: Biological Action. In E. S. E. Hafez and T. N. Evans (Eds.), *Human Reproduction.* New York: Harper & Row, 1973.
11. Nissen, E., and Kent, D.   Liver tumors and oral contraceptives. *Obstetrics and Gynecology* 46:460, 1975.
12. Pisani, B.   Rhythm—Thermal Application. In Mary Steichen Calderone (Ed.), *Manual of Family Planning and Contraceptive Practice.* Baltimore: Williams & Wilkins, 1970.
13. Profile of a typical patient seeking legal abortion given. (Editorial.)   *Medical Tribune,* November 10, 1971.
14. Silverberg, S., and Makowski, E.   Endometrial carcinoma in young women taking oral contraceptive agents. *Obstetrics and Gynecology* 46:503, 1975.
15. Synthetic hormone could improve fertility control. (Editorial.)   *Journal of the American Medical Association* 217:757, 1971.
16. Tietze, C.   Joint program for the study: Early medical complications of legal abortion. *Studies in Family Planning* 3:97, 1972.
17. Tietze, C.   Intrauterine Devices: Clinical aspects. In E. S. E. Hafez and T. N. Evans (Eds.), *Human Reproduction.* New York: Harper & Row, 1973.
18. Tyler, E. T.   Frozen semen banks. *Medical Tribune,* March 22, 1972.
19. Wiehe, V.   Psychological reactions to infertility: Implications for nursing in resolving feelings of disappointment and inadequacy. *Journal of Obstetric, Gynecologic and Neonatal Nursing* 5:28, July/August, 1976.

FURTHER READING

Calderone, M. S. (Ed.).   *Manual of Family Planning and Contraceptive Practice.* Baltimore: Williams & Wilkins, 1970.
Dodds, D. J.   Reanastomosis of the vas deferens. *Journal of the American Medical Association* 220:1498, 1972.
Gilbert, S.   Artificial insemination. *American Journal of Nursing* 76:259, 1976.
Hafez, E. S. E., and Evans, T. N. (Eds.).   *Human Reproduction.* New York: Harper & Row, 1973.
Hale, R. W., and Pion, R. J.   Laminaria: An underutilized clinical adjunct. *Clinical Obstetrics and Gynecology* 15:829, 1972.
Herbst, A. L., Poskanzer, D. C., Robboy, S. J., Friedlander, L., and Scully, R. E.   Prenatal exposure to stilbestrol. *New England Journal of Medicine* 292:334, 1975.
Manisoff, M. T.   *Family Planning: A Teaching Guide for Nurses.* New York: Planned Parenthood—World Population, 1969.
Menning. B.   Resolve—a support group for infertile couples. *American Journal of Nursing* 76:258, 1976.
Shinzo, I., Tien, S. L., and Yoshio, A.   Immunologic analysis of sperm-immobilizing factor found in sera of women with unexplained sterility. *American Journal of Obstetrics and Gynecology* 101:677, 1968.
T-mycoplasmas and male infertility. (Editorial.)   *Science News* 109:37, 1976.
Zipper, J.   Metals as intrauterine contraceptives. *Contemporary Ob/Gyn* 4:85, 1974.

Chapter 5 Anticipating Parenthood

MOTIVATIONS FOR REPRODUCING

Each society has accepted customs surrounding the sexual behavior, marriage, and reproduction of its members. Socially accepted sexual behavior has differed through periods of history, according to one's sex, cultural background, religion, and social class. In many societies the standard of sexual conduct is established as a way to ensure that a man's possessions are passed on only to legitimate heirs.

Likewise, the accepted customs surrounding marriage are influenced by much the same factors as those controlling sexual conduct. While the ceremonies or rites involved may differ from society to society, their function of publicizing the union is the same. The marriage gives the individuals social acceptance to bear children, thus legitimizing them as future parents. The society acknowledges not only the individuals' acceptability as parents, but also their duty to reproduce.

Society is motivated to have its members reproduce since its very survival depends on it, but what about the motivations of the individuals themselves? Often a basic, biologically innate reproductive drive is assumed to be the motivational force, particularly by psychoanalysts. The strongest argument against this theory is that if man, as other mammals, were motivated solely by such a drive, reproduction would have to continue throughout all of a woman's childbearing years [51]. However, the number of children born to a couple can be a matter of choice in the present day. If the biological drive were as forceful as is claimed, then the social and personal consequences of having children—strained finances, additional responsibility and work, and restraints on time and freedom—would not have as much influence as they do. The fact is, however, that the most common reasons for limiting the number of children are the mundane realities involved in having and rearing them [51].

Most of the psychoanalytic theories of motivation for reproduction begin with Freud. He theorized that a little girl, noticing that she has no penis, wishes to obtain one from her father. The penis becomes equated with a child and therefore she wishes for a child by her father. This wish, suppressed as she grows older, eventually becomes the wish for a child in an adult sexual relationship [16].

Helene Deutsch sees the woman's desire for a child as being related to vaginal sensations and to experiences of eating, holding food inside, and finally expelling it [51]. With maturity, these experiences are synthesized and projected to the image of having a baby.

Therese Benedek believes that the reproductive wish is triggered by the menstrual cycle. She theorizes that the hormonal changes associated with ovulation periodically prepare women for motherhood and constitute the physiological stimuli for desiring a child [16]. Benedek sees "motherliness" as independent of hormonal control; however, it is through interaction with the hormonal cycle that the ego matures. This is a necessary step in the development of a person's ability to care for others [4, 7].

Motivations formulated by Lerner include gratification of infantile needs for affection and repair of a damaged body image by identification with a perfect fetus and by overcoming a sense of castration with a swelling abdomen. He also contends that with pregnancy women strengthen their sense of female identity by competing with other psychologically significant female rivals, and that women may use pregnancy as a means of self-punishment for guilty thoughts and deeds [16].

In addition to the psychoanalytic theories, a number of other explanations of the motivations of women in bearing children should be examined. In American society, childbearing is still emphasized as a primary function of women. This aspect of the feminine role is communicated at an early age, and women who choose not to conform to this expectation often feel guilt and self-doubt.

Having children can satisfy a number of needs: confirmation of feminine identity, a sense of recognition and adequacy as a mature woman, a substitute for unachieved career aspirations, and a means for easier participation in the activities of friends and relatives who already have children. A couple may look forward to having their own characteristics reflected and passed on in a child. For some parents, childbearing may represent an opportunity to compensate for their own inadequacies by rearing a child who will achieve what they have not been able to accomplish. If their own childhood was not happy, they may look forward to the opportunity of demonstrating their own abilities to be good parents. Other individuals may want to reproduce the kind of environment and happy experiences they had as children.

Many people anticipate satisfaction and fulfillment from parenthood. The child may be someone the parent can cuddle, love, nurture, and teach; on the other hand, the child may be thought of as a burden, causing the sacrifice of freedom and a restriction on financial independence.

The appraisal of one's own competence for motherhood or fatherhood affects the decision to have children, as does the relationship with one's younger siblings. The relationship with one's mate may affect childbearing motivations; e.g., whether or not he or she is seen as a potentially good parent and is interested in having children. A couple may anticipate that a child will bring them closer together. Positive influences are provided by the special attention that accompanies pregnancy and the curiosity that is satisfied by it.

An individual's relationship with his own parents becomes an important consideration. Becoming a parent may symbolize independence from one's own parents; at the same time, it provides an opportunity to satisfy the desire of one's own parents for grandchildren.

Before their reproductive years end, older couples may be highly motivated to have children, as are couples who have been childless because of difficulties in reproducing.

While all of the foregoing factors may be positive motivations for having children, they may have negative aspects that serve as deterrents [16].

ASPECTS OF THE PARENTAL ROLE

Whatever their motivations may be, a couple contemplating having children soon realizes, as Rossi notes, that there are some aspects of this role that are unique when compared to their other major roles as adult members of society, the roles of marriage partner and worker [39]. Educational preparation for parenthood is often minimal. For 12 years, most Americans prepare formally for further education or for employment, spending little or no time learning about how to prepare for parenthood. During this time, some individuals also do reality testing of their future work role, exploring their likes and dislikes as part-time workers before the responsibility of working full time falls upon them.

In the United States most couples date or are engaged for variable periods of time before marriage; during this courtship, aspects of the husband-wife relationship can be tested. This may range from enjoying each others company for long periods of time, socializing as a couple, and finding housing and buying furniture, to living and loving together. In so doing, many of the assumptions they hold about what it will be like to be married can be verified or rejected; the choice is still open.

Other than babysitting, care of young siblings, or possibly the buying of baby equipment, for parents there is no such preparatory period for reality testing. With the birth of the baby, the transition to parenthood on a 24-hour basis occurs abruptly. The options for rejection of the role at this point barely exist.

According to many authorities, another unique feature of the parental role is the absence of objective standards by which success or failure can be measured during childrearing. Definite criteria exist by which satisfactory role fulfillment as a worker can be judged, and there are popular conceptions of what constitutes a successful marriage, but the objective criteria for parents to judge their success or failure while their children are growing are much more elusive.

Unlike beginning a job or entering into marriage, both of which, for the most part, are entered into voluntarily, pregnancy may be the result of pleasure-motivated sexual activity with no conscious desire to become a parent. Certainly the number of induced abortions, estimated at one million a year, reflects this difference. Likewise, society's attitude toward terminating a potential parental role by abortion differs greatly from its attitude toward terminating one's job or marriage. Certainly this is also true with terminating an actual parental role. Even children who have been legally adopted often become involved in trying to locate or be located by natural parents. The energy and emotion involved here is far greater than that involved in trying to reestablish ties with former mates or jobs.

Society's pressure to assume the parental role is perhaps the common factor that unites the other major adult roles. Women, particularly, are supposed to like children and want babies. Contrary opinions and feelings are still generally met with disapproval. While most people do want children, not all children are wanted. One study [12] of over 200 American mothers from a low income group reported that slightly over half clearly wanted their children. A Scottish study [41] reported that in a sample of almost 300 primigravadas, 41 percent did not want the pregnancy, 41 percent wanted it, and 18 percent did not mind. In a sampling of over 200 student wives, 64 percent stated they were happy about their pregnancies [36]. Still another study [19] reports that 80 percent of the sampled women were happy about their first one or two children, but only 31 percent were happy about the fourth or more. Other studies reflect higher percentages being happy about the fourth child, but these studies are based on subjects from favored economic groups and also from data obtained sometime after the children were born. Data collected from women while they are pregnant yield more negative responses [42].

FEELINGS DURING PREGNANCY

There have been few objective large-scale studies to identify common patterns of emotional response in fathers and mothers throughout childbearing. Nevertheless, pregnancy is generally regarded by psychologists and other health care workers as a period of increased susceptibility to crisis. It is a time when preventive intervention can do much to influence the attitudes and functioning of prospective parents.

During childbearing, the couple is faced with the challenges of redefining their present roles, working through old and possibly forgotten conflict relationships, and entering the parent role. In addition, it is a period that can encourage further development of the couple's mutual concern, tenderness, and intimacy. The emotional and physical adjustments required of the parents cause varying levels of stress and anxiety; these levels may change from one pregnancy to another in the same couple.

Some of the specific factors that contribute to the psychological response of the parents include body image changes, cultural expectations, relationships with and support of parents and close relatives, emotional security and positive relationships within the marriage, economic security, adequacy of housing, number of other children, and the interval between pregnancies. While pregnancy has been characterized by some as a period of dependency and possibly regression in the mother, this tendency is reduced by a secure life situation, a harmonious environment, and emotional support. In the past pregnant women have frequently been labeled dependent or regressed without a realistic appraisal of the stresses placed on them and of the resources available that might help them cope more effectively.

Expectant Mother

Because it is a time when so many strange, threatening, and seemingly unpredictable things are happening to her, the pregnant woman has much she would like to talk about, yet hesitates to do so for fear of being reprimanded or appearing abnormal or ignorant. According to Caplan [10], there is a shift in the woman's intrapsychic equilibrium; old conflicts and fantasies that were repressed in the unconscious come to the surface. It is as though a weakening of the normal defense forces has occurred, allowing previously unacceptable, irrational thoughts and impulses to surface. The accompanying free-floating anxiety is fixed to various objects and situations in the form of phobias, fearful forebodings, and dreams. The dreams, which may indicate apprehension, involve the infant, misfortunes, environmental threats such as being attacked, and, later in the pregnancy, the process of labor and delivery.

Pregnant women, according to one study [30], identify more tangible sources of anxiety in the prenatal period, such as physical discomfort, medical complications, fatigue and irritability, depression, fear of an abnormal baby, and fear for themselves. These anxieties, along with their emotional lability and their thoughts about death and dying, cause them on occasion to question their own sanity and their ability to cope. Reassurance that these are normal reactions is an essential part of prenatal care. Pregnant women need an attentive listener, one who displays more than a casual interest in how they are doing, and who will encourage them to verbalize their anxieties.

Expectant Father

For the expectant father, the changes caused by pregnancy influence his self-concept, his relationship to the woman, and his role in the social world outside the home. While the baby's birth is perhaps the most spectacular moment, a man's psychological involvement in pregnancy is shown in many ways.

Some men have physical complaints similar to the common symptoms of pregnancy, with the more anxious expectant fathers having the greater number of symptoms. Some have nausea and vomiting, constipation or diarrhea, or headaches and dizzy spells. Studies have shown nausea and vomiting are the most common symptoms, along with loss of appetite and toothache [46]. Symptoms may appear at any time but usually do not appear before the end of the second to the middle of the third month; they are, it is believed, most likely to be the result of feelings of ambivalence toward or identification or empathy with the woman.

Stresses for the expectant father may include coping with the woman's increasing dependency, particularly when the extended family members are far away, and coping with the threat of the loss of the woman's undivided attention and the threat to the couple's economic stability [38]. In addition, as he reflects on and evaluates the role his father played when he was a child, he begins to wonder what kind of a father he will be. Even an expectant father who has other children may feel ambivalence, evaluating his past fathering and projecting what it will be like with an additional child. Thus, pregnancy is frequently a period of insecurity for men.

The most comprehensive review of parents' reactions to childbearing is provided by the Colmans in their book, *Pregnancy: The Psychological Experience* [13]. They, as well as other authorities, differentiate the emotions predominate in each trimester.

First Trimester

The most important task for the woman during the first trimester is accepting the reality of her pregnancy and understanding its implications. Perhaps because of the physical discomforts during this period and the feelings of insecurity about new or additional responsibilities, ambivalence is the primary emotion now. Initial positive reactions are more likely to be found in primigravidas. Because initial negative attitudes may be replaced by more accepting ones later in the pregnancy, unplanned babies are not always unwelcomed babies. Likewise, planned babies are not always welcomed once the woman faces the realities of pregnancy and motherhood.

Many factors are involved in the woman's reactions to and ambivalence about the pregnancy. For most women, the focus in the first trimester is on themselves, since there is little tangible evidence of the baby's growth. Physical discomforts and subtle changes within her body demand her attention. She must cope with things such as nausea, vomiting, tender and swollen breasts, irritability, headache, fatigue, depression, and anxiety. The sudden and inexplicable mood swings contribute to the day-to-day difficulties faced by many pregnant women.

Sexual drive may vary in the first trimester. For some women there is a decrease in sexual desire, perhaps caused by nausea and fatigue or by changes in body image (e.g., breast enlargement and weight increase), which may seem great even at this early stage. Intercourse after conception may produce guilt for those who feel that its purpose is for childbearing. Other reasons for a decrease in sexual desire include fear of injuring the baby, insecurity, and financial and personal worries. However, some women feel more sensual during pregnancy and show an increased sexual drive, wanting to be cuddled, played with, and cared for. Even the most stable relationship may be upset by the changes now taking place. Therefore, it is important for a couple to understand and be prepared for what might happen.

Toward the end of the first trimester and into the second trimester, the primigravida concerns herself with her relationship with her own mother. She now becomes concerned with the kind of mother she will be and begins forming her own maternal identity, incorporating the good qualities to which she has been previously exposed. In doing so, she reviews those facets of her own childhood that produced pleasant and unpleasant feelings. Multigravidas generally review their past experience of mothering in light of an additional child.

For expectant fathers also, the main task during the first trimester is the acceptance of the reality of the pregnancy. This is generally accompanied by mixed emotions. Even those men who dread the responsibility of childrearing may take pride in this proof of their masculinity.

Whatever he feels, his wife will probably be seeking reassurance that he is pleased, that he will not reject her. . . . A husband may at first be pleased with the demands made upon him. . . . But if she is unable to get up every morning or falls asleep each time he wants to make love, it is likely that he will lose his warm protective feelings toward her and become more resentful and demanding. [13]

By the end of the first trimester, he begins to feel the responsibilities of fatherhood and questions his competence. He is now involved with the realistic particulars demanded by an enlarging family: need for additional room, financial concerns, and emotional stress and strain. At the same time, he senses the woman's involvement with herself and may feel excluded.

It is still too early for common issues of parenthood to unite husband and wife. If there is to be a mutual alliance during the pregnancy, it must begin to be forged at this stage, before the uniqueness of their experiences creates obstacles too great to be bridged. [13]

Second Trimester

Caplan and other authorities view the second trimester as a time when the mother becomes increasingly introverted, passive, and dependent. Caplan [10] sees the woman as a taker instead of a giver, a situation often requiring family adjustment. Hanford [24] reports that conflicts decline during the second trimester; by this time many women have come to accept the pregnancy. In interpreting data, however, one must remember that acceptance does not necessarily imply happiness. While many women are happy about their pregnancy, some regard it as a stress for as long as six months post partum or longer [33].

The highlight of the second trimester is feeling the baby move, and the baby now becomes conceptualized as a separate individual. Perhaps more than in the previous trimester, the woman feels a loss of control as her pregnancy becomes more visible. The fact of intercourse can no longer be hidden; sexually inhibited women may feel shame or disgust. As one woman describes her feelings:

You are quite obviously pregnant; then it is a queer naked feeling to walk along the street and feel no longer anonymous, realizing that there is one secret of your life that everyone who looks can know—that at least one private incident of your past has become almost incredibly public and that you can bear, as it were, the stigma of past passion wherever you go. [31]

Some women may feel more erotic now. There is, according to Masters and Johnson [32], a physical basis for this. Vaginal lubrication and the blood flow to the pelvic region increase. This causes the erogenous areas to become engorged more rapidly and excitement to linger after orgasm. This erotic feeling may make the woman more sexually demanding than her partner can cope with, especially with the obstacles of her changing shape and mood swings. Some couples may achieve better sexual relationships now; however, if they cannot discuss their sexual feelings, the entire relationship may deteriorate.

The man takes on new importance in the woman's eyes during this trimester, and she becomes very concerned for his safety. The woman's closeness to her partner is more evident if her mother or other close relatives or friends are not available to help care for her or plan for the baby.

Feeling the baby move is also a dramatic high point for the expectant father, intensifying the reality of his coming fatherhood. He may become preoccupied with childhood memories about his mother's or a relative's pregnancies, or even dream of becoming pregnant himself. He may become upset as he recognizes his own nurturant qualities or feels envy or jealousy toward the mother of his child. The woman's dependence on him and her concern about him and his safety may be a threat to his independence. In an effort to cope with these increased demands, expectant fathers may now develop new hobbies or devote more time to their work.

Third Trimester

During the third trimester, women feel a sense of accomplishment as well as anxiety about the coming labor and delivery. The anxiety shows a definite increase in the last half of the third trimester, according to Grimm [21]. In several studies [30, 49] multigravidas show higher anxiety levels than primigravidas; therefore, as the Colmans note, it is not valid to assume that multigravidas feel they have proved themselves or know what it is all about [13].

In addition to labor and delivery, the baby becomes the pregnant woman's main focus in the last trimester. Much of her time and thoughts are consumed with making the final preparations for the baby, naming him, and dreaming of how he will appear. The end of pregnancy can be a very sentimental time as she thinks of the special privileges that have been hers for the past months. Despite this, she looks forward to the end of pregnancy, for it is more difficult to sleep, eat, and carry out many of her daily activities. For some, careers end temporarily as they are forced to leave their jobs.

It is a time when the pregnant woman questions her self-image since she seems so large and her shape is so different. She needs reassurance that she is still loved. Attempts at intercourse may now pose a problem.

The wife's abdomen may present an insurmountable obstacle for a couple whose sex practices have always been conservative. Guilt or regression may result from experimentation with alternate modes of gratification which rely on exotic postures or oral and manual manipulation. [13]

It is especially important that the couple be close and communicate well with each other because of the experimentation that lovemaking may require or the fact that abstinence may be the choice of some couples.

By the third trimester the expectant father has had to cope with some of the problems brought on by the pregnancy. Men who have avoided dealing with the pregnancy in the past will continue to do so, spending their time and energies at work, with hobbies, or perhaps with other women [26].

Men actively involved with the pregnancy are drawn into practical activities such as helping with final preparations for the baby, planning for the trip to the hospital, and dealing realistically with financial issues. Some expectant fathers may participate in childbirth education classes with the woman and learn specific ways to care for her. Some may share the woman's increasing anxiety, and, in working together, their relationship may become more intense. Since some men may feel a sense of responsibility for the pregnancy, they may feel more tender or protective toward the woman. A man's own ideas about fathering now become more concrete.

FAMILY SUPPORTS

The type of family structure a woman has can be a valuable source of support during childbearing. In our society the nuclear family (mother, father, and children) is the best known family form. The Industrial Revolution has been considered the turning point from which the nuclear family evolved from the extended family, although some historical evidence indicates that it was the prevailing residential unit long before that time [20]. The nuclear family has been considered the center of emotional support, responsible for the growth of privacy in the family, and a way of better training the young in an isolated and controlled setting [20].

Within the nuclear family, members are not influenced as much by the limits and standards of older generations but rather have the opportunity to test things on their own. Stereotyped masculine and feminine roles are not as workable, since both partners must work together as an intimate team. Of necessity, the myriad of family needs are satisfied by few family members. In the nuclear family the pregnant woman has her husband for support. Unless she has sufficient money or close friends or relatives nearby, her support system may be limited to him.

The nuclear family has been criticized for the above reasons, and because of the intense relationship that develops among the family members and the fact that its children have few adult role models. Some critics feel that society has gradually usurped many of the functions of the nuclear family, e.g., as a recreational facility, as a socializing group for children, and for personal fulfillment of its members.

The extended family (mother, father, children, and one or more relatives) has a number of advantages. The daily work may be shared, as well as the economic cost of maintaining the household. According to some authorities, children who are cared for by several loving adults may be able to relate more easily to others. They may develop their male or female identities with less difficulty because they have been exposed to more role models. In general, they receive better socialization than those confined to two parents in the nuclear family. For some adults, the extended family provides security; for others, it requires conformity, limiting the opportunity to develop new life-styles [37].

The resurgence of the communal movement in America represents an attempt to allow for new ways of living and approaches to problem-solving, while incorporating the more positive aspects of the extended family. The communal movement in urban as well as rural settings has assumed a number of different forms. In some instances, the commune retains nuclear family units within it, and couples simply live in the same residence. In other communes, there are no identifiable smaller family units and everything is shared in common. Members may or may not hold jobs in the outside world.

The more stable, longer-lived communes are usually highly structured and tend to be centered around a common ideology, values, and goals. Decision-making is usually done by the group according to majority rule; responsibility for daily work, expenses, and childrearing is shared. Less stable communes seem to lack a strong cohesiveness and organization. While its members espouse a philosophy of closeness and involvement, they function fairly independently, often leaving group conflicts unresolved and work unfinished [27].

Home delivery with the father and midwife or doctor present is popular in some communes, since it reduces medical intervention and allows the childbirth experience to be shared more fully. The child is with the mother from the moment of birth and may be breast-fed for several years. In more radical communes birth certificates may be scorned, since the individual is then registered and will become a likely candidate for taxation and compulsory public education [45].

THE SINGLE PARENT

In contrast to the support offered in the extended family and some communal systems, the responsibilities of family life in the one-parent family fall for the most part on a lone individual [29]. Single-parent families result from single-parent adoptions, loss of one parent through death or divorce, or illegitimacy.

A small but growing number of single-parent families result from the change in adoption policies since the mid-1960s. These changes took place in response to the difficulties in finding homes for children with physical handicaps, older children, and children of a minority or mixed race. It is now recognized that a single parent can adequately raise children if given sufficient support from the parent's friends, relatives, and from community resources.

In the past one of the concerns of adoption agencies about single individuals adopting children was the lack of a suitable role model for the development of sexual identity. Today they look for a male or female figure in the adopting single parent's circle of friends or relatives. Even without one, they recognize that with an emotionally mature mother or father, a child can be expected to develop an appropriate sexual identity.

Single individuals adopting children appear to be emotionally mature, self-aware, self-confident, and able to tolerate a great deal of frustration. They tend to pursue an independent life and are not overly concerned about what other people think. While they do not have to be well educated, studies show that they are intelligent. They are motivated more by what they can contribute toward the child's normal development than by the fulfillment of their own needs [8].

Single-parent families, resulting from divorce, desertion, separation, or death, have always been with us. Because the remaining parent must develop a life-style that is different from his previous life-style, he is initially faced with a period of adjustment. He has to adjust to parenting for 24 hours a day without the assistance from the other parent that he once had. Other problems involve finding day-care centers and housekeepers and a need to work and to provide the additional emotional support to the child that was formerly supplied by the other parent. According to the Eglesons [15], the children often react by developing closer ties and being more sympathetic to the remaining parent. However, some children feel they must assume more responsibility at home and resent the fact that the parent's job takes him away.

A major source of single-parent families is unmarried mothers who keep their babies. There has been a steady rise in the number of illegitimate births (Table 5-1) and it is projected that this increase will continue [53].

UNMARRIED MOTHERS

The causes of illegitimacy have been attributed to many things. Theories advanced by everyone from psychiatrists, psychologists, and sociologists to the man on the street have attempted to characterize and in many cases stereotype women who have become pregnant outside of marriage. However, this same stereotyping has not been applied to the unmarried father.

A recurrent theme is that illegitimacy reflects an underlying family pathology; this pathology may include lack of love, understanding, and security at home, broken homes, a poor parent-child relationship, conflicts between parents, and a dominating mother or father [52]. Other theories emphasize the unwed woman's immature personality, her increased dependency needs, emotional disturbances,

Race and Age	Year					
	1945	1950	1960	1965	1968	1970
By race of mother						
White	56.4	53.5	82.5	123.7	155.2	175.1
Nonwhite	60.9	88.1	141.8	167.5	183.9	223.6
By age of mother						
Under 15	2.5	3.2	4.6	6.1	7.7	9.5
15–19	49.2	56.0	87.1	123.1	158.0	190.4
20–24	39.3	43.1	68.0	90.7	107.9	126.7
25–29	14.1	20.9	32.1	36.8	35.2	40.6
30–34	7.1	10.8	18.9	19.6	17.2	19.1
35–39	4.0	6.0	10.6	11.4	9.7	9.4
40 and over	1.2	1.7	3.0	3.7	3.3	3.0
Total number	117.4	141.6	224.3	291.2	339.2	398.7
Percent of all births	4.1%	3.9%	5.3%	7.7%	9.7%	10.7%

Source: Modified from U.S. National Center for Health Statistics. *Vital Statistics of the United States.* Washington, D.C. (published annually).

Table 5-1. Number (in Thousands) of Illegitimate Live Births in the United States, by Race and Age of Mother

rebellion against authority, and weak ego being responsible for sexual acting-out. Each of these theories has been taken to task. Wimperis [48] pointed out that extramarital affairs and premarital intercourse are fairly common. Should all who have these relations be regarded as emotionally disturbed, or would this designation apply only to those who have a child as a result? Studies by Clark Vincent [47] show that there are many unmarried mothers who apparently have mature personalities and who have come from stable homes with good parent-child relationships. A girl is more apt to come from a broken home if she happens to come from the lower socioeconomic class, where broken homes occur more frequently. Emotional deprivation is not inevitable for a person from a broken home, since there are often strengths in the situation which compensate for the absence of a parent.

Other theories attribute illegitimacy to the woman's need to be pregnant and to have a child. Sometimes women fear and doubt their femininity and even question their ability to produce children. Pressure from the peer group may also be a powerful influence in causing illegitimacy. However, in some cases of illegitimacy peer group contacts are limited, with few social contacts, few permanent friendships and few male contacts, causing the woman to feel a need to establish a close relationship with someone.

Another belief is that the illegitimacy rate reflects a decrease in religious conviction. In one study [11], however, one-third of a group of Canadian unwed mothers considered themselves fairly religious or strongly religious, which is similar to the proportion of religious adherence in the general population. In addition, Cutright [14] notes that in the United States church membership rose from 49 to 64 percent between 1940 and 1965. During that same period the illegitimacy rate more than doubled.

Sex Education

A major problem facing youth today is the contradictory messages they receive from society. On one hand, it is chic and desirable to be as sensual and sophisticated as possible, with an emphasis on having fun and developing one's sexual responses. On the other hand, part of the "sophistication" is knowing when to stop so that one does not become a parent before being ready to fill the role. Somewhere in between, youth is expected to learn how to do this by some kind of magic. Sex education is a beginning. Arnold [5] aptly notes "legislators and schools say 'it' should be taught in church or at home. Church and home 'pass the buck' back to the school. Consequently sex education is taught by anyone a year older than the one learning or by anyone who could sneak into an X-rated movie." While many schools do have sex education in the curriculum, the majority deal only with the biological aspects of reproduction. For the most part no one cares to deal with the affective component of sexual relations and methods of coping with the emotions involved. Young people are left to determine for themselves how to deal responsibly with sexual drives, either by controlling situations that end in unplanned pregnancy or by using birth control measures to prevent pregnancy.

Nurses should be involved in programs to help young people deal with their sexuality. Because illegitimacy is likely to be around for some time to come, nurses also need to be aware of those services that are most beneficial to unmarried mothers. In providing support for these women, programs designed to deliver comprehensive care have been structured around three main problem areas: medical care, social service, and education.

Problems and Comprehensive Services

It is a well-established fact that pregnancy in unwed mothers is accompanied by distinct hazards, including higher rates of prematurity, increased susceptibility to complications of pregnancy, and a resulting increased infant and maternal mortality [34]. The age, parity, and social conditions of many women in this group may be, in part, responsible for the increased risks. Whatever the reason, the fact remains that this high-risk group is in need of early and continuous prenatal care.

A number of deterrents prevent many of these women from receiving the care they need. Some women seek care late, in an attempt to conceal their pregnancy out of fear, guilt, or denial. Others tend to wait because of inadequate information about resources available to them, the cost of medical care, or disillusionment with medical clinics and the response of many personnel. If staff members fail to recognize that their own values and standards may not be the same as the patient's, they may tend to assume that she has certain feelings and will react in a certain way. This obstacle to effective care and communication is hard to overcome. As a result, the needs felt by the patient are often not met as the staff attends to meeting the needs they have identified.

Cahill [9], for instance, noted that personnel in one hospital made various invalid assumptions about patients: They assumed that the unmarried mother was embarrassed, had a negative attitude toward her pregnancy, and inevitably faced the decision of whether to keep or relinquish her baby. They tried to provide complete privacy and avoided any discussion of her unwed motherhood, and the problems, if any, that it presented for her.

For many teenage mothers, in addition to the medical risks of unwed pregnancy, there is the added problem of the interruption of their education, which decreases the likelihood of their ultimate independence. Many drop out of high school because of personal embarrassment, family pressures, and school policy. Eighty-five percent of those who drop out do not continue their schooling.

According to the National Alliance Concerned with School Aged Parents [28], an organization advocating better educational programs for pregnant teenagers, only 240 school systems in 37 states either permit pregnant girls to continue in classes or enroll them in special classes. Of the 37 states, 33 require that the girl drop out after the fifth month when she begins to look pregnant. Only 4 allow her to return to regular classes after the baby is born. This provides education to only 25 percent of the pregnant school girls in the United States. Most of the programs are concentrated in large cities.

Many school districts still disapprove of pregnant girls attending classes with other students, holding to the idea that pregnancy is "catching." Many believe that if the school allows the girl to continue her education normally, it appears that the school is approving premarital pregnancy and that soon "everyone will be doing it." Some school districts even expel the father if his identity becomes known [28]. Often girls are expelled on the pretext that pregnancy will interfere with their learning, yet a majority of the adolescents in one study [6] said that they were able to study better, concentrate harder, and retain more knowledge when they were pregnant, particularly in the second trimester.

In addition to the medical and educational problems the unmarried mother must cope with, she is often in need of practical assistance in dealing with the stresses of daily life and the plans that must be made for her and the baby's future. In one study [40], mothers identified a number of their needs—housing, financial aid, baby care, employment or job training, help with personal or social adjustment, medical care, and legal aid. Health care workers also felt the mothers had implicit needs for friendship, an independent life, and the respect of others for their personal worth.

Unwed teenage mothers especially need help in crisis periods throughout the pregnancy [43]. Health workers might not have dealt directly with the first and most acute crisis—that of being confronted with the actuality of the pregnancy and the need to inform parents and other authority figures. However, they must deal with the unwed mother's feelings and reactions to the pregnancy. A second period of crisis might develop about the time the teenage mother drops out of school and experiences isolation from her peers. A third crisis may develop when the mother's personal freedom is curtailed as she cares for the baby on a 24-hour basis at home.

For the adolescent now faced with caring for a baby, the developments of normal adolescence are interrupted. Pregnancy interferes with important psychosexual maturation. For example, changes in body image, a problem in normal adolescence, become more difficult to cope with as they are intensified by pregnancy. At the same time she is establishing an identity as a woman, she must assume the task of establishing an identity as a mother. Likewise, the emotional instability of adolescence is compounded by the emotional lability of pregnancy. For most adolescents, pregnancy decreases their choice of a vocation and their ability to separate from their parents. Because they are still adolescents, the expectation to fulfill demanding adult roles at this time often leads to frustration and failure.

One approach to solving the myriad of problems faced by a pregnant unmarried mother is to provide comprehensive services aimed at the major problem areas. Often, care in existing medical facilities is fragmented, depersonalized, and so time-consuming that it frustrates even the most mature adult. In an attempt to counteract this deficiency, some agencies have made efforts to personalize their patient care by instituting an appointment system, having the patients relate to the same staff members at each visit, and arranging clinic time to include evening hours.

Some national agencies attempting to solve or combat problems faced by the unmarried mother are the Florence Crittenton Homes, the Salvation Army's Booth Memorial Homes, and homes under the auspices of Catholic Charities. In recent years comprehensive programs, such as Young Mothers' Educational Development (YMED) in New York State, Delaware Adolescent Program in Wilmington, Yale-New Haven's Young Mothers' Program, and the federally funded Maternal-Infant Care (MIC) Project, have been established. The medical services of all of these agencies generally include prenatal care, hospital care, postpartum checkups to mothers, newborn care in the hospital, and well-baby care for varying periods after birth.

These social agencies attempt to help girls solve their personal problems that may have led to or been caused by their pregnancy, thereby increasing their potential for a more satisfying future. These agencies also provide assistance with practical aspects of housing, finances, and baby care centers. Finding adequate housing can be a problem for unmarried mothers, since public housing may be reluctant to give her space, viewing her as a social liability, and landlords often exploit her [44].

The educational services are aimed at providing a continuing formal education, with the hope that the mothers will continue their schooling following childbirth or that they will seek vocational or job training. Such programs may or may not be residential. Usually they are located fairly close to the mother's home and encourage involvement of her basic family and the father of the baby. Ideally, their services do not end with delivery of the baby but continue to function as a source of support to the mother until she is able to assume an independent role.

While the number of programs providing comprehensive care is increasing, some still feel that such attention inevitably encourages promiscuity; this remains an obstacle to more rapid progress. Such reasoning may also include denials that the problems exist and insistence that existing facilities can handle the problems of pregnant women of all ages and that there is a lack of financial resources for such projects [18].

Unmarried Fathers

Unlike the pregnant unmarried mother, who has been the focus of research and comprehensive supportive programs, the unmarried father remains virtually ignored. Vincent [47] cites several reasons for this. The double standard has led to a harsher judgment for the female than the male for sexual misbehavior. The presumption of innocence until proved guilty offers more protection for the male. Sexual misbehavior that threatens the mores supporting legitimacy is very evident in the female; therefore, her behavior is censured. Since the unmarried mother and the illegitimate child constitute a potential economic burden for society, they generate more public interest. Unwed mothers also are easier to identify and study as a group than are unwed fathers.

The most comprehensive work that has been reported was done at Vista Del Mar Child Care Service in Los Angeles by Ruben Pannor and his associates [35]. Data were collected on 222 unmarried mothers and 96 unmarried fathers. Contrary to the widely held stereotype, the relationship between the mother and father was more than a casual one. When the pregnancy became known, most of the fathers were very willing to take part in the mother's planning and decision-making, especially when she requested it. Pannor's data reinforced Vincent's findings that the fathers and mothers were approximately the same age and from a similar social, economic, cultural, and educational background.

Interviews of the fathers revealed seemingly contradictory ideas. Although most subscribed to the "sex is fun" ethic, many reported their actual experiences to be unsatisfactory, leaving them feeling guilty, depressed, and scared. The majority of the fathers and mothers did not use contraception, although they were knowledgeable about it and did not feel they would have difficulty in obtaining it. Almost 50 percent of the fathers stated that they did not like contraceptives; 24 percent stated that intercourse was not planned; 12 percent acted on the faith that nothing would happen. A commonly recurring comment was to the effect that the use of contraceptives debased the act: "she wasn't that kind of girl."

There appeared to be a widespread lack of concern for the consequences to the partner. "When neither sexual partner possesses a strong identity and neither is responsible and mature, each reinforces the other to satisfy personal needs" [35].

Pannor and associates [35] list ways in which the unmarried father can best participate when pregnancy becomes a reality:

1. Giving support to the unmarried mother. This lends some dignity to the relationship and is important to the mother.
2. Helping to plan for the child's care and future.
3. Acknowledging and meeting financial responsibility. (Fathers in the study were willing to do this.)
4. Looking at the problems revealed by the pregnancy.
5. Understanding the meaning and responsibilities of marriage and parenthood.
6. Examining his attitude toward the child's mother.
7. Identifying his attitude toward sex and understanding the meaning of sexual relations.
8. Understanding his attitude toward fatherhood. (Holding their babies after birth helped the fathers toward this goal.)

The fathers in Pannor's study had the social workers' help in working toward the above goals. When the fathers were involved throughout the pregnancy, the final decision about the child's future was made either jointly by the father and mother, or, as in most of the other cases, was made by the mother and reinforced by the father. This seemed to leave both parents with a more positive feeling about their choice.

Parents of the unwed couples also were participants in the study. Since Pannor and his associates felt that they had a right and a responsibility to assert themselves. The couples needed to be aware of the parents' thoughts and feelings, as well as the extent of the practical supports that they were willing to offer. In addition, the parents needed to help in understanding and coping with the situation.

Whether or not to keep the baby is a decision that is made by the mother alone or with the support of the baby's father, relatives or friends. In some cultural groups it is the accepted norm to keep the baby; in these cases, for the most part, the decision is ready-made. When a mother decides to place her baby for adoption, she should have explored all the alternatives open to her and have chosen the one that is best for her. It is important that she be supported in her decision by health care personnel; the mother should not have the additional burden of having to cope with the expression of opposing attitudes and values of the staff. As one young mother stated, "I found myself giving support to nurses who would say, 'I don't see how you can give up such a beautiful baby,' or 'I can't be here when you leave. It will be so sad because I know you're giving up the baby.'"

The first few days after delivery can be particularly trying as additional details concerning adoption procedures must be finalized at a time when the mother feels fatigued, isolated, and unable to make decisions. Following the relinquishment of the baby, the mother may begin to feel guilt and loneliness. She may undergo a grieving process as she works through what the separation from the baby has meant to her. For some, this will take a considerable amount of time.

ADOPTION

Adoption has a long history. Early Romans, Egyptians, and Greeks used adoption as a means of providing an heir or successor. The Bible mentions the adoption of Moses and Esther. It is only since the 1850s in the United States that adoption has had legal restrictions placed on it [2].

Recent statistics have shown that the demand for adoptions is rising. At the same time the supply of white babies available for adoption has decreased, mainly because of better birth control methods, liberalized abortion laws, and the increasing number of unmarried mothers who decide to keep their babies. Fewer than one-third of the babies born out of wedlock in a year are adopted. According to the Child Welfare League of America, for every 100 white babies awaiting adoption, there are 116 prospective homes. For every 100 nonwhite babies awaiting adoption there are 39 prospective homes [17]. This has caused an increase in the number of nonwhite or mixed race children being adopted by white families, as well as an effort to help more black families adopt black children. More black families might adopt if there were not misunderstandings of adoption requirements regarding age, economic status, and proof of sterility. Other deterrents have included a reluctance to be questioned about personal matters, the expectation of rejection, anxiety about filling out required forms, and inability to meet the legal fees [1, 17, 23].

About half of the children adopted each year are adopted by relatives. Of the other 50 percent, well over half involve children born out of wedlock. About two-thirds of these adoptions by nonrelatives are arranged by social agencies, while the other third result from independent adoptions (Table 5-2). In the latter instance, the child is placed directly with the adoptive parents, either by the mother herself, or through an unlicensed intermediary, such as a physician, lawyer, or minister.

In agency adoptions, the child is first placed with an agency and from there with the adoptive parents. While agency adoptions seem to be more controlled, there are still a number of associated problems. Often there are unnecessary delays and restrictive policies. Substandard legal and health services may be a problem if there is inadequate legal and medical staff supervision [2].

A service provided by some agencies is the collection of detailed information about the natural father as well as the mother, which they can make available to the adoptive parents. This effort is directed toward providing many more adoptive children with a realistic and more complete picture of their biological heritage, and with the reasons their natural parents chose adoption for them [3].

Problems associated with independent adoptions are far more numerous. This type of adoption can foster a "black market" in baby-selling. There is no assurance that the intermediary is competent or willing to do the studies of prospective parents usually completed by agencies. It is also unlikely that the natural mother will receive casework help, and there is a greater likelihood that she will try to get her baby back. Frequently the child is not legally free for adoption at the time he is placed and at the time the adoption should be completed [2].

The best professional service is provided when lawyers, social workers, and doctors work cooperatively to represent the best interests of the child, whose rights supersede those of the natural or adoptive parents. It is paramount in importance that the child is placed in a family evaluated by qualified persons as having emotional, physical, mental, financial, and spiritual qualities that will best implement the child's maximum development [50].

At the same time the natural mother has the right to medical, legal, religious, and financial assistance during her confinement, delivery, and recovery. She also has the right to decide about the disposition of her child under a minimum of pressure. When the child is illegitimate, generally only the mother's consent is necessary for purposes of adoption. Once she has relinquished the child for adoption, she loses her

Table 5-2. Number (in Thousands) of Child Adoptions in the United States, by Type

Type of Adoption	1955	1960	1965	1968	1970	1971
By relatives	45	49	65	80	86	86
By nonrelatives	48	58	77	86	89	83
Placed by social agencies	27	33	53	64	69	66
Total number of adoptions	93	107	142	166	175	169

Source: Modified from U.S. National Center for Health Statistics. *Vital Statistics of the United States.* Washington, D.C. (published annually).

right to have a voice in the child's future, except to ask that he be placed in a family whose religion is similar to hers [47]. (This exception seems to be becoming less common [22].)

The general rule appears to be that the mother's right to the illegitimate child supersedes the father's, but the father's right is superior to that of all other persons. However, the father, unless married to the mother, has no legal right to the child and cannot stand in the way of the adoption unless he sues in court for a declaration of paternity. If it is granted, then his signature is also necessary in order for the adoption to take place [25].

The adoptive parents have a right to know the physical, social, mental, and emotional makeup of the natural parents of the child. They also have a right to be protected against the possibility that the natural parents might change their minds about the adoption. There is a period of 6–12 months during which the child is placed in the adoptive home before the legal adoption can take place. Once the adoption has been finalized, the child and the adoptive parents experience the same legal rights as any other family.

REFERENCES

1. Adoption, 1975. *Contemporary Ob/Gyn* 5:35, 1975.
2. American Academy of Pediatrics. *Adoption of Children.* Evanston, Ill., 1967.
3. Anglim, E. The adopted child's heritage—Two natural parents. *Child Welfare* 44:339, 1965.
4. Anthony, E. J., and Benedek, T. (Eds.). *Parenthood: Its Psychology and Psychopathology.* Boston: Little, Brown, 1970.
5. Arnold, L. T. Teenage pregnancy. *Journal of the Tennessee Medical Association* 64:1054, 1971.
6. Barglow, P., Bornstein, M., Exum, D., Wright, M., and Visotsky, H. Some psychiatric aspects of illegitimate pregnancy in early adolescence. *American Journal of Orthopsychiatry* 38:672, 1968.
7. Benedek, T. The organization of the reproductive drive. *International Journal of Psychoanalysis* 41:1, 1960.
8. Branham, E. One parent adoptions. *Children* 17:103, 1970.
9. Cahill, I. Facts and fallacies about illegitimacy. *Nursing Forum* 4:30, 1965.
10. Caplan, G. Psychological aspects of maternity care. *American Journal of Public Health* 47:25, 1957.
11. Clamen, A. D., Williams, B., and Wogan, L. Reaction of unmarried girls to pregnancy. *Canadian Medical Association Journal* 101:328, 1969.
12. Cobliner, W. G. Some maternal attitudes toward conception. *Mental Hygiene* 49:550, 1965.
13. Colman, A., and Colman, L. *Pregnancy: The Psychological Experience.* New York: Herder and Herder, 1971.
14. Cutright, P. Illegitimacy: Myths, causes, and cures. *Family Planning Perspectives* 3:26, 1971.
15. Egleson, J. and Egleson, J. *Parents Without Partners.* New York: Dutton, 1961.
16. Flapan, M. A paradigm for the analysis of childbearing motivations of married women prior to birth of the first child. *American Journal of Orthopsychiatry* 39:402, 1969.
17. Gallagher, U. Adoption resources for black children. *Children* 18:49, 1971.
18. Garell, D. C. DAPI—when no one else will take you. *Delaware Medical Journal* 42:77, 1970.
19. Gordon, E. M. Acceptance of pregnancy before and since oral contraception. *Obstetrics and Gynecology* 29:144, 1967.
20. Gordon, M. *The Nuclear Family in Crisis.* New York: Harper & Row, 1972.
21. Grimm, E. Psychological tension in pregnancy. *Psychosomatic Medicine* 23:520, 1961.
22. Gustin, K. The Adopting Family. In D. Hymovick and M. Barnard (Eds.), *Family Health Care.* New York: McGraw-Hill, 1973.

23. Hammons, C. The adoptive family. *American Journal of Nursing* 76:251, 1976.
24. Hanford, J. Pregnancy as a state of conflict. *Psychological Reports* 22:1313, 1968.
25. Holder, A. The illegitimate and his father. *Journal of the American Medical Association* 216:1909, 1971.
26. Jarvia, W. Some effects of pregnancy and childbirth on men. *Journal of the American Psychoanalytical Association* 10:689, 1962.
27. Kanter, R. Communes. In M. Gordon (Ed.), *The Nuclear Family in Crisis*. New York: Harper & Row, 1972.
28. Kiester, E., Jr. The bitter lessons too many of our schools are teaching pregnant teenagers. *Today's Health* 72:54, 1972.
29. Klein, C. *The Single Parent Experience*. New York: Walker, 1973.
30. Larsen, V. Stresses of the childbearing year. *American Journal of Public Health* 56:32, 1966.
31. Lewis, A. *An Interesting Condition*. New York: Doubleday, 1950.
32. Masters, W. H., and Johnson, V. E. *Human Sexual Response*. Boston: Little, Brown, 1966.
33. Nilsson, A. Para-natal emotional adjustment: A prospective investigation of 165 women. Part 1. *Acta Psychiatrica Scandinavica* 220 (*Supplement*):9, 1970.
34. Paavola, A. The illegitimacy rate and factors influencing the pregnancy and delivery of unmarried mothers. *Acta Obstetricia et Gynecologica Scandinavica* 47:1, 1968.
35. Pannor, R., Massarik, F., and Evans, B. *The Unmarried Father*. New York: Springer, 1971.
36. Poffenberg, S., Poffenberg, T., and Landis, J. T. Intent toward conception and the pregnancy experience. *American Sociological Review* 17:616, 1952.
37. Rayner, E. *Human Development*. London: Allen & Unwin, 1970.
38. Retterstol, N. Paranoid psychoses associated with impending or newly established fatherhood. *Acta Psychiatrica Scandinavica* 44:51, 1968.
39. Rossi, A. S. Transition to Parenthood. In I. L. Reiss (Ed.), *Readings on the Family System*. New York: Holt, Rinehard, & Winston, 1972.
40. Sauber, M., and Rubinstein, E. *Experiences of the Unwed Mother as a Parent*. New York: Community Council of Greater New York, 1965.
41. Scott, E., Illsley, R., and Biles, M. E. A psychological investigation of primigravidae. Part 3. Some aspects of maternal behavior. *Journal of Obstetrics and Gynaecology of the British Commonwealth* 63:494, 1965.
42. Sherman, J. *On the Psychology of Women*. Springfield, Ill.: Thomas, 1971.
43. Signell, K. The crisis of unwed motherhood: A consultation approach. *Community Mental Health Journal* 5:304, 1969.
44. Singer, A. *A program for young mothers and their babies. Social Casework* 52:567, 1971.
45. Smith, D., and Sternfield, J. The hippie communal movement: Effects on childbirth and development. *American Journal of Orthopsychiatry* 40:527, 1970.
46. Trethowan, W. H. The Couvade Syndrome. In J. G. Howells (Ed.), *Modern Perspectives in Psycho-Obstetrics*. New York: Bruner/Mazel, 1972.
47. Vincent, C. *Unmarried Mothers*. New York: Free Press, 1961.
48. Wimperis, V. *The Unmarried Mother and Her Child*. London: Allen & Unwin, 1960.
49. Winokur, G., and Werhoff, J. The Relationship of Conscious Maternal Attitudes to Certain Aspects of Pregnancy. *Psychiatric Quarterly* 30 (*Supplement*):61, 1956.
50. Wolff, S. The fate of the adopted child. *Archives of Disease in Childhood* 49:165, 1974.
51. Wyatt, F. Clinical notes on motives of reproduction. *Journal of Social Issues* 23:29, 1967.
52. Young, L. *Out of Wedlock*. New York: McGraw-Hill, 1954.
53. Yurdin, M. Recent trends in illegitimacy—implications for practice. *Child Welfare* 49:373, 1970.

Chapter 6 The Development of the Placenta and Fetus

FERTILIZATION

The process of fertilization involves the penetration of the ovum by a spermatozoon and the mingling of the nuclear material of each, resulting in a one-celled *zygote,* a term that is also loosely applied to later stages of cell division. This initiates cellular division, leading to the formation of a new individual. In the union of egg and sperm, which usually takes place in the ampulla of the tube, there are several significant biological implications: (1) The diploid number of chromosomes (46 chromosomes) is restored; (2) the sex of the zygote is determined by the spermatozoon through its contribution of an X or a Y chromosome; and (3) a series of mitotic divisions begins that result in cleavage and further development of the zygote.

Although only one of the many millions of spermatozoa deposited in the female genital tract actually fertilizes the ovum, the others may aid the fertilizing sperm in penetrating the ovum. Presumably their enzymatic action helps to detach the corona radiata. In so doing, some sperm become embedded in the zona pellucida (Figure 6-1). Soon after the spermatozoon enters the ovum, the ovum finishes its second maturational division and its chromosomes arrange themselves in a vesicular nucleus known as the female pronucleus. Meanwhile, the head of the spermatozoon swells, forming the male pronucleus. The fusion of the two pronuclei restores the diploid number of chromosomes to the new individual (Figure 6-2). A series of mitotic divisions now begins.

Following the two-celled stage, the zygote continues its division into an increasingly larger number of cells, but these cells become smaller with each cleavage division. Therefore, while the number of cells increases rapidly, the total mass increases little. The dividing cells in this stage are known as *blastomeres.*

During this cell division, the zygote passes down the tube. Transport of the cleaving egg along the tube is brought about by ciliary activity and tubal peristalsis, which probably act on the fluid in the tube rather than directly on the egg. During this phase, the egg lives mainly on the meager nutritional store of the blastomeres themselves. It is also possible that it derives some nutritional elements, such as amino acids and monosaccharides, from the breakdown products of tubal secretions [2].

On the third or fourth day after ovulation, the zygote, containing 12–16 cells and called the *morula* at this stage, enters the uterus. The morula consists of an *inner cell mass,* which develops into the embryo, and a surrounding *outer cell mass,* which forms the *trophoblast* and later develops into the placenta. During the next two or three days, as the morula continues to divide, fluid from the uterine cavity passes into the intercellular spaces of the inner cell mass. As the fluid continues to increase,

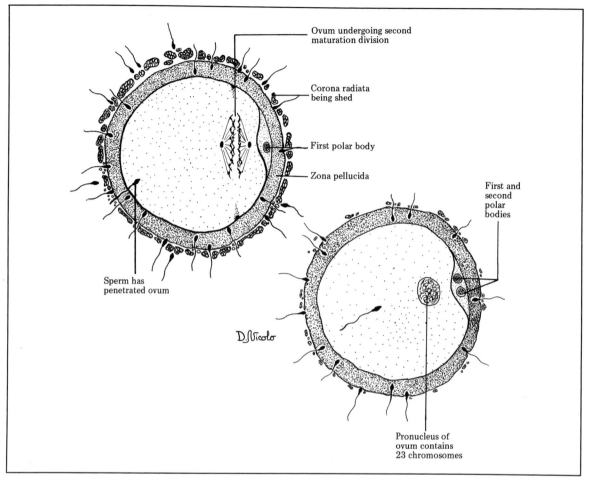

Ovum undergoing second
maturation division

Corona radiata
being shed

First polar body

Zona pellucida

First and
second
polar
bodies

Sperm has
penetrated ovum

D.Nicolo

Pronucleus of
ovum contains
23 chromosomes

*Figure 6-1. Ovum being
fertilized.*

these spaces form a single cavity, the *blastocele*. The zygote is now known as the *blastocyst, blastula,* or *blastodermic vesicle*. The inner cell mass, now known as the embryoblast, is located on one pole, while the outer cell mass (trophoblast) forms the wall of the blastocyst. The blastocyst, now floating free in the uterine cavity, derives its nutrition from the uterine glands, which secrete a mixture of mucopolysaccharides, glycogen, and lipids [2]. During this period the zona pellucida is lost, and the trophoblast is then able to become attached directly to the surface of the endometrium.

Around the eighth day, a second cavity, the primitive yolk sac, forms in the area of the blastocyst cavity. Although it does not store yolk, it is important for several reasons [6]. Apparently the yolk sac has some role in the early transport of nutrients to the embryo while uteroplacental circulation is being established. Blood forms on the walls of the yolk sac in the third week and continues to form there until hematopoiesis begins in the liver. Primitive germ cells appearing in the wall of the yolk sac in the third week subsequently migrate to the developing gonads, where they be-

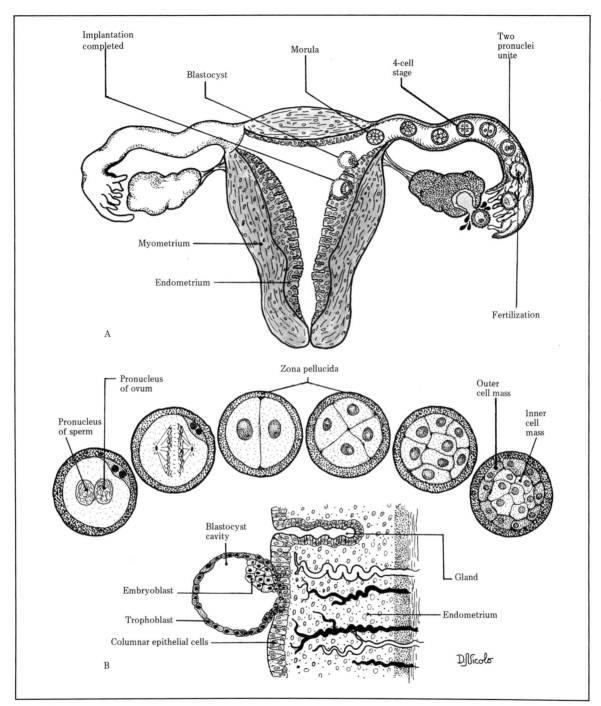

Figure 6-2. Implantation of the blastocyst. A. Serial representation of ovum from ovulation to implantation. B. Blastocyst beginning implantation (*zona pellucida has been lost*).

come germ cells. During the fourth week, the dorsal part of the yolk sac becomes the primitive gut of the embryo.

After the twelfth week, the yolk sac is located in the chorionic cavity between the amnion and the chorionic sac; it now begins to shrink and solidify as pregnancy advances. It may sometimes be seen on the fetal surface of the placenta at the time of delivery.

OUTER CELL MASS

Implantation

The trophoblast begins implanting in the endometrium six to seven days after fertilization. This occurs most often on the upper part of the posterior uterine wall. The trophoblastic cells burrow between the columnar epithelial cells, and these epithelial cells soon begin to degenerate. By the eighth day the blastocyst is partially embedded in the endometrium. At the embryonic pole of the blastocyst, the trophoblast forms a solid disc composed of an inner layer, the *cytotrophoblast,* and an outer layer, the *syncytiotrophoblast* or *syncytium.* At this time the endometrium adjacent to the implantation site is edematous and increasingly vascular, and its large tortuous glands secrete glycogen and mucus. The syncytial layer has the ability to erode maternal tissues, and once the process begins it advances rapidly.

Spaces known as trophoblastic lacunae appear by the ninth day in the proliferating syncytium. Soon the syncytium invades small, irregular capillaries in the uterine mucosa, forming maternal sinusoids. Blood oozes from the sinusoids into the lacunae, thus establishing a rudimentary uteroplacental circulation. As the trophoblast continues to invade more sinusoids, the lacunae eventually become continuous with maternal arterial and venous capillaries. Because of the difference in pressure between these capillaries, maternal blood begins to flow through the lacunar complex (Figure 6-3).

By this time (the twelfth day) the uterine epithelium has usually healed over the area through which the trophoblast eroded its way into the mucosa. Occasionally, bleeding may occur at the implantation site as a result of increased blood flow into the lacunar spaces in this area. (The pregnant woman may think that the resulting vaginal bleeding is her menstrual period, since it occurs around the thirteenth day after ovulation. This may cause confusion in determining the expected date of delivery.)

Placental Formation

The lacunae and the syncytial strands surrounding them, which were arranged irregularly at first, now begin to radiate out from the cytotrophoblast. Cytotrophoblastic cells project into the organized syncytial strands, forming *primary villi.* The villi, surrounded by lacunae, have a cytotrophoblastic core covered with syncytium. By the beginning of the third week, the trophoblast, also referred to as the chorion, has developed many primary villi (Figure 6-4).

Figure 6-3. Blastocyst embedded in the endometrium approximately 12 days after fertilization. Syncytium invades maternal sinusoids.

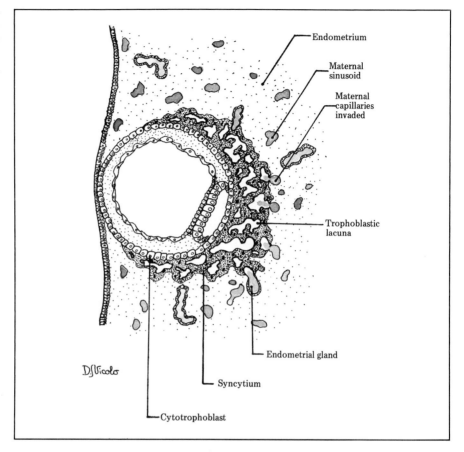

The primary villi enter into the stage in which they are called secondary villi when they develop central cores of mesenchyme. Small capillaries begin to arise in the villous core, branch out into the villus (which by this stage is now a tertiary villus), and during the fourth week of development make contact with the intraembryonic circulatory system. The primary villi become anchored deep in the uterine endometrium, and soon numerous small fingerlike projections branch from existing villous stems into surrounding *lacunar,* or *intervillous, spaces.* These are known as *free,* or *terminal villi.* Some researchers have stated that the fetus relies on free, or terminal, villi for exchange between fetal capillaries and maternal blood in the intervillous space [2]. By the fourth month, these terminal villi have only syncytium and the endothelial wall of the capillaries to separate maternal and fetal circulations.

Villi cover the entire surface of the chorion early in pregnancy. Soon those villi beneath the embryo continue to grow and form the *chorion frondosum* or bushy chorion. At the same time the villi on the side opposite the embryo degenerate, leaving that side smooth by the third month. This portion of the chorion is known as the *chorion laeve,* or bald chorion (Figure 6-5).

The thickened uterine endometrium is known as the *decidua* during pregnancy.

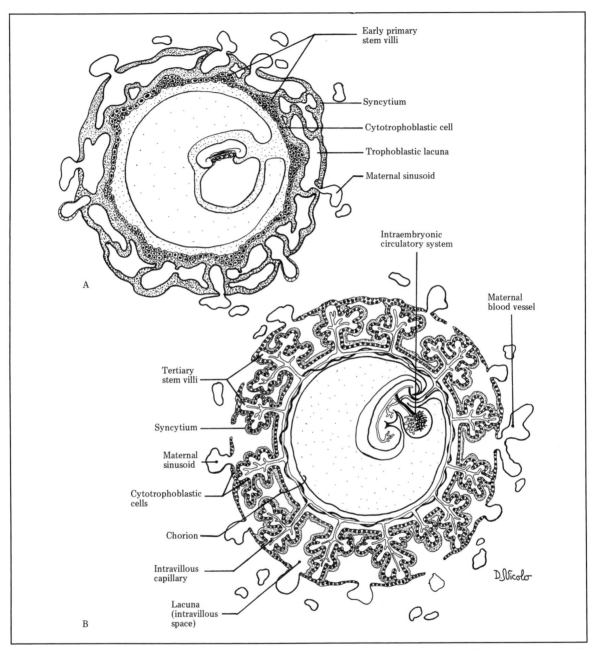

Early primary
stem villi

Syncytium

Cytotrophoblastic cell

Trophoblastic lacuna

Maternal sinusoid

A

Intraembryonic
circulatory system

Maternal
blood vessel

Tertiary
stem villi

Syncytium

Maternal
sinusoid

Cytotrophoblastic
cells

Chorion

Intravillous
capillary

Lacuna
(intravillous
space)

B

D. Nicolo

*Figure 6-4. A. During the second week of embryonic development cytotrophoblastic cells begin to form primary stem villi.
B. At four weeks of development there are many villi. Capillaries have formed within them and have made contact with
the intraembryonic circulatory system.*

Figure 6-5. Uterine decidua and developing chorion.

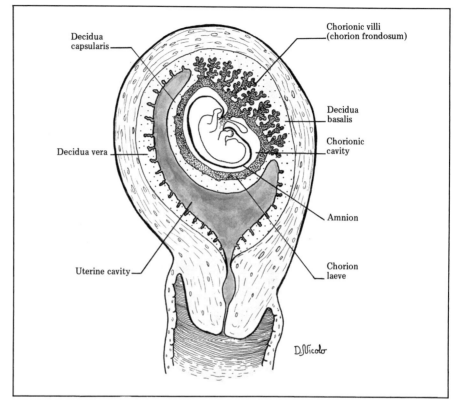

The layer in contact with the chorion frondosum is called the *decidua basalis*. It is composed of a compact layer tightly connected to the chorion and a spongy layer with dilated glands and spiral arteries. The placenta is formed from the decidua basalis and the chorion frondosum (the only functional part of the chorion). The decidual layer covering the chorion laeve is known as the *decidua capsularis*. Early in its development the decidua capsularis has a structure similar to the decidua basalis. Later, the growing conceptus causes it to project into the uterine cavity; the decidua capsularis becomes stretched and degenerates by the third month. The chorion laeve then comes in contact with the epithelium of the *decidua vera* on the opposite side of the uterus. By the fourth month the two fuse, obliterating the uterine cavity (Figure 6-6).

Another important membrane, the amnion, begins to develop by about the seventh to eight day after ovulation. It begins as a small vesicle and grows into a small sac that eventually surrounds the embryo. Further growth of the sac brings the amnion into contact with the chorion, and the two, although slightly adherent, can be separated at term.

Figure 6-6. Fusing of the decidua vera and the chorion laeve occurs by the fourth month of embryonic development. The uterine cavity is now obliterated.

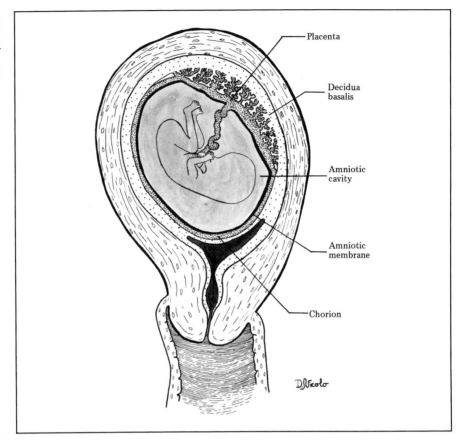

In early pregnancy the normally clear alkaline fluid that collects within the amniotic cavity is primarily a product of the amnion. Its functions are to cushion the fetus against injury, provide a medium in which it can move, and maintain a relatively constant temperature. The amount and constituents of the fluid change as pregnancy progresses. During the first half of pregnancy, the fluid is similar in composition to maternal plasma but has less protein and little solid material. In the latter half of pregnancy it contains varying amounts of desquamated fetal cells, lanugo, scalp hair, and vernix caseosa, as well as other solutes. Also in the latter half of pregnancy the fetus contributes to amniotic fluid composition and volume by both urinating and swallowing large amounts of fluid. The fetal urine raises the concentration of urea, creatinine, and uric acid. Although the total volume may vary, there is an average of about 1000 milliliters of amniotic fluid at term.

Maturing Placenta

The placenta continues to increase in both size and weight throughout pregnancy. At term it weighs approximately 450–680 grams (1–1½ pounds), or about one-sixth of the weight of the baby. It has a discoid shape, and the appearance of its two surfaces is markedly different. The fetal surface is covered by the shiny amnion. The rough, red maternal surface is divided into an average of 22 lobes, or *cotyledons,* which develop between the fourth and fifth months as a result of septum formation by the decidua basalis (Figure 6-7).

The placenta's functions, many of which begin soon after implantation, include fetal respiration, nutrition, excretion, and hormone exchange. It also synthesizes hormones and probably has an immunological and protective role. As the placenta grows and the fetal demands increase, certain necessary changes alter placental efficiency. The syncytium thins and the number of blood vessels close to its surface increase, facilitating transport of materials to and from the fetus. Later in pregnancy its efficiency is decreased by other changes, including the obliteration of certain vessels and deposits of fibrin and calcium in the placenta.

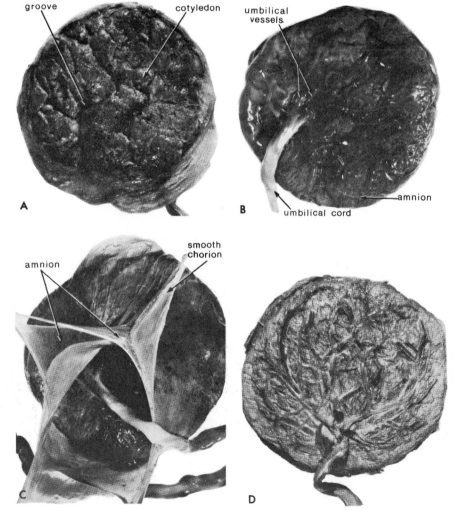

Figure 6-7. Full-term placentas. A. Maternal surface, showing cotyledons and grooves. B. Fetal surface, showing blood vessels running under the amnion and meeting at the umbilical cord. C. Inner amnion and outer smooth chorion. D. Marginal attachment of cord, often called battledore placenta. (*From K. L. Moore.* Before We Are Born. *Philadelphia: Saunders, 1974.*)

Table 6-1. Placental Transport

Substance	Mechanism	Characteristics
Oxygen and carbon dioxide	Simple diffusion	Dependent on rate of maternal blood flow in intervillous space and flow of fetal blood in chorionic villi and on thickness and surface area of placental barrier
Water	Diffusion	Peak in transfer at 36th week, when it is $3\frac{1}{2}$ liters/hour to and from fetus—70 times as great as at the 9th week
Sodium and potassium	Diffusion and active transfer	Less than 0.1% of sodium that reaches fetus is retained. Equal amounts in mother and fetus
Calcium	Active transfer	Fetus obtains calcium at expense of maternal reserves. Maternal calcium metabolism increased in pregnancy. Placental barrier offers little resistance. Higher in fetus than in mother
Iron	Active transfer	Fetus obtains iron at expense of maternal reserves. Higher in fetus than in mother
Phosphates	Active transfer	Inorganic phosphates twice as high in fetal blood as in maternal blood
Fluoride	Unknown	Readily crosses placental barrier. Appears to be concentrated in the placenta and this perhaps regularizes its transfer
Iodide	Similar to that of iodide concentration by thyroid gland	Taken up by fetal thyroid gland as early as 14th week of gestation. Readily crosses placental barrier
Carbohydrates	Diffusion and active transport	Principal source of energy for the fetus. Concentration of glucose in fetal blood is 20–30% lower than that of mother, perhaps due to utilization by placenta itself
Lipids fats and fatty acids	Not resolved. May be diffusion, active transport, pinocytosis	Concentration greater in maternal blood than in fetal blood. Absorption of fat, fatty acids, and glycerol in placenta may be similar to absorption in intestinal canal
Amino acids, polypeptides, and proteins (antibodies and antigens)	Probably active transport; pinocytosis	Amino acids used in fetal circulation for synthesis of plasma and tissue proteins. Higher in fetus than in mother. Significant levels of gamma globulin antibodies reached between 22nd–30th week. Increase to equal maternal level at 9th month
Vitamins	Very complex; probably active transport	Most known vitamins present in the placenta although precise localization indefinite. Water soluble vitamins cross more readily than fat soluble vitamins. Levels of vitamin A and E lower in fetus than in mother; B complex, C, and D higher in fetus; B, C, D, E stored in placenta

Table 6-1 (Continued)

Substance	Mechanism	Characteristics
Drugs and antibiotics	Diffusion; some active transport	Placenta is permeable to most drugs; the higher the molecular weight, the slower the passage. Passage of insulin controversial
Infectious agents	Unknown	Some bacteria, protozoa, viruses, rickettsiae. Permeability of placenta to *Treponema pallidum* increased after the 5th month

PLACENTAL EXCHANGE.

Placental exchange of substances between mother and fetus occurs across the *placental barrier,* or *membrane,* which is composed of a layer of syncytium and fetal capillary endothelium. The exchange is dependent on adequate maternal blood flow in the intervillous space and fetal blood in the chorionic villi.

Studies have shown that passive transfer through a semipermeable membrane is not the only method of placental exchange. It is believed that some antibodies are transported by pinocytosis [5]. Many substances, such as calcium, sodium, iron, inorganic phosphates, and amino acids, are present in greater concentrations in fetal blood than in maternal blood; it appears that they have crossed the placental membrane via active transport. Although it was once assumed that the placental membrane remained a complete barrier, current theory indicates that there may be a limited exchange of fetal and maternal blood cells, hormones, and immunological substances in normal pregnancy (Table 6-1) [2].

HORMONE PRODUCTION

Presently only five hormones are known to be produced by the placenta: the protein hormones, namely human chorionic gonadotropin (HCG), human chorionic somatomammotropin or human placental lactogen (HPL), and thyrotropin; and the steroid hormones, namely estrogen and progesterone. It is generally believed that the syncytium is the site of hormone production (Table 6-2) [7].

Since the placenta must be considered a homograft, one wonders why the products of conception do not habitually provoke an immune response in the mother; the reason (or reasons) that they do not remains a mystery. The most acceptable explanation for the survival of this homograft is that the placental membrane results in a fairly complete anatomic separation of maternal and fetal circulations [5].

INNER CELL MASS

Embryonic Period (Two to Eight Weeks)

From the beginning of the second week until the eighth week, the embryo undergoes morphogenesis (i.e., all major features of the external body take recognizable form), and organogenesis (i.e., the main organ systems are laid down). During the long fetal period that follows, the organs undergo little more than maturation.

SECOND WEEK

By the eighth day of development, the cells of the growing embryo (embryoblast) differentiate into two distinct cell layers. The layer of small flattened polyhedral cells is known as the entodermal germ layer, and the layer of high columnar cells is

Table 6-2. Placental Hormones[a]

Hormone	Source	Characteristics, Values, and Functions
Human chorionic gonadotropin (HCG)	Syncytium	Chemical and biological properties similar to pituitary luteinizing hormone. Appearance in urine is used as test for pregnancy Detected in blood and urine soon after implantation (10 days after conception). Peak between 50–70 days of gestation—20,000–100,000 IU/24 hours. Low level maintained thereafter (4000–11,000 IU/24 hours). Disappears within four days postpartum. Stimulates and prolongs existence of corpus luteum
Human placental lactogen (HPL) chorionic somatomam- motropin)	Syncytium	Composition similar to human pituitary growth hormone. Present in urine Detected during fourth week after conception. Concentration rises rapidly throughout pregnancy, reaching peak (serum level) in last trimester 2–10 mcg/ml at term. Rapidly disappears from maternal circulation within one day after delivery Plays possible role in mammary development. Might be synergistic with HCG in maintenance of corpus luteum. Significant physiological antagonist of insulin. May be "diabetogenic" factor in pregnancy
Progesterone	Syncytium	Necessary for maintenance of pregnancy. Transition from dependence on ovarian production to dependence on placental production at 6–8 weeks of gestation Daily production in late pregnancy is about 250 mg Principal metabolite is pregnanediol (found in urine). Fetus contributes little to production directly or by the provision of precursors
Estrogen	Syncytium	By seventh week of gestation, more than 50% of estrogens in maternal circulation produced by the placenta Increased amounts of estriol excreted in urine during pregnancy; 24–28 mg/24 hours is the average excretion at term Significant fetal contribution to placental production of estrogen. Maintenance of fetal circulation essential to adequate placental function. Fetus provides estrogen precursors from adrenal gland and liver. Therefore, determination of urinary estriol during pregnancy can be test of placental function and fetal well-being
Thyrotropin	Syncytium	Thyroid-stimulating properties

[a]Evidence for the synthesis of other hormones, such as melanocyte-stimulating hormone, adrenocorticotropic hormone, relaxin, corticosteroids, and aldosterone is not conclusive.

known as the ectodermal germ layer. The ectodermal and entodermal cells form the *bilaminar germ disc.* The ectodermal cells are initially attached to the growing cytotrophoblast. With further development, spaces that have appeared between the two layers form the amniotic cavity. The entodermal disc shows a slight thickening by the end of the second week. This thickening is located in the midcephalic region of the embryonic disc and is called the *prechordal plate;* it is this structure that establishes a cephalocaudal axis (Figure 6-8).

THIRD WEEK

Approximately at the beginning of the third week, ectodermal cells in the caudal region of the germ disc multiply and move toward the midline, forming a narrow groove with small bulges on either side. This structure is known as the *primitive streak.* It appears to mark the main axis of the embryo, along which the spinal cord will later develop. Research indicates that modified ectodermal cells travel to the region of the primitive streak and eventually pass between the ectodermal and entodermal layers. There they form a new germ layer, the mesoderm, which is the last embryonic layer to develop (Figure 6-9).

By the middle of the third week, the embryonic disc has become elongated and pear-shaped, with a broad cephalic end and a narrow caudal end. Growth takes

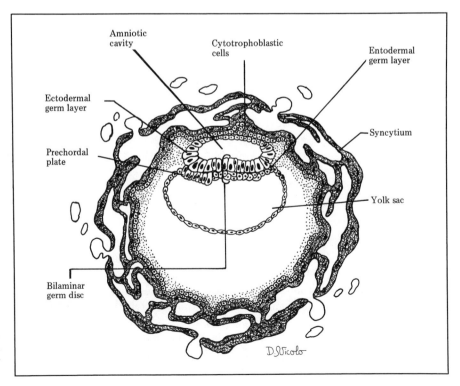

Figure 6-8. During the second week of embryonic development the ectoderm and entoderm are formed. The prechordal plate develops, establishing a cephalocaudal axis in the embryo.

Figure 6-9. Developing mesoderm at the beginning of the third week of embryonic development.

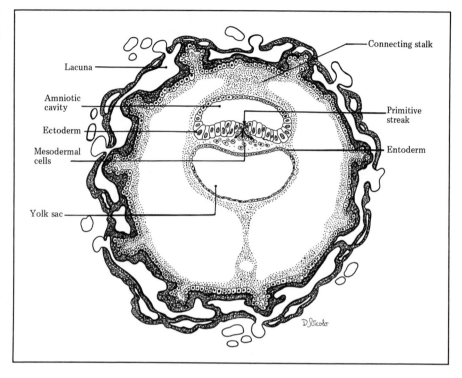

place particularly in the cephalic region, where the three germ layers begin further specific development, whereas in the caudal part this development will not occur for approximately another week. Thus, a maturational developmental pattern (i.e., one of cephalic priority) for all later growth is set. By the end of the third week the three basic layers of the embryo proper, entoderm, ectoderm, and mesoderm, have been formed (Figure 6-10).

Also by the end of the third week, a series of mesodermal blocks, known as somites, appear on each side of the midline. They appear in a craniocaudal sequence and by the end of the first month approximately 40 pairs have formed. Their formation shapes the contours of the embryo, and during this time the size of the embryo is usually expressed in terms of the number of somites. The 33 pairs of vertebrae that form the spinal column develop from these somites (Figure 6-11).

FOURTH WEEK

By the end of the first month, the embryo is 6 millimeters ($\frac{1}{4}$ inch) long and its head comprises one-third of its total length. Externally there is no distinguishable face; however, outlines of the eyes can be seen on the side of the face just above a large opening, the primitive mouth cavity. The foundations for the brain, spinal cord, and entire nervous system have been established. Most organs are just beginning to form. The heart, an S-shaped bulb, is now pulsating rhythmically. The liver, stomach, intestines, pancreas, lung buds, and primordia of the thyroid gland are definable.

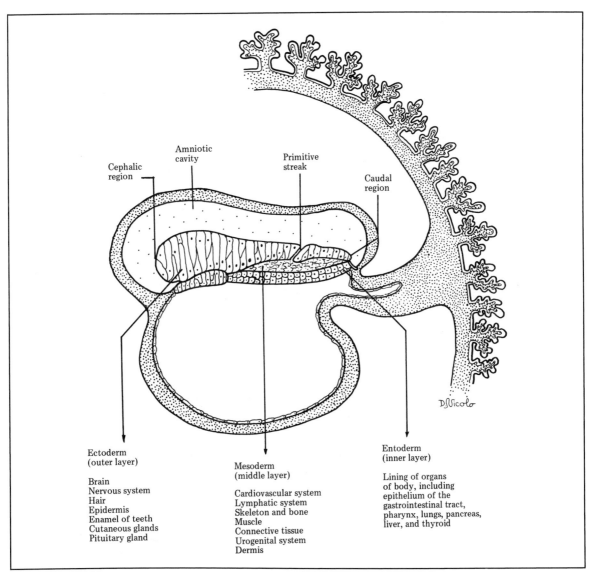

Labels in figure:

Cephalic region

Amniotic cavity

Primitive streak

Caudal region

Ectoderm (outer layer)

Brain
Nervous system
Hair
Epidermis
Enamel of teeth
Cutaneous glands
Pituitary gland

Mesoderm (middle layer)

Cardiovascular system
Lymphatic system
Skeleton and bone
Muscle
Connective tissue
Urogenital system
Dermis

Entoderm (inner layer)

Lining of organs
of body, including
epithelium of the
gastrointestinal tract,
pharynx, lungs, pancreas,
liver, and thyroid

Figure 6-10. By the end of the third week of embryonic development, three germ layers have evolved that later form various body systems.

During the second month, the external appearance of the embryo begins to look more human. Even though somites are still visible, the age of the embryo at this stage is expressed as crown-rump (C.R.) length (the measurement from the vertex of the skull to the midpoint of the buttocks).

FIFTH WEEK

In the fifth week the arm and leg buds become visible. The ear pits appear on the side of the head and the jaws begin to form, giving the face a more humanlike appearance. The pituitary gland is forming, as are the pharyngeal branches that will later

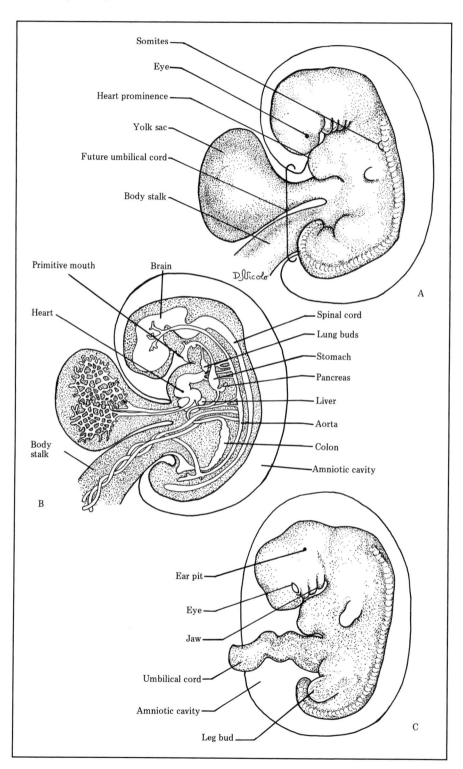

Somites

Eye

Heart prominence

Yolk sac

Future umbilical cord

Body stalk

DSNicolo

A

Primitive mouth

Brain

Heart

Spinal cord

Lung buds

Stomach

Pancreas

Liver

Aorta

Colon

Amniotic cavity

Body
stalk

B

Ear pit

Eye

Jaw

Umbilical cord

Amniotic cavity

Leg bud

C

*Figure 6-11. Four- and
five-week-old embryos
with formed somites (size
is now expressed by the
number of somites).
A. Embryo at four weeks.
B. Internal structures of
embryo at four weeks.
C. Embryo at five weeks.*

give rise to the bronchi. The neural mechanisms for vestibular function and hearing are developing. The umbilical cord is now a distinct structure that connects the embryo to the placenta (Figure 6-11C).

The umbilical cord develops from the attaching body stalk that is readily distinguishable in the 21-day embryo; the body stalk usually grows from the center of the implantation site. Since an equal amount of trophoblastic proliferation occurs on either side of the implantation site, the umbilical cord is most often centrally located on the placenta [10]. In the early somite stage a chain of vessels in the body stalk provides circulation between the developing embryo and the chorionic villi. These vessels are soon reduced to four main stems, two on the right and two on the left. The right vein degenerates early, thus leaving the cord with one large vein and two smaller arteries. The vessels of the cord are supported by a specialized connective tissue known as Wharton's jelly, and both the vessels and Wharton's jelly are surrounded by a membrane of amniotic tissue. Cords vary in length; at term the umbilical cord averages 2 cm (1 inch) in diameter and 55 cm (22 inches) long. Because the vessels are longer than the cord itself they must coil and twist, which frequently results in false knots. With fetal movement, a long cord is likely to become wrapped around the baby's neck. A short cord may be instrumental in detaching the placenta if traction is put upon it. About 1 percent of cords lack one of the arteries, a condition which is associated with congenital fetal malformations. While all fetal organ systems are subject to malformation, studies have indicated that genitourinary defects, esophageal atresia, and imperforate anus occur most frequently [1, 3].

SIXTH WEEK

During the sixth week the eye muscles form, the eyes become pigmented, the basis for the sensation of smell is established, and the teeth and facial muscles begin to form. Paddlelike rudiments of hands develop, while cartilage centers for later bone formation take shape. The embryonic kidney is in the process of developing and the urethra becomes patent at this time, establishing a communication with the amniotic cavity. The penis is forming in the male, and the testes can be distinguished from ovaries. The liver is beginning to take over the job of forming blood cells (Figure 6-12).

SEVENTH WEEK

During the seventh week, the eyes and ears continue rapid development. The retinal nerve cells and the semicircular ear canals become established, and the palate and tongue take form in the mouth. The neck now becomes distinct, connecting the head with the body. The cartilage of the jaws, ribs, and vertebrae begin to be replaced by bone, and most muscles become well organized. The urogenital and rectal passages become completely separate (Figure 6-13).

EIGHTH WEEK

By eight weeks, the embryo weighs 1 gram (0.04 ounce) and is 3 centimeters (1.2 inches) long (C.R.). The hands and feet are well formed. The eyes have moved to the

Figure 6-12. Six-week-old embryo with paddlelike hands.

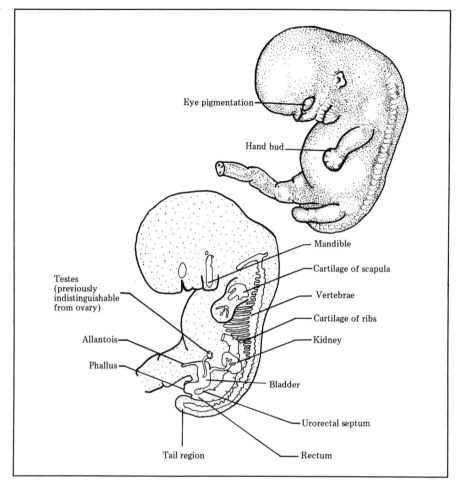

Eye pigmentation

Hand bud

Mandible

Cartilage of scapula

Vertebrae

Cartilage of ribs

Kidney

Testes (previously indistinguishable from ovary)

Allantois

Phallus

Bladder

Urorectal septum

Tail region

Rectum

front of the head, giving a more human look to the face. Bone is now rapidly replacing cartilage, and the major blood vessels are forming their final pattern. The heart, which is now functionally complete, has attained the form it will have during fetal life. The thyroid, thymus, and adrenal glands are developing, and the taste buds are forming. Intestinal villi are beginning to develop. The clitoris appears in the female fetus, and the ovaries or testes begin their descent toward their final location in the male. The gasp reflex, a primitive breathing movement, is now present, and somatic movements can be seen although they are not felt by the mother at this time.

Thus, the end of the embryonic period is marked with a certain degree of completeness. Because all major organ systems have been started, if not already established, the fetus is not as susceptible to the effects of disease, drugs, radiation, and other external threats. Although the fetus is not out of danger, the above factor plus its larger body size increases its resistance.

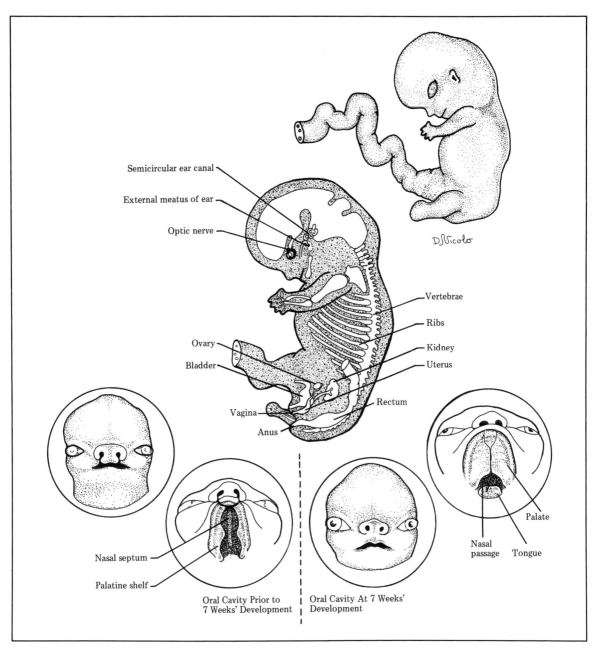

Figure 6-13. Seven-week-old embryo. Palate and tongue have now formed.

Semicircular ear canal

External meatus of ear

Optic nerve

Ovary

Bladder

Vagina

Anus

Vertebrae

Ribs

Kidney

Uterus

Rectum

Nasal septum

Palatine shelf

Oral Cavity Prior to 7 Weeks' Development

Oral Cavity At 7 Weeks' Development

Palate

Nasal passage

Tongue

Fetal Period (9–40 Weeks)

The developmental phase from the beginning of the third month until delivery is called the *fetal period*. It is primarily a time of rapid body growth, although some further tissue differentiation does occur (Table 6-3). The age of the fetus is now expressed as C.R. length or as crown heel (C.H.) length, the measurement from the vertex of the skull to the heel. (Haase's rule is often used to determine the C.H. length of a fetus of known gestation. Up to the fifth month, the number of the month is squared, thus giving the C.H. length in centimeters. Following the fifth month, the number of the month is multiplied by 5. Thus a 4-month old fetus would have a C.H. length of 16 centimeters, or 6 inches.) During the first half of the fetal period, the fetus grows rapidly in length, particularly during the fourth and fifth months. The weight of the fetus, however, increases relatively little during this period. During the latter half of the fetal period, particularly during the last two and one-half months, the fetus gains about 50 percent of its full-term weight.

THIRD MONTH

During the third month, the limbs reach their relative length in proportion to the rest of the body, with the lower limbs a little shorter and less developed than the upper ones. Fingernails, toenails, and hair follicles begin to form, and the thumb develops opposition. The eyelids form and seal shortly thereafter, remaining closed for three months (Figure 6-14).

Tooth buds now appear for all 20 temporary teeth, making this a particularly important time for the fetus to receive an adequate amount of calcium and minerals. The swallowing and sucking reflexes are better developed, taste buds are numerous, and salivary glands begin to form. The thyroid and digestive glands are complete. The pancreas forms insulin and the gallbladder secretes bile into the fetal intestine, where villi are more definable and peristalsis of the small intestine can be observed. The kidneys begin to form urine, which passes into the bladder and from there into the amniotic fluid.

The ill-defined genital structures of both sexes begin to take recognizable shape. The prostate gland is forming in the male, as are the fallopian tubes, uterus, and vagina in the female. The lungs have taken shape and respiratory movements can be observed. Now the vocal cords are beginning to form, and bone marrow is a site for blood production. Numerous connections develop between muscles and nerves, and

Table 6-3. Average Fetal Length and Weight

Age (weeks)	Length	Weight
8	4 cm (1.6 in)	1–4 gm (0.04–0.1 oz)
12	9 cm (3.5 in)	30–40 gm (1.1–1.4 oz)
16	16 cm (6.3 in)	120–130 gm (4.2–4.6 oz)
20	25 cm (10 in)	300–400 gm (10–14 oz)
24	30 cm (12 in)	600–700 gm (1.3–1.5 lb)
28	35 cm (14 in)	1000–1200 gm (2.2–2.6 lb)
32	43 cm (17 in)	1800–2000 gm (4.0–4.4 lb)
36	46 cm (18 in)	2500–2700 gm (5.5–6.0 lb)
40	50 cm (20 in)	3100–3400 gm (6.8–7.5 lb)

Figure 6-14. Three-month-old fetus.

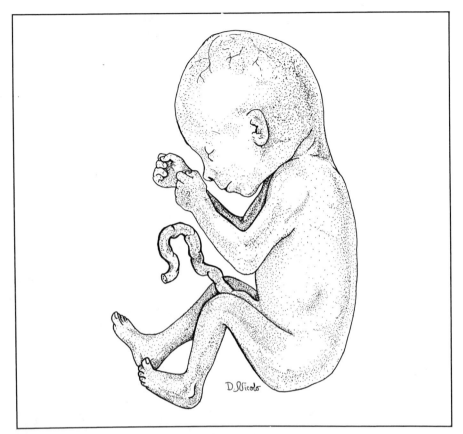

the fetus at this time becomes responsive to a touching stimulus. During the third and fourth months, specialized sensory endings begin to develop in the skin. It is questionable, however, if distinct senses of pain, touch, or temperature exist in prenatal life. Similarly, there is no evidence that the fetus has a sense of position [11].

FOURTH MONTH

The fetus is more erect at this time, since its back has become more muscular and its bony skeleton more developed. It stretches and exercises its arms and legs. Its skin is pink or red, thin, loose, and wrinkled; lips have formed on the mouth and fingerprints have developed.

The basal metabolic rate begins to show a progressive increase. The surface of the fetal brain has many convolutions. The sealed eyes are sensitive to light, but sound evokes little reaction from a four-month-old fetus. If the maternal abdominal wall is thin enough, the heartbeat of the fetus can be heard. Oocytes are developing in the ovaries of the female fetus.

Meconium, a sterile, viscid, odorless, dark green substance, is present in the fetal intestinal tract. At term, meconium contains desquamated epithelial cells, hair, and

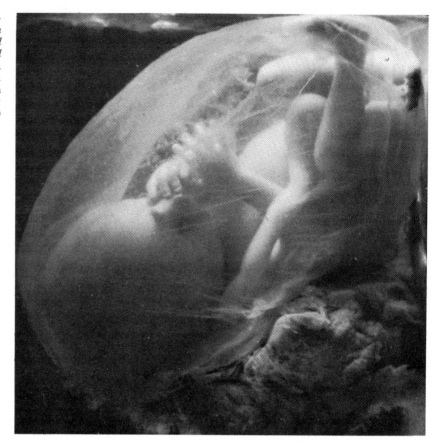

vernix from the amniotic fluid swallowed by the fetus, and mucus, bile, and other secretions of the intestinal glands. This comprises the first stool of the newborn.

During the fourth month, the fetus makes sucking motions and swallows some amniotic fluid. (Some babies are born with calluses on their thumbs from sucking them in utero.) It has been suggested that the sugars and proteins swallowed may contribute nutritionally to the fetus, and that amniotic fluid provides the fetus with some gamma globulin and antibodies [11]. There is some evidence that fetal taste buds may be activated in utero by sweetening the amniotic fluid. One study seemed to indicate that sweetening the amniotic fluid with saccharine enticed the fetus to swallow greater quantities [11]. There have also been attempts to feed the fetus in utero by injecting assimilable proteins into the amniotic fluid. The injection of dye into the amniotic fluid is sometimes used as a diagnostic tool, since the fetus swallows it and it lodges in the stomach and intestines, where it can be viewed on x-ray (Figure 6-15).

FIFTH MONTH

By this time the fetus has settled into a favorite lie or resting position. Fetal movements can now be recognized as kicking or turning. Sleeping habits begin to appear, and the fetus responds to loud noises or music. The firm hand grip (grasp reflex) denotes muscular strength, coordination, and reflex action.

Sweat glands are forming, and the sebaceous glands are secreting a fatty substance that forms a protective, cheeselike paste, known as *vernix caseosa.* At this stage, the fetus is covered with fine hair, or *lanugo,* and has baby hair on its head and eyebrows and has a faint fringe of eyelashes. Nipples appear over the mammary glands.

During the fifth month, adult hemoglobin can be identified in fetal blood. In the early months of gestation, fetal blood contains fetal hemoglobin, which is progressively replaced by adult hemoglobin as term approaches. Fetal hemoglobin has a greater affinity for oxygen and a constant, high oxygen-carrying capacity. Gamma globulin, identified in fetal blood as early as 20 weeks, reaches a concentration at term that either equals or exceeds that found in maternal blood.

SIXTH MONTH

During the sixth month the skin begins to thicken on the hands and feet; the body skin appears reddish and wrinkled, with little or no subcutaneous fat. The hair on the head is growing long, and the fetus is covered with abundant vernix. The grasp reflex has strengthened; the startle reflex is present at the end of the sixth month. The eyes are structurally complete, and the lung alveoli are beginning to develop.

Ossification is advancing; the first true bone formation has occurred in the breastbone. At six months the fetal bones contain as little as 12 percent calcium, compared to calcium content of 90 percent in adult bone [11]. At this time the bony fetal skeleton can be seen on x-ray.

SEVENTH MONTH

At this point the fetus has a 10 percent chance for survival if born prematurely. During this time, the brain makes tremendous strides in its development, and the localization of functional areas occurs. The nervous system has developed enough to make rhythmic breathing movements possible if air is available; swallowing is possible if food is put in the mouth, and body temperature can be regulated. By the seventh month, the lanugo has begun to fade, appearing primarily on the back and shoulders. The testes begin to descend into the scrotal sac of the male fetus.

The lungs have reached the stage of development at which the expansion of air passages will permit them to function in oxygenating the blood. Pulmonary surfactant, a phospholipid-rich substance with very low surface tension, now coats the alveolar epithelium [8]; this helps to prepare the alveoli for expansion by air at birth.

EIGHTH MONTH

If born during the eighth month, the fetus will have a 70 percent chance of survival. Its weight gain at this time results from an increase in subcutaneous fat, the insulating properties of which help to control the body temperature of the fetus. The skin, which is now pink (or pale in dark-skinned babies), has lost its wrinkled appearance.

NINTH MONTH

During the ninth and last calendar month of gestation, the fetus is less active than previously, perhaps because it is so large and there is so little space left in the uterus. The remaining vernix caseosa appears mostly on the back. The fetus has firm breasts. The eyes are blue since the eye pigmentation needs a period of exposure to light before it is fully developed. The gums are ridged. Considerable meconium is in the large intestine. The fetus has acquired maternal antibodies that will protect it for approximately the first six months after birth, until the immune system begins functioning. The immunities include measles, rubella, mumps, whooping cough, and scarlet fever.

FETAL CIRCULATION

Since the fetal lungs are not called upon to function independently while in utero, oxygenation of the fetus depends on a specialized circulatory flow. Aspects of the fetal circulation, which become altered after birth, include the umbilical vessels, the ductus venosus, foramen ovale, and ductus arteriosus (Figure 6-16).

The umbilical vein carries oxygenated blood from the placenta to the fetus, and the umbilical arteries carry blood with a low oxygen content from the fetus to the placenta. The umbilical vein divides into two branches just below the liver; the larger branch becomes the ductus venosus and empties directly into the inferior vena cava, while the smaller branch unites with the portal vein to empty blood into the liver. After the blood from the smaller branch circulates through the liver, it enters the inferior vena cava through the hepatic vein. Thus the inferior vena cava above the hepatic vein contains oxygenated blood from the placenta and unoxygenated blood returning from the lower portion of the fetus. The superior vena cava contains unoxygenated blood returning from the fetal head, neck, and arms.

Blood coming into the heart from the inferior vena cava is for the most part immediately deflected by a fold of endocardial tissue from the right atrium into the left atrium; it flows through the foramen ovale, an opening between the two chambers. From the left atrium, blood flows into the left ventricle. Eighty percent of this blood comes from the inferior vena cava and 20 percent from the fetal lungs via the pulmonary veins. The heart, brain, and upper portion of the fetus are supplied by 25 percent of the left ventricular output into the aorta, while the other 75 percent goes directly to the descending aorta.

Little or none of the less oxygenated blood from the superior vena cava normally passes through the foramen ovale, but rather passes into the right ventricle and from there into the pulmonary artery. This blood, for the most part, is shunted to the descending aorta through the ductus arteriosus, a wide channel connecting the two vessels. Only a small volume of blood goes through the lungs before the onset of respiration, therefore making the pressure in the left atrium low. From the descending aorta, most of the deoxygenated blood flows through the hypogastric arteries to the umbilical arteries and back to the placenta. The remainder flows into the inferior vena cava, where it mixes with blood returning from the placenta via the umbilical vein.

Figure 6-16. Fetal circulation.

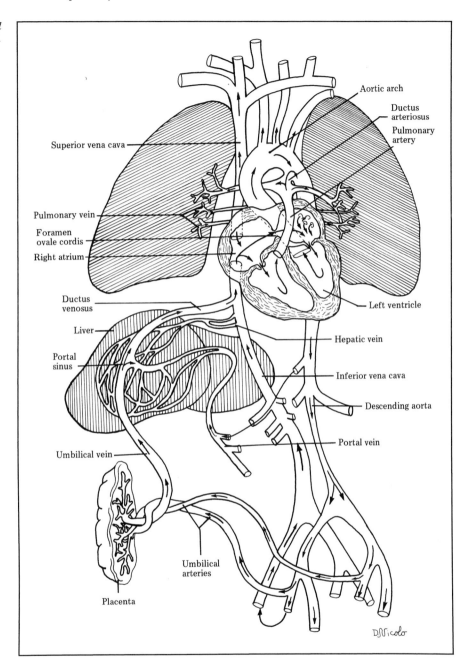

REFERENCES

1. Ainsworth, P. and Davies, P. A. The single umbilical artery: A five-year survey. *Developmental Medicine and Child Neurology* 11:297, 1969.
2. Boyd, J. D., and Hamilton, W. J. *The Human Placenta*. Cambridge, England: Heffer and Sons, 1970.

3. Feingold, M., Fine, R. N. and Ingall, D.   Intravenous pyelography in infants with single umbilical artery. *New England Journal of Medicine* 270:1178, 1964.

4. Hellman, L. M., and Pritchard, J. A.   *Williams Obstetrics* (14th ed.). New York: Appleton-Century-Crofts, 1971.

5. Langman, J.   *Medical Embryology*. Baltimore: Williams & Wilkins, 1963.

6. Moore, K. L.   *The Developing Human: Clinically Oriented Embryology*. Philadelphia: Saunders, 1973.

7. Reid, D., Ryan, K., and Benirschke, K.   *Principles and Management of Human Reproduction*. Philadelphia: Saunders, 1972.

8. Reynolds, E. O., and Strang, L. B.   Alveolar surface properties of the lung in the newborn. *British Medical Bulletin* 22:79, 1966.

9. Rugh, R., and Shettles, L. B.   *From Conception to Birth: The Drama of Life's Beginnings*. New York: Harper & Row, 1971.

10. Thomsen, K., and Hiersche, H.   The Functional Morphology of the Placenta. In A. Klopper and E. Diczfalusy (Eds.), *Foetus and Placenta*. Oxford: Blackwell Scientific, 1969.

11. Windle, W. F.   *Physiology of the Fetus*. Springfield, Ill.: Thomas, 1971.

FURTHER READING

Allan, F. D.   *Essentials of Human Embryology*. New York: Oxford University Press, 1969.

Fetus's vulnerability to foreign chemicals. *Science News* 109:72, January 31, 1976.

Klopper, A., and Diczfalusy, E. (Eds.).   *Foetus and Placenta*. Oxford: Blackwell Scientific, 1969.

Tuchman-Duplessis, H., David, G., and Haegel, P.   *Illustrated Human Embryology,* Vol. 1, *Embryogenesis*. New York: Springer, 1972.

Wang, H.   *An Outline of Human Embryology*. London: Heineman Medical, 1968.

Chapter 7 Normal Pregnancy

The primary aim of obstetrical care is to ensure a healthy and happy outcome for families experiencing pregnancy and birth. The goal encompasses more than just preventing or minimizing physical complications for mother and infant; since childbearing is such a significant and personal experience, obstetrical care must include the teaching and support necessary to make this event as positive and rewarding as possible. The experiences a man and a woman encounter during the period of pregnancy, labor, delivery, and the early days after birth, have far-reaching effects, not only on their own self-images but also on their relationships with their newborn. Their own ability to cope, plus the teaching, guidance, and support they receive from health care personnel, can do much to make this a period that will either foster or inhibit their personal growth.

Nursing, because of its focus on the interpersonal process and on the prevention of and adaptation to stress, makes an unquestionable contribution to the goals of obstetrical care. Whether it is as members of health teams or as independent practitioners, nurses who have learned their skills well can be invaluable to families during childbearing.

CONFIRMATION OF PREGNANCY

Some women initially visit a doctor or clinic because they believe they are pregnant and want the pregnancy confirmed. Pregnancy is most often tested for by seeking evidence of the presence of human chorionic gonadotropin (HCG) in the woman's urine. In the past, many of these tests required the sacrificing of laboratory animals, and results were not available for several days and sometimes up to a week or more. Currently these methods have been replaced by the use of immunological tests, which use either red blood cells or latex particles coated with HCG. When exposed to antiserum containing antibodies against HCG, these red blood cells or latex particles agglutinate. The antiserum is first mixed with the urine of the woman who is being tested for pregnancy. If she is pregnant, the HCG in her urine and the antibodies in the antiserum are bound together. The subsequent addition of the red blood cells or latex particles results in no agglutination. They precipitate out, yielding a positive pregnancy test (Figure 7-1). If the woman is not pregnant the antibodies against HCG remain unbound and are agglutinated when the red blood cells or latex particles are added. The method using red blood cells takes approximately two hours and has been reported to be 98 percent accurate, while the one using latex particles takes about two minutes and its accuracy is reported to be about 92 percent [8].

Figure 7-1. Positive pregnancy test shows no agglutination. Negative reaction shows agglutination, which appears as solid dots.

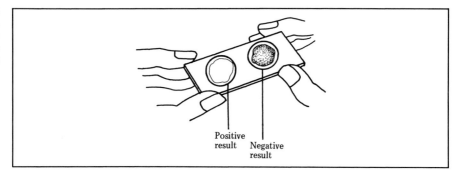

Positive result

Negative result

Figure 7-1. Positive pregnancy test shows no agglutination. Negative reaction shows agglutination, which appears as solid dots.

The immunological tests currently being used vary in their sensitivity or reactivity with HCG. While the more sensitive tests can detect pregnancy from as early as six to eight days after conception [13] to three to four days after the first missed period [5], they also tend to yield false positive results because they also can react with urinary follicle-stimulating hormone (FSH), luteinizing hormone (LH), or both. The tests will react with LH during ovulation and with the high levels of FSH during the menopause. Most of the tests generally yield few false negatives after 14 days following the first missed menstrual period.

False negative reactions will occur early in pregnancy (first 20 days after the first missed menstrual period) with the less sensitive tests or with dilute urine specimens. For this reason, women are asked to bring the first voided morning urine to be tested, since the levels of HCG in it should be high. Specimens allowed to stand 8 hours or longer at room temperature may cause loss of HCG activity and produce false negative reactions. The less sensitive tests may also yield negative reactions during the second and third trimesters, when the HCG levels are low [5, 13].

The use of these pregnancy tests provides just one indication of pregnancy; a positive result from such a test is a probable but not positive sign of pregnancy. Other signs and symptoms indicative of pregnancy may be elicited during a history and physical examination (Table 7-1).

HISTORY AND PHYSICAL EXAMINATION

As part of the physical examination, an internal pelvic examination is usually done. Nurses can provide valuable support to a patient in a number of ways. If the patient has not had a vaginal examination previously, the nurse should provide a skillfully worded explanation, depending on the patient's level of understanding, anxiety, and knowledge of her own body. When the examination is being performed, it will help to provide privacy and to explain what is happening and what is about to happen. It will be important to communicate to her the significance of relaxation. She may be asked to keep her buttocks on the table while letting her legs fall loosely apart or to breathe deeply through her mouth to help relax her abdominal muscles.

In addition to the pelvic examination, a thorough history and physical examination (as mentioned previously) are essential to provide quality care to the woman and her family. The format generally includes the items shown in Figure 7-2. Unfortunately, in many instances the data gathering stops here. The woman is given an

*Table 7-1. Signs and
Symptoms of Pregnancy*

Signs or Symptoms	Appearance after Conception	Other Possible Causes
Presumptive signs or symptoms		
Amenorrhea	Usually reliable 14 or more days after date period expected	Emotional disturbance, chronic disease, hormone imbalance
Breast changes		
Enlargement	Usually after 10 weeks	Hormonal therapy or imbalance, various
Tenderness	After 4 weeks	tranquilizers, intracranial tumors
Nausea and vomiting	Usually after 4–6 weeks	Emotional disturbance, drugs, infections, gastrointestinal irritations
Fetal movement (quickening)	Usually 14–17 weeks	Intestinal gas
Blueness of vagina, vulva, and cervix (Chadwick's sign)	Usually 6–12 weeks	Pelvic tumors, obesity, heart disease
Skin pigmentary changes	8 weeks until term	Hormonal imbalance, drugs
Urinary frequency	Usually 8–12 weeks	Infection, drugs
Fatigue	First trimester	Increased activity, infection, anemia, drugs
Probable signs or symptoms		
Enlarged abdomen	Usually after 4th month	Weight gain, abdominal tumor
Soft uterine isthmus (Hegar's sign)	After 6 weeks in multigravida; 8 weeks in primigravida	Uterine tumors
Soft cervix (Goodell's sign)	4–6 weeks	Pelvic infection
Braxton Hicks contractions	May begin as early as 6–8 weeks	
Fetal outline	After 6th month	Uterine tumors
Ballottement	4th to 5th months	
Pregnancy tests	Reliable by 4 weeks	Endocrine imbalance
Positive signs		
Fetal heart sounds	By Doppler, 10 weeks; by stethoscope, 20–22 weeks	Funic souffle, uterine souffle, maternal pulse, intestinal gas
Fetal movements felt by an examiner	Usually after the 5th month	
Fetal outline by:		
X-ray	Usually 4 months or later	
Sonography	6 weeks or later	

evaluation of her condition (usually she is told that her condition is good), and she is advised to report any of the following unusual signs:

1. Swelling or puffiness of the face and/or hands and fingers
2. Persistent headaches
3. Blurred vision, double vision, or spots before the eyes
4. Fainting or dizziness
5. Abdominal pain or cramps
6. Persistent vomiting
7. Pain on urination
8. Chills or fever
9. Bleeding or loss of fluid from the vagina
10. Epigastric pain

PRENATAL RECORD

Hospital		Doctor				Date

Hosp. No.	Office No.	Insurance		

Pts. Name		Age	Race	Relig.	Country of Birth	Occupation

Address		Phone	Marital Status S M W D Sep.	Years Married	Education

Name of Father of Child		Age	Ht.	Wt.	Significant disease

Business Address		Business Phone	Occupation	Education

FAMILY HISTORY: (Tbc, Hypertension, Heart D., Diabetes, Neuro-Psych., Epilepsy, Allergies, Mult. Births, Congenital Anom.)

MENSTRUAL HISTORY: Onset at	Yrs.	Interval	Days	Duration	Days	Amt.

Months Preg. Attempted	L.M.P.	Normal?	E.D.C.

PRIOR MEDICAL HISTORY	√ Pos.	Remarks (Include date and time of Rx)	HISTORY SINCE LAST MENSTRUAL PERIOD	√ Pos.	Remarks (Include date and time of Rx)
Kidney Disease			Nausea		
Heart Disease			Vomiting		
Hypertension			Indigestion		
Rheumatic Fever			Constipation		
Tuberculosis			Headache		
Venereal Disease			Bleeding (Specify)		
Gyn. Disorder			Vaginal Discharge		
German Measles			Edema		
Nervous & Mental			Abdominal Pain		
Diabetes			Urinary Complaints		
Thyroid Dysfunction			German Measles		
Phlebitis, Varicosities			Other Virus		
Epilepsy			Radiation (Specify)		
Drug Sensitivity			Accidents		
Allergies			Medications		
Blood Dyscrasia					
Blood Transfusions					
Rh, ABO Sensitivity					
Operations, Accidents					

SUMMARY OF PREVIOUS PREGNANCIES	Full Term	Premature	Abortions	Now Alive	Mult. Births

No.	Year	Place of Confinement	Dur. of Gestation	Dur. of Labor	Type of Delivery	Born A or D	Weight	Complications	
								Maternal	Child

Figure 7-2. Form for antepartal history and physical examination. (Form developed jointly by the Committee on Maternal and Child Care of the American Medical Association and the American College of Obstetricians and Gynecologists.)

Figure 7-2 (Continued)

Patient's Name: _____ Date of Birth: _____

PHYSICAL EXAMINATON:

| T. | P. | R. | B.P. | Hgt. | Pres. Wt. | Wt. at L.M.P. |

Eyes _____ Teeth _____ Thyroid _____ Throat _____ Skin _____

Heart _____

Lungs _____

Breasts _____ Nipples _____ Tumors _____

Abdomen _____ Height of Fundus _____

Fetal Heart _____ Presentation and Position _____

Extremities _____ Varicosities _____ Edema _____

General Body Type _____

PELVIC EXAMINATION (bi-manual and speculum): _____

Vulva _____

Vagina _____

Perineum _____

Cervix _____

Uterus _____

Adnexae _____

Rectal Exam. _____

Diag. Conj. _____ cm. | Trans. Diam. Outlet _____ cm. | Shape Sacrum _____

Arch _____ Coccyx _____ S.-S. notch _____

Ischial Spines _____

Inlet:	Mid Pelvis:	Outlet:	Prognosis for Delivery:
☐ Adequate	☐ Adequate	☐ Adequate	
☐ Borderline	☐ Borderline	☐ Borderline	
☐ Contracted	☐ Contracted	☐ Contracted	

LABORATORY EXAMINATIONS: For Syphilis _____ Type _____ Date _____ Result _____

Blood Type and Rh: Patient _____ Father of Child _____

Hemoglobin _____ Hematocrit or RBC _____

Urinalysis: Albumin _____ Sugar _____ Microscopic _____

Exam. for Tbc: Type _____ Date _____ Result _____

(Cytology, Chemistry, etc.)

FACTS OF SPECIAL IMPORTANCE:
Initial Over-all Evaluation of Patient:

Sensitivities _____ Nutritional Status _____

Type of Del. planned _____ Anesthesia planned _____

Physician to call if attending M.D. not available _____

M.D. who will attend infant _____ Is breast feeding planned? _____

Date _____ Signed _____

(Original to be submitted to hospital upon completion.)

Figure 7-2 (Continued)

	Name						Hosp.				Hosp. No.			Office No.	

SUBSEQUENT PRENATAL VISITS

Date	SYMPTOMS						Blood Pressure	Weight	Ht. of Fundus	Position & Presentation	Fetal Heart	Albumin	Urine		Nutrition	Rx and Remarks	Initials
	Headache	Dizziness	Edema	Nausea & Vomiting	Bleeding								Sugar	Hemoglobin			

Date	Progress Notes & Consultation	Date	Progress Notes & Consultation

Rh antibody titer followup: date: result:

date: result: ; date: result:

Speculum examination in third trimester, including cytologic examination, if made:

Date		Signed	

(Original to hospital at approximately 38 weeks.)

American Medical Association 1968
Printed in the U.S.A.

Price: Single copy, 25¢ each; 50-99, 23¢ each; 100-499, 21¢ each; 500-999, 19¢ each; 1000 or more, 17¢ each. Prices are subject to change.

0138-366H; 671-150M

(OP-65)

She is told to return for her next visit in a specified period of time. In general, this is about every four weeks until the seventh month, then every two weeks until the eighth month and every week during the last month. On these return visits, her general health, including eating and sleeping habits and discomforts of the pregnancy, are discussed. A history of the woman's normal daily diet forms the basis for assessment of her specific dietary needs. Usually vitamins and supplementary iron are prescribed routinely. Her weight, blood pressure, fundal height, fetal heart tones, and urinary sugar and protein are checked, and she is examined for signs of complications. All too often the visits are quick ones and are generally oriented only to the physical needs of the woman.

PSYCHOSOCIAL CONSIDERATIONS

In order to provide first-rate care, information on the psychosocial needs of the woman must be obtained from the very beginning if this is to be an experience that supports the personal growth of the woman and her family. While this information may be gathered by other health care workers, nurses, because of their educational background and orientation to psychological needs, are assuming a larger role in this area.

Before meeting the woman, the nurse must know what information needs to be gathered, and she must know and be able to apply the basic principles of interviewing. First and most important in this process is establishing a relationship with the woman, which begins on the initial visit and sets the tone for subsequent meetings. It is now that the nurse must communicate a caring attitude—one which shows she respects and values the patient as a person. A relaxed atmosphere makes it easier to establish such a rapport.

The nurse might begin the interview with an introduction, explaining the purpose of the meeting, and eliciting the pregnant woman's expectations. The nurse should explain that the information discussed will be used to help plan the woman's care in the months ahead. During the meeting she should be encouraged to talk freely; the nurse should use reflective technique and open-ended questions to allow the woman to lead the conversation as much as possible. In the initial visit the nurse should provide as much information as the woman wants in order to answer her immediate questions.

In order to formulate a comprehensive plan of care, nurses might want to investigate the following areas during subsequent visits (Table 7-2). What is the woman's reaction to being pregnant? Was it a planned pregnancy? Does her nonverbal communication coincide with her verbal communication as she discusses being pregnant? What is her facial expression? Does she wear maternity clothes (and how early in the pregnancy)? When appropriate, has she begun making preparations for the baby (clothes, a bed, bottles)?

The woman's knowledge of pregnancy and reproduction has far-reaching effects on her reactions now. What is her knowledge? Has she been pregnant before (Table 7-3)? How did her mother view pregnancy? Does she view it in the same way? What has been her past experience in caring for children? What changes in her life

Table 7-2. Antepartum Assessment and Teaching

Areas of Assessment

1. What is the couple's or woman's adaptation to the pregnancy?
   a. Was this a planned pregnancy?
   b. Is the woman wearing maternity clothes?
   c. Are preparations being made for the baby?
   d. Is there a preferred sex? a preferred name?
   e. Are there characteristics and features attributed to the fetus (fantasized child)?
2. What is the support system—emotional and financial? What are the feelings of significant others to the pregnancy?
3. What are the expectations of pregnancy and delivery? How difficult was labor for the woman's mother?
4. What was the quality of the parents' parenting?

Areas of Teaching

1. General hygiene, discomforts of pregnancy, normal daily activities, feelings about pregnancy
2. Fetal growth and development
3. Physiological changes of pregnancy
4. Nutrition
5. Anesthesia and analgesia
6. Labor and delivery
7. Tour of labor and delivery area
8. Routines of the agency
   a. Routines during labor
   b. How significant others can become involved
   c. Routines on the postpartum unit
9. Birth control
10. Child care
    a. Newborn care
    b. Sibling rivalry
    c. Normal responses while adjusting to new roles and responsibilities
    d. Community groups and agencies offering supporting services

situation will this pregnancy initiate? Will her career plans be interrupted or altered? Will a change in body image be a problem for this woman?

The strength of a woman's support systems can be a crucial factor. Does she have personal stability? Has she been able to cope successfully with stress in the past? Are there others in her life (the baby's father, other family members, friends) who

Table 7-3. Definition of Terms Applied to Pregnancy

Term	Definition
Gravidity	Number of pregnancies regardless of duration
Gravida	A woman who is or has been pregnant
Primigravida	A woman who is pregnant for the first time
Multigravida	A woman who has been pregnant more than once
Nulligravida	A woman who has never been pregnant
Para	Number of pregnancies that have continued to the period of viability
Primipara	A woman who has had one pregnancy that reached the period of viability
Multipara	A woman who has had more than one pregnancy that reached the period of viability
Nullipara	A woman, either primigravida or multigravida, who has not yet delivered a viable infant

can support her now? (This is important not only financially but also when she needs rest from the rigors of daily living.) Does the woman fall into the high-risk group because of age, physical complications, or other reasons, which will require more intensive health care? Is there someone who might be able to help with the work at home? Is there someone nearby with whom she can talk?

Every effort should be made to include the baby's father in the meetings. How is he coping with the pregnancy? Who is answering his questions and supporting him? Is it possible to actively involve him in planning the family's care?

The above data, of course, will be collected over a number of visits. After the first meeting, it is important to assess the situation to see what information has already been obtained and how much is still needed in order to plan the best possible care with the patient. The information should be part of her chart, so that it is available to all members of the health team who will be providing continuing care to her.

DURATION OF PREGNANCY

The average duration of pregnancy from conception to birth is 266 days. If counted from the first day of the last menstrual period, as it often is, the average duration of pregnancy is approximately 280 days or 40 weeks. Fifty percent of all live births occur within 40–41 weeks; however, pregnancies extending two to three weeks beyond the expected date of delivery are fairly common and are generally regarded as within acceptable limits (Table 7-4).

Nägele's rule, based on a 28-day menstrual cycle, is generally used to estimate the expected date of delivery, or expected date of confinement (EDC). This is done by counting back three months from the first day of the last menstrual period and adding seven days. For example, if the patient's menstrual period began December 2 (12/2), the EDC would be September 9 (9/9). While this method is only an approximation, it has been found to be highly dependable.

Table 7-4. Number and Percentage of Births Related to Gestational Interval (Weeks 26–52)

Week	Number of Births	Percentage of Total Births	Week	Number of Births	Percentage of Total Births
26	1	0.03	40	745	25.18
27	0	0	41	818	27.64
28	4	0.14	42	397	13.42
29	3	0.10	43	152	5.14
30	4	0.14	44	41	1.39
31	7	0.24	45	16	0.54
32	6	0.20	46	12	0.41
33	13	0.44	47	3	0.10
34	22	0.74	48	1	0.03
35	21	0.71	49	2	0.07
36	49	1.66	50	0	0
37	92	3.10	51	2	0.07
38	160	5.40	52	2	0.07
39	386	13.04			
			Total	2959	100

Source: Modified from A. Treloar, B. Behn, and D. Cowan. Analysis of gestational interval. *American Journal of Obstetrics and Gynecology* 99:36, 1967.

Pregnancy is sometimes divided into 10 lunar months. A lunar month consists of 28 days, or a period coinciding with the average menstrual cycle. The first lunar month of pregnancy is calculated from the first day of the last menstrual period. Pregnancy is also divided into trimesters, or periods of approximately three calendar months. The first trimester begins from the time of conception, and pregnancy then consists of a total of three trimesters or approximately $8\frac{3}{4}$ calendar months.

PHYSIOLOGICAL ASPECTS OF PREGNANCY

Uterus and Cervix

The most marked changes in a pregnant woman's body occur in the uterus. From a small, almost solid organ, weighing between 30–60 grams (1–2 ounces), it enlarges to a thin-walled muscular sac, weighing between 700–1000 grams (1.5–2.2 pounds), increasing its capacity by between 500–1000 times. During the first trimester the uterus becomes almost spherical in shape. During the second and third trimesters it changes from a globular to an ovoid shape.

Uterine enlargement is most marked in the fundus, with the greatest growth occurring in the first half of pregnancy. In the first trimester, uterine enlargement is due primarily to tissue hypertrophy, stimulated principally by increased levels of estrogen and perhaps progesterone. Even in those pregnancies that are extrauterine, the uterus itself may double in size during the first trimester due to this hormonal stimulation. During the second and third trimesters, further uterine enlargement is due to mechanical stretching and thinning of the uterine wall caused by the growing fetus.

The uterine musculature hypertrophies considerably; although the growth of new muscle fibers is quite limited, there is a great increase in the amount of fibrous and elastic tissue. All of these changes strengthen the uterine wall.

During the first half of pregnancy, uterine lymphatics and blood vessels, particularly veins, hypertrophy. Blood vessels become increasingly coiled and later uncoil as the uterus stretches, thus supplying the expanded surface area. Uterine oxygen consumption, as well as blood flow, is increased, and the nerve supply, like the blood vessels, hypertrophies.

The mechanism of uterine contractions is not fully understood. The general consensus is that progesterone reduces the excitability of the uterus, possibly by affecting the membrane potential of the myometrium, particularly over the placental site. This effect is antagonized somewhat by estrogen. The gradual increase in contractility has been attributed to increased concentrations of actomyosin in the uterine muscles.

During the first 30 weeks, uterine activity consists of slight contractions of low intensity occurring about every minute and localized to small areas in the uterus. At the same time, other contractions (Braxton Hicks contractions) occur over a larger area approximately every hour but with a greater intensity. It is thought that they aid placental function by enhancing circulation in intervillous spaces. As term approaches, Braxton Hicks contractions become more frequent and intense. Because of this, they may be the cause of false labor, in which these contractions are mistaken for the contractions of true labor. At this time they also pull the muscle fibers that surround the internal cervical os and contribute to effacement (thinning of the cervix), particularly in the primigravida. If Braxton Hicks contractions cause discomfort to the woman, abdominal breathing may help.

During the fourth month, the uterus rises out of the pelvic cavity and partially fills the abdominal cavity (Figure 7-3). As this happens, tension is placed on the broad ligaments, and the round ligaments begin to hypertrophy and elongate. The round ligaments now help to stabilize the upper part of the mobile uterus, while its lower portion remains anchored by cervical connections.

Because the upper portion of the uterus is free in the abdominal cavity, when the woman stands it falls forward and rests on her anterior abdominal wall, thus altering her center of gravity. To compensate for this, she walks with her head and shoulders thrust backward and chest protruding. The walking stride she now assumes is called "the pride of pregnancy."

This posture may cause a lordosis, resulting in backache. If the backache is mild,

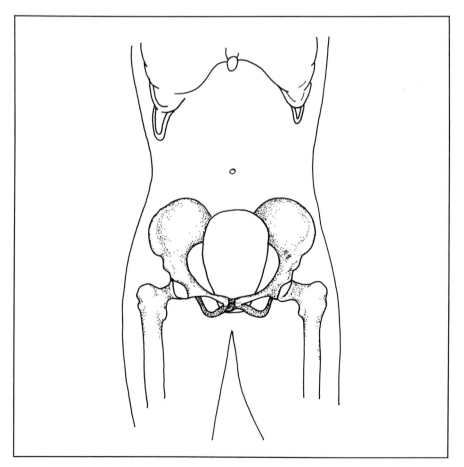

Figure 7-3. By the end of the fourth month the uterus has risen out of the pelvic cavity.

it may be relieved by the use of a light maternity girdle, maintenance of good posture, pelvic rocking exercises, or possibly a bed board. It is important that she wear well-fitting, comfortable shoes with good arch supports. The shoes need not be low-heeled, unless the woman develops a backache or is unable to maintain good balance with high-heeled shoes.

When she is supine, her uterus falls backward and rests on her vertebral column and anterior large vessels. The compression of these vessels leads to a decrease in venous return to the heart, possible decrease in cardiac output, and hypotension, a condition sometimes referred to as the "inferior vena cava syndrome." When it does occur, a change to the left lateral position removes the pressure of the uterus from the vessels.

As the uterus fills the abdominal cavity, it gradually pushes the intestines to the sides and upward. It elevates the diaphragm, causing dyspnea and shifting the position of the heart. Because of the position of the sigmoid colon on the left, the uterus tends to turn toward the right.

The cervical portion of the uterus undergoes pronounced softening (Goodell's sign) and cyanosis as early as one month after conception. These changes are due to increased vascularity, hyperplasia of cervical glands (which increases their secretion), and edema. The glands of the cervical mucosa proliferate, and, as a result, a meshlike mucosal structure, the mucous plug, is formed. This helps to seal the uterine contents from contamination (Figure 7-4).

The uterine changes cause a number of common complaints during pregnancy. The enlarged uterus causes pressure on the pelvic blood vessels, impairing circulation to the lower extremities, which may be responsible for muscle cramps in the legs. The actual cause of these cramps is not certain; however, they have also been attributed to inadequate or impaired absorption of calcium, parathyroid deficiency, hyperventilation, or excess loss of chloride from the body. Immediate relief from the cramps may come by standing up with feet flat on the floor, or dorsiflexing the foot, while straightening the leg by downward pressure on the knee (Figure 7-5). Suggested preventive measures include exercise and good body alignment in order to improve circulation.

Effective utilization of calcium depends on a proper ratio of calcium to phosphorus. When large quantities of milk are taken in, the calcium-phosphorus ratio is disturbed since more phosphorus is absorbed than calcium. Therefore, a pregnant woman with muscle cramps may be asked to decrease her milk intake. A calcium preparation taken at bedtime will elevate ionizable calcium levels in her plasma. Another suggestion is to take aluminum hydroxide with milk to remove some of the phosphorus.

The enlarging uterus contributes to bladder irritability in the first trimester. Increased anteflexion displaces the cervix and stretches the base of the bladder. This feeling simulates that of a full bladder, resulting in urinary frequency. The frequency disappears as the uterus rises into the abdomen, only to reappear at or near the end of pregnancy, when the fetal head descends into the pelvis. If a woman finds frequency a real problem in the first trimester, it has been suggested that she limit her fluids in the evening so that her sleep will not be repeatedly disturbed by nocturia.

Figure 7-4. The mucous plug during pregnancy helps to seal the uterine contents from contamination.

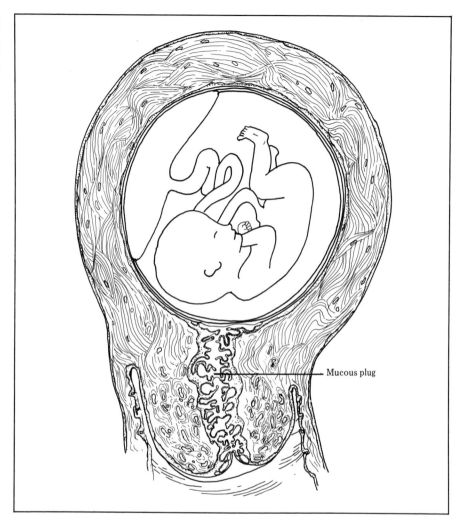

Mucous plug

Vagina

During pregnancy, under the influence of increased estrogen, the vaginal walls show a thickening of the mucosa, a loosening of connective tissue (to facilitate expansion), and a hypertrophy of smooth muscle cells. Increased vascularity gives the vagina its violet color (Chadwick's sign). Copious thick white secretions result from increased production of lactic acid from the glycogen in the vaginal epithelium. The acid pH (3.5–6.0) helps to keep the vagina free from pathogenic organisms; however, all these changes contribute to an increased incidence of vulvovaginitis in pregnancy.

Two infections in particular, moniliasis and *Trichomonas vaginalis,* appear frequently. Moniliasis, a yeast infection caused by *Candida albicans,* may cause a profuse, cheesy, white irritating discharge. This organism has been cultured from the vagina in about 25 percent of women approaching term; this is not surprising

Figure 7-5. The woman can relieve leg cramps by dorsiflexing her foot while straightening her leg, with downward pressure on her knee.

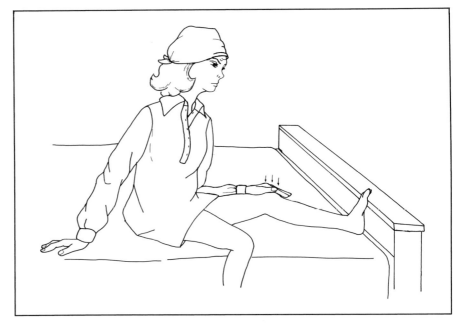

since the vaginal mucosa has a high glycogen content, which serves as an excellent growth medium. The treatment of moniliasis in the past consisted of local applications of gentian violet. Currently the fungicide nystatin (Mycostatin) is used without known fetal effects.

T. vaginalis, a protozoal infection, is characterized by a foamy white or yellow leukorrhea with irritation and pruritis. This infection is currently treated by the use of metronidazole (Flagyl) orally and vaginally. There are no reported adverse effects on the fetus following its use after the first trimester. A vinegar douche (3 tablespoons of white vinegar in 2 quarts of water) is sometimes recommended. A man may likewise be infected with *Trichomonas* organisms and should be examined and treated; in this way reinfection of the woman is avoided.

Most cases of increased vaginal discharge during pregnancy have no pathological cause. If the secretions are troublesome, a vinegar douche is often recommended. Douching during pregnancy, however, should be kept to a minimum; it should never be done with a bulb syringe, to avoid a possible air embolism. When a douche bag is used, it should not be placed more than 2 feet above hip level to prevent high fluid pressure. The nozzle should not be inserted more than 3 inches into the vagina.

Vulvar pruritis and discomfort may also be relieved by keeping the area as free from discharge as possible by washing frequently with water and a mild soap. In addition, the combination of panty hose and nylon panties can prevent the evaporation of normal perspiration and retain heat, thus providing a good environment for the incubation of organisms.

Ovaries and Fallopian Tubes

During pregnancy, ovulation ceases and maturation of new follicles is suspended. Ovarian veins hypertrophy. The corpus luteum of pregnancy probably functions maximally during the first month of pregnancy, primarily producing progesterone. This serves to maintain an adequate uterine environment necessary for proper implantation and retention of the pregnancy. The tubal musculature probably undergoes little or no hypertrophy during pregnancy; under the influence of progesterone, its activity is at a low ebb.

Abdominal Wall

Occasionally the muscles of the abdominal wall are unable to withstand the tension caused by the growing uterus, and the *recti* separate in the midline. This creates a *diastasis,* which can result in the anterior uterine wall being covered by only a thin layer of skin, fascia, and peritoneum. This diastasis can actually be felt in the postpartum period (see page 258).

Breasts

Mammary growth during pregnancy is stimulated by the continued presence of progesterone and estrogen and by the lactogenic properties of chorionic somatomammotropin. Estrogen enhances development of the breast ductal system, and progesterone, the development of the alveolar system. Increased blood supply con-

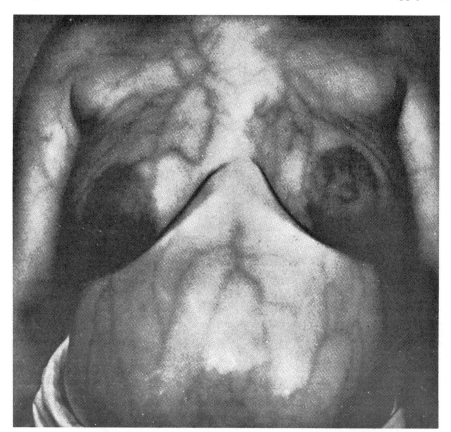

Figure 7-6. Infrared photograph of woman one month before term, showing accentuated venous pattern over breasts and abdomen. (From L. M. Hellman and J. A. Pritchard. Williams Obstetrics [14th ed.], 1971. Courtesy of Appleton-Century-Crofts, Publishing Division of Prentice-Hall, Inc.)

tributes to initial breast enlargement. After the second month, hypertrophy of mammary alveoli causes the breasts to continue to increase in size and become nodular. As the breasts enlarge further, veins become visible just below the skin (Figure 7-6). With extensive enlargement, stretch marks (striae gravidarum) may develop.

Nipples become larger, more deeply pigmented, and more erectile. After the first few months, a thick yellowish fluid, colostrum, may be expressed from them with gentle massage.

At the same time the areolae become broader and more deeply pigmented. The depth of the pigmentation varies with the woman's complexion: the darker her complexion, the deeper the pigmentation (Figure 7-7). Scattered throughout the areolae are a number of small elevations, hypertrophied sebaceous glands called Montgomery's glands (Montgomery's tubercles). Their secretions protect the surrounding skin and keep it pliable.

Special breast care is often advised to enhance the ability to nurse, to toughen the nipples (and thereby decrease the incidence of cracking), and to enhance erectility and eversion of the nipples. Daily cleansing with warm water and a soft clean cloth, followed by careful drying, is important. Using soap may remove protective natural skin oils and leave the nipple more subject to damage. Since the skin on the surface of the nipples is thin, measures such as rubbing them gently with a washcloth are used to toughen them. When crusts form as a result of breast secretions, they may be softened by applying a suitable nipple cream or lanolin.

Occasionally inversion of the nipples occurs. If the woman plans to breast-feed,

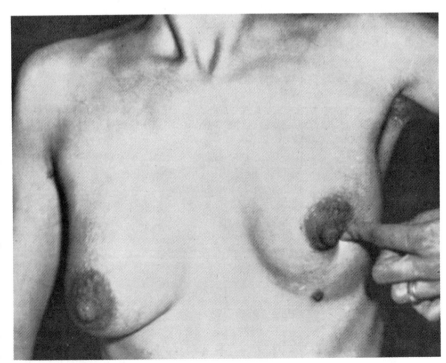

Figure 7-7. Breast changes of pregnancy. Note the deep pigmentation of the areolae and nipples and the prominence of Montgomery's glands. The accessory nipple beneath the left breast is also pigmented. (From J. R. Willson, C. T. Beecham, and E. Carrington. Obstetrics and Gynecology [5th ed.]. St. Louis: Mosby, 1975.)

Figure 7-8. Technique of correcting inverted nipples. The nipples may be everted by placing the thumbs on opposite sides of the areola close to the nipple and applying firm but gentle pressure into the tissue and then pushing away from the areola.

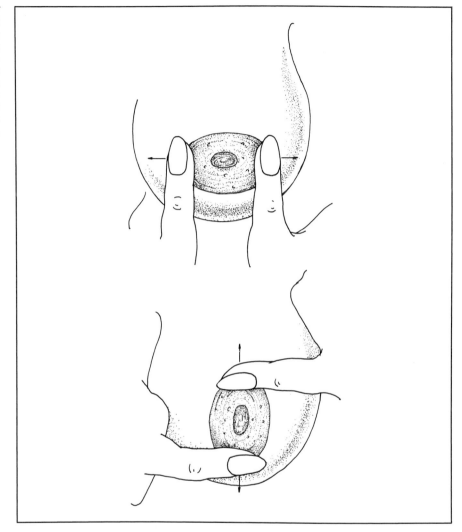

this inversion can be counteracted by placing the thumbs on opposite sides of the areola close to the nipple (Figure 7-8). The woman then presses firmly but gently into the breast tissue, gradually pushing away from the areola; she then releases pressure but keeps her thumbs in position. This is done four or five times in succession in both the horizontal and vertical directions and is carried out daily.

Nipples can be made more erect by rolling them between the thumb and forefinger, applying even, gentle pressure for 15–30 seconds. Cream may be massaged into the tissue by using this method.

Any of the above conditions may be discovered as the nurse makes careful examination of the woman's breasts. This is usually a good time to teach the mother the technique of breast self-examination and to stress the importance of doing it monthly when she is no longer pregnant (Figure 7-9). She should also be alerted to

Figure 7-9. Breast self-examination. A. Stand with hands on hips and observe for symmetry or changes, looking in a mirror. B. Follow same procedure with hands in air. C. Squeeze palms together to contract pectoral muscles. Breasts should project outward. Observe for bilateral motion and signs of dimpling. Tumors on the pectoral muscle may cause dimpling and uneven projection. Squeeze nipples to see if fluid may be expressed, which would indicate possible lesions in the ductal system. D. Palpate breast in a circular motion much like following the spokes on a wheel. E. While lying on side, palpate the breast and axilla area for lumps.

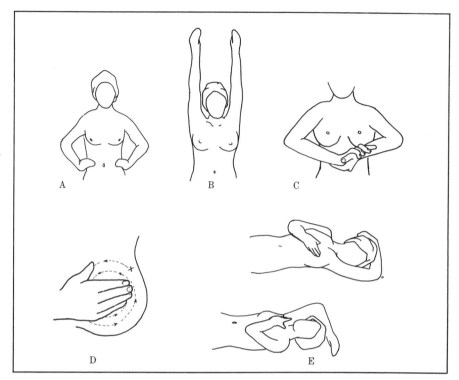

the nodular breast changes that occur during pregnancy and regress afterward.

In addition the nurse should check the fit of the woman's brassiere. Since the increasing size of the breasts may make them pendulous, a well-fitting supporting brassiere is very important. The brassiere should fit smoothly below the breasts, supporting and lifting them so that the nipples are on a line with the midpoint of the upper arm (Figure 7-10). Wide adjustable shoulder straps will be more comfortable and should keep the brassiere from riding up in the back or slipping down in the front. Usually the cup size should be one size larger than before pregnancy.

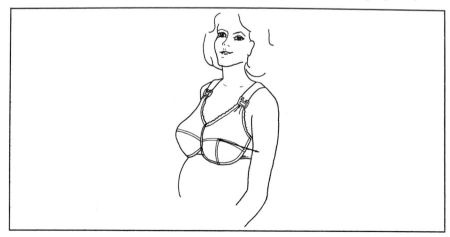

Figure 7-10. Maternity brassiere. A well-fitting maternity brassiere supports the breasts so that the nipples are on a line with the midpoint of the upper arm.

Skin

In the last trimester, about 50 percent of all pregnant women develop slightly depressed red streaks over the abdomen and sometimes over the breasts (Figure 7-11). These stretch marks (striae gravidarum) fade and become silvery two or three months after delivery, but the silvery markings persist indefinitely. Several theories have been advanced to explain the cause of striae, ranging from hyperactivity of the adrenal cortex to stretching of the skin with rupture of underlying elastic fibers. Occasionally such stretch marks are seen in cases of abdominal distention or increased fat tissue. Although various ointments have been suggested to prevent striae, there is no known effective prevention.

The woman's umbilicus, which is usually still deeply indented during the first trimester, becomes steadily more shallow as pregnancy advances. At term it may be level with the surface or protrude somewhat. There is increased vascularity of the skin and muscles of the perineum, as well as softening of the connective tissue.

From the second trimester, there is increased pigmentation of the breast areolae (as mentioned previously). In addition, a line of increased pigmentation, the *linea nigra,* may appear over the lower abdomen from the umbilicus to the symphysis pubis. The woman's forehead and cheeks may become more darkly pigmented, resulting in *chloasma,* or the butterfly mask of pregnancy. This effect, which may be exaggerated by exposure to the sun, disappears or regresses after delivery.

Little is known about the etiology of these pigmentary changes. It is known,

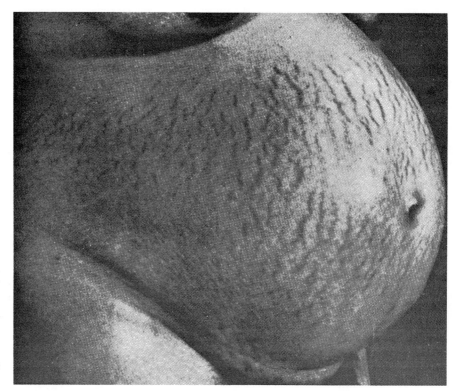

Figure 7-11. Woman at term with marked abdominal striae. (From L. M. Hellman and J. R. Pritchard. Williams Obstetrics *[14th ed.], 1971. Courtesy of Appleton-Century-Crofts, Publishing Division of Prentice-Hall, Inc.)*

however, that the level of melanocyte-stimulating hormone (MSH) is increased from the end of the second month of pregnancy until term. In addition, estrogen and progesterone are reported to have a melanocyte-stimulating effect.

Many Caucasian women (though fewer black women) develop palmar erythema and/or spider angiomas (vascular spiders). These angiomas are dilated precapillary vessels radiating out from a central dilated arteriole, probably as a result of high estrogen concentrations.

Because perspiration is more profuse during pregnancy and activity of sebaceous glands may increase, daily baths are advisable. In the last two months of pregnancy, when keeping her balance becomes more of a problem, the woman may find getting in and out of a bathtub awkward. It is for this reason, rather than the avoidance of vaginal contamination, that tub baths are discouraged at this time, since it is now generally accepted that tub water does not enter the vaginal canal, as was once believed.

Digestive System

During the first two trimesters of pregnancy, there is a decrease in the production of gastric acid and pepsin. The large amounts of progesterone produced by the placenta contribute to a relaxation of the alimentary tract, resulting in decreased tone and motility, delayed gastric emptying, and an increased absorption of nutrients. Constipation commonly occurs in pregnancy, as a result of decreased tone and motility of the intestines and displacement and pressure from the enlarging uterus. Lack of exercise and inadequate intake of fluids and roughage can be important contributing factors in constipation; these should be explored before remedies are suggested. If a laxative is necessary, prune juice, bulk-producing agents, stool softeners, or milk of magnesia may be used. The use of mineral oil is discouraged, since it tends to interfere with the absorption of the fat-soluble vitamins.

Heartburn may also be a problem in pregnancy. The enlarging uterus puts pressure on the stomach and alters its position. This effect, in addition to the decreased gastric motility, which can cause a reverse in peristaltic waves, results in a reflux of stomach contents into the lower esophagus. To relieve heartburn, local antacids, such as aluminum hydroxide gels, may be used to soothe the mucosa and neutralize the acid reflux. Sodium bicarbonate, a systemic antacid, should not be used, since it results in absorption of excessive sodium. In addition to the use of antacids, smaller, more frequent meals may help.

During pregnancy, the increased progesterone production may cause the gums to become hyperemic and softened. Mouth secretions may become acidic, and many women mention an increase in salivation. Occasionally, a vascular swelling of the gums, known as an *epulis* of pregnancy, may develop; it regresses after delivery. Because of these changes and the incidence of nausea and vomiting in early pregnancy, good oral hygiene is essential. If the gums bleed, brushing may be done with a softer toothbrush and a mild toothpaste; an alkaline mouthwash may be used.

Contrary to the popular notion that "each pregnancy costs a tooth," there is no demineralization of teeth during pregnancy. What seems like an increased incidence of dental caries during pregnancy may be due to their discovery through a more thorough health examination at this time. However, acid content of the mouth, a change in eating habits, and the increased blood supply to the teeth may contribute to tooth decay during pregnancy. Dental work is not contraindicated; however, if dental x-rays are necessary, they are postponed until the latter half of pregnancy. In addition, a lead apron should be used to protect the abdomen.

Nausea and vomiting are common occurrences during pregnancy, appearing for the most part in the morning. These symptoms occur in about 50 percent of all pregnant women, beginning between the fourth and sixth weeks and generally easing by about the twelfth week. The cause is unknown. Negative feelings about her pregnancy (e.g., ambivalence, uncertainty, and anxiety), may play a role in causing these symptoms. On a physiological note, hypoglycemia has been suggested as a cause, as has the decreased gastric motility and the relaxation of the alimentary tract. It has also been noted that the period of nausea and vomiting coincides with the period of high levels of chorionic gonadotropin. Eating smaller meals or having a rapidly absorbed carbohydrate, such as orange juice, toast or crackers, before arising or when nauseated may help. Dry high-carbohydrate foods seem to work better than liquids. Avoiding greasy foods and strong food odors may also help. Anti-emetics may be prescribed if these measures fail.

Pregnancy has also been described as a period of cholestasis. The gallbladder may become atonic and distended, with the bile quite thick, which predisposes to gall-stone formation.

Eating patterns may change during pregnancy; for example, there may be an increase in appetite and thirst, particularly in early pregnancy. Later in pregnancy, a reduced capacity for large meals leads to frequent snacking. Many women report a desire for highly flavored foods such as pickles, perhaps related to a dulling of the sense of taste in pregnancy. Some women may experience pica (a desire to eat bizarre substances), leading to the eating of such items as clay, coal, solid laundry starch, and refrigerator frost. Clay and laundry starch eaten in sufficient quantities cause anemia, weight loss, and other problems related to nutritional deficiencies.

Dirt-eating, or geophagia, seems to be the result of a superstition handed down from the past. In Africa warriors carried earth from their homeland with them into distant battles, where the earth was eaten for strength. Other people believed that eating dirt stimulated sexual prowess. During pregnancy, eating clay was supposed to benefit bowel evacuation, aid in proper positioning of the fetus, prevent syphilis, and help avoid nausea and dizziness. Starch ingestion supposedly aided in blood clotting and made the delivery easy [12].

Respiratory System

The pregnant woman's P_{CO_2} is lowered by the increase in progesterone production. It has been reported that the respiratory centers are far more sensitive to stimulation by CO_2 during pregnancy, causing the woman to hyperventilate. She breathes more deeply and has an increased tidal volume and alveolar ventilation. Her hyperventilation causes a respiratory alkalosis, which is compensated for by the kidney through an increase in bicarbonate excretion and a corresponding decrease in plasma sodium concentration. Because of this mechanism, there is little or no change in blood pH.

Later in pregnancy, the enlarged uterus causes elevation of the diaphragm. For the same reason, the lower ribs flare out and may not recover their normal position after pregnancy. The transverse diameter of the rib cage increases, probably due to increased mobility of the rib attachments.

The changes in the respiratory system interfere with sleep and comfort. Good body mechanics and good erect posture (both standing and sitting) alleviate discomfort. In order to get some relief (by increasing space within the rib cage), a woman might raise both arms above her head; when lying down, she should use two or more pillows under her head and shoulders.

Cardiovascular System

Blood volume at term rises to about 45–50 percent above nonpregnant levels. This increase begins in the first trimester, is most rapid during the second trimester, peaks at approximately 32–36 weeks, and then plateaus. Some studies [17] report a drop in volume in the 36- to 40-week period, although this may be related to testing methods and the position of the woman. The increased volume serves to meet the demands of the enlarging uterus, helps to maintain adequate circulation when the woman is standing or lying down, and acts as a reserve for blood loss at delivery. The blood volume increase is several hundred milliliters higher in multigravidas than primigravidas; the reasons for this are unknown.

The uterus receives the greatest proportion of the increased blood flow; early in pregnancy the kidney receives a significant increase. Blood flow to the skin and mucous membranes increases by 70 percent by the thirty-sixth week, causing peripheral vasodilatation and complaints of "feeling the heat," sweating, and nasal congestion. As a result of the nasal congestion, some women snore when they are pregnant. The increased blood flow to the hands may explain the increased rate of fingernail growth during pregnancy. Also in pregnancy, there is a rise in the proportion of growing hairs, with fewer at a resting stage prior to falling out. Thus, the pregnant woman reaches term with many over-age hairs, accounting for the loss of hair that often occurs following delivery.

The heart is pushed upward by the diaphragm and is rotated forward. Heart sounds heard now, such as pulmonic and apical systolic murmurs, might be considered pathological in the nonpregnant state. During pregnancy the mean cardiac output rises from 4.5 liters per minute to a maximum of about 6 liters per minute, an increase of about 33 percent. The heart rate increases from 70 to 85 beats per minute, an increase of only about 20 percent. To compensate for the difference, the stroke volume must increase also. It has been reported that the peripheral resistance of the vessels is reduced, possibly because of the effects of estrogen and progesterone. This results in venous dilatation in the pulmonary vascular bed and in the legs. Capillary engorgement may occur throughout the respiratory tracts, affecting the larynx and vocal cords; this may temporarily change the voice.

The increase in plasma volume is followed by an increase of about 30 percent in the production of red blood cells. It should be noted that the increase in red cell volume is proportionately less than the increase in plasma volume. This results in a physiological anemia, or pseudoanemia, most evident in the second trimester of pregnancy. The hemoglobin may fall to an average of 11–12 grams per 100 milliliters of blood, from an accepted norm of 13.7–14.0 grams per 100 milliliters. The hematocrit may drop to an average of about 34 percent from an accepted norm of 40–42 percent.

Because of the increased number of red blood cells, the iron requirement also rises. The increased need, though slight in the first half of pregnancy, is great during the second half of pregnancy, when the woman needs approximately 6–7 milligrams of iron per day to meet the demand of her own body and that of the growing fetus. If these demands are not satisfied, the fetus can receive iron from the placenta, but the woman suffers a drop in hemoglobin.

In addition to the increase in red blood cells, there is a rise in white blood cells, platelets, globulins, cholesterol, and sedimentation rate, while albumin and total proteins decrease. Some clotting factors show an increase during pregnancy. Fibrinogen levels may be increased by as much as 50 percent or more, and Factor VIII is also markedly increased. There are also significant rises in Factors VII, IX, and X, although the reasons for these increases are unknown. Controversy exists with regard to changes in the fibrinolytic system in late pregnancy, normal labor, and postpartum period, but it is generally believed this system is depressed in pregnancy and enhanced in the postpartum period [1, 4].

During the later part of pregnancy, there is a decrease in venous return from the lower extremities, partly caused by pressure from the enlarged uterus on the pelvic veins and inferior vena cava. This commonly results in dependent edema, leg cramps, and the development or aggravation of varicosities in the legs, vulva, and anal area. When this occurs, the woman should be encouraged to rest more during the day, with her legs elevated if possible. When she is in bed, a pillow under the mattress will maintain the elevation more consistently than a pillow placed under the legs. Constricting clothing, such as garters or rolled stockings, should be avoided. Support stockings may be helpful, but should be put on after the legs have been elevated for several minutes, or preferably before the woman gets out of bed in the morning. Activities that require prolonged standing should be avoided.

Varicosities in the anal area (hemorrhoids) may be painful and may itch and/or bleed. The woman may be instructed to use her finger (lubricated with a substance such as petroleum jelly) to push protruding hemorrhoids back inside the rectum. In addition, cold or witch-hazel compresses may relieve the discomfort and itching. The woman should also be told that hemorrhoids may be aggravated by constipation, and that she should take measures to avoid constipation. Hemorrhoids usually regress after delivery; if surgical removal is necessary, it is usually delayed until that time.

Vulvar varicosities may be relieved by placing a pillow under the buttocks or by elevating the hips for frequent rest periods (Figure 7-12). The presence of vulvar varicosities may make it difficult to choose the site for an episiotomy.

In the latter months of pregnancy women will notice that their feet swell, especially around the ankles, after normal activity. This dependent edema is common,

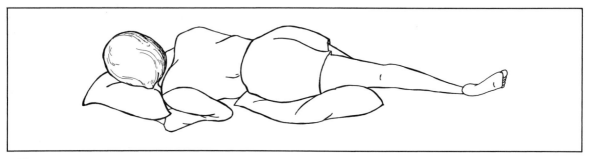

Figure 7-12. Position for relief of vulvar varicosities.

whereas edema of the hands and face is not common and should be reported to the obstetrician. Dependent edema will be relieved somewhat when the woman goes to bed at night. As she assumes a horizontal position, venous return from the legs will increase. This often causes nocturia, since the body now rids itself of the extra fluid that has collected in the legs during the day.

Endocrine System

The pituitary changes during pregnancy are not great. The pituitary gland enlarges somewhat, and there is increased activity of the posterior pituitary hormone, oxytocin. The anterior pituitary hormones FSH and LH are decreased. The reported low blood levels of pituitary somatomammotropin (growth hormone) may perhaps be due to increased levels of chorionic somatomammotropin. The blood level of MSH is also increased.

The thyroid, like the pituitary, enlarges during pregnancy. The basal metabolic rate rises progressively during pregnancy as a result of the increasing growth of the fetus. The increased amount of estrogen causes a rise in the concentration of thyroid hormone; since most thyroid hormone is protein bound, the amount of unbound active hormone does not rise appreciably.

During pregnancy, there is some increase in the level of adrenal corticosteroid, which has been implicated as the cause of abdominal striae, glycosuria, hypertension, and heavier facial features during pregnancy. Early in the second trimester, significant amounts of aldosterone are secreted, and the level becomes even higher in the third trimester. Some studies [6, 7] suggest that these elevated levels protect the women from the natriuretic effects of progesterone.

The level of ionized or active calcium is not significantly lower during pregnancy as compared to its level during the nonpregnant state.

Urinary System

During pregnancy the glomerular filtration rate is increased 50–60 percent without an increase in tubular reabsorption. This results in the excretion of many solutes, e.g., urea, uric acid, creatinine, amino acids, folic acid and other water-soluble vitamins, and glucose. Progesterone is believed to cause relaxation of the smooth muscle in the renal pelvis, ureters, and bladder, which contributes to dilatation of the pelvis and ureters and results in urinary stasis. The dilated ureters also elongate and in so doing tend to curve or coil (Figure 7-13). Dilatation of the ureters is always greater

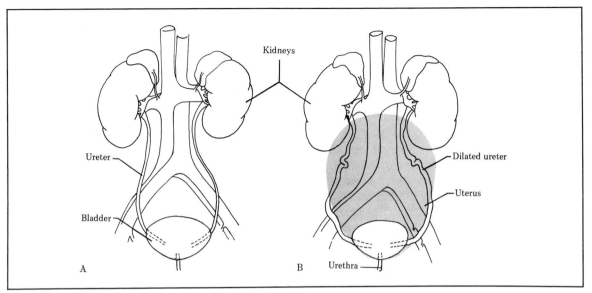

Kidneys

Ureter

Bladder

A

Dilated ureter

Uterus

Urethra

B

Figure 7-13. A. Normal urinary system. B. Urinary system during pregnancy. The ureters dilate, elongate, and coil, increasing the collecting space of the urinary tract and adding to urinary statis. These changes increase the incidence of urinary tract infections during pregnancy.

on the right side above the pelvic brim, due to the dextrorotation of the pregnant uterus; the left ureter may be cushioned somewhat by the sigmoid colon. These changes regress following pregnancy.

Because of the increased collecting space of the urinary tract and the resulting urinary stasis, pregnant women are more likely to have large numbers of bacteria in their urine, even in the absence of symptoms. Cystitis and upper urinary tract infections are common.

Musculoskeletal System

A very important part of prenatal care is a thorough examination of the woman's bony pelvis, since its diameters must be large enough to accommodate the fetal head as it passes through the birth canal.

The pelvis is made up of four bones: the two innominate bones (or hip bones), which form the sides and the front, and the sacrum and the coccyx, which form the back. The pelvic bones are held together by the fibrocartilage of the symphysis pubis and several ligaments.

The bony pelvis is divided into two parts, the false pelvis and the true pelvis, separated by a line referred to as the linea terminalis, or pelvic brim. The false pelvis lies above the line and is bounded by the lumbar vertebrae posteriorly, the iliac crests to the sides, and the lower portion of the abdominal wall anteriorly. The false pelvis provides support for the abdominal organs, including the pregnant uterus (Figure 7-14).

The true pelvis lies below the linea terminalis; its walls are formed by the sacrum, coccyx, and the lower portion of the hip bones. Because the true pelvis forms the passage through which the baby must travel during birth, it is of great obstetrical significance.

The true pelvis is divided into three parts: the inlet, the midpelvis, and the outlet.

Figure 7-14. Bony pelvis. The false pelvis lies above the linea terminalis, the true pelvis below.

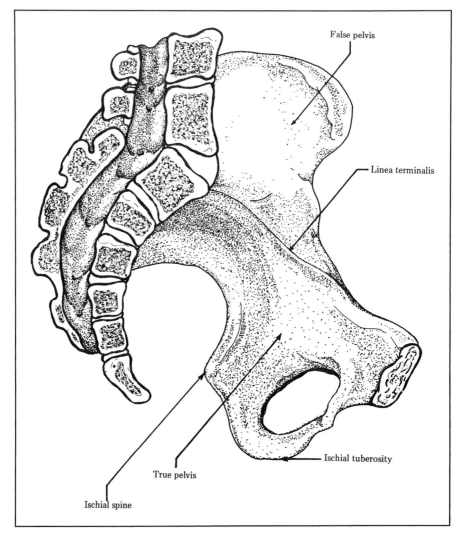

Figure 7-14. Bony pelvis. The false pelvis lies above the linea terminalis, the true pelvis below.

The inlet is the uppermost boundary of the true pelvis and is bounded by the upper margin of the symphysis pubis in the front, the linea terminalis on the sides, and the first sacral vertebra or sacral promontory (an important obstetrical landmark) in the back. The largest diameter of the inlet is the transverse diameter. Its smallest diameter (anterior-posterior) is the most important measurement and is measured three different ways, depending on the point on the symphysis from which the measurement is made. The *true conjugate* is the distance from the top of the symphysis to the middle of the sacral promontory. It usually measures 11 centimeters (4.3 inches) or more; the minimum acceptable measurement for most vaginal deliveries is 10 centimeters.

The *obstetrical conjugate,* the distance between the inner surface of the symphysis and the sacral promontory, is a few millimeters shorter than the true conjugate.

Exact measurement of the obstetrical conjugate may only be obtained by x-ray, but it can be estimated by subtracting 1.5–2 centimeters (0.6–0.8 inch) from the third diameter, the *diagonal conjugate* (usually 12.5 centimeters, or 4.9 inches). The diagonal conjugate is the distance from the lower margin of the symphysis to the sacral promontory. The physician usually measures this diameter by placing his first two fingers in the vagina and touching the sacral promontory (Figure 7-15). This process may be uncomfortable for the woman, requiring preparation and support from the nurse. It may also be deferred until the second trimester, when vaginal and perineal tissues are more easily stretched.

The diameters of the midpelvis cannot be measured clinically. The smallest diameter of the midpelvis, the distance between the ischial spines, averages 10.5 centimeters (4.1 inches). The spines themselves are another obstetrical landmark and are palpated on pelvic examination to determine their prominence. Prominent ischial spines may indicate a contracted pelvis.

Figure 7-15. Measuring the diagonal conjugate from the lower margin of the symphysis to the sacral promontory.

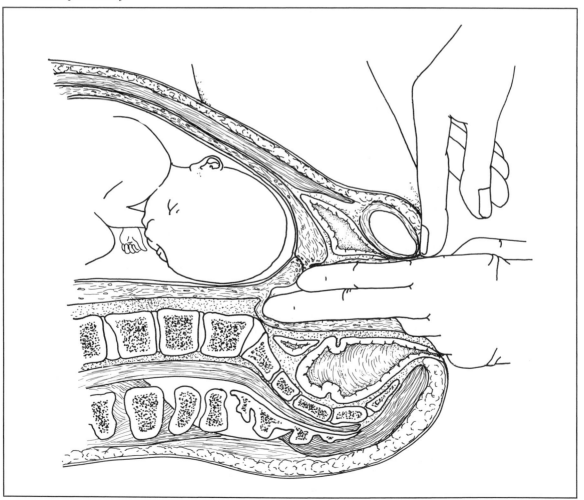

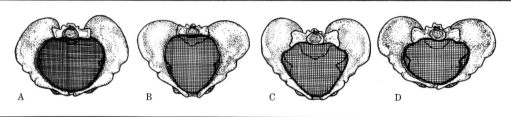

Figure 7-16. Four main types of pelvic shapes: A. Gynecoid. B. Anthropoid. C. Android. D. Platypelloid.

The outlet is the lowest boundary of the true pelvis. It is bounded by the lower margin of the symphysis anteriorly, the ischial tuberosities to the side, and the tip of the sacrum posteriorly. Its most critical diameter is between the ischial tuberosities; ideally this diameter should be 9 centimeters (3.5 inches) or more. The minimum acceptable measurement that will allow vaginal delivery is 8 centimeters (3.1 inches). Since this diameter is shortened when the pubic arch is narrow, the arch is always checked during the pelvic examination.

In addition to these measurements, the coccyx is checked for mobility. If it is fixed, it may shorten the diameters of the outlet and may fracture during delivery.

VARIATIONS IN PELVIC SIZE AND SHAPE

Pelvic size and shape can be influenced by a number of things: sex, racial characteristics, general body build, nutritional status (especially conditions such as rickets during childhood), congenital defects, and disease or injury of the spine, pelvic bones, or lower extremities. There are four main types of pelvic shapes. The gynecoid pelvis (the normal female pelvis) is found in about half of the obstetrical population. Since important diameters may be smaller in the other pelvic shapes, they may be the source of difficulty at the time of delivery (Figure 7-16).

As a result of hormonal increases (possibly estrogen, progesterone, and relaxin), the pelvic joints begin to relax in the first half of pregnancy and become increasingly mobile in the last three months. As a result, walking may become difficult and uncomfortable. These changes tend to regress within three to five months after delivery.

During the last trimester, women sometimes experience aching, weakness, and numbness in the upper extremities. This may be a result of the traction placed on ulnar and median nerves by the anterior flexion of the neck and by the slumping of the shoulders characteristic of the pregnancy posture.

COMMON CONCERNS

Exercise, Rest, and Sleep

A woman's prepregnancy exercise pattern forms the basis for her level of activity during pregnancy. In general, it is not felt to be necessary to limit exercise, provided the woman does not become excessively fatigued. However, she should remember that it will take her longer to become rested following exercise and that her balance and coordination may be impaired. For these reasons, if a woman is not used to exercising or active sports, now is not the time for her to begin. Activities or sports that have a risk of bodily injury (such as skiing and snowmobiling) should be considered very carefully with each woman, in terms of her individual history and the length of her pregnancy.

An adequate amount of rest is very important, especially during the last six weeks. Sometimes several short periods of rest are more convenient than longer ones; each woman's daily activities should be taken into consideration when suggestions are being made. Generally half-hour rest periods in the morning and afternoon are recommended. A woman who works should use her break periods to best advantage by sitting with her legs elevated, if possible, and perhaps closing her eyes for a few minutes. Whenever possible women should be encouraged to sit rather than stand.

The sleep center is probably a central site of action for progesterone so that it is common for pregnant women to be listless, tired, and sleepy [4, 9]. During pregnancy, women should try to get at least 8 hours of sleep a night.

The most comfortable relaxation position for some pregnant women is lying on the side with a pillow under the flexed upper knee or with a pillow under the abdomen. If she is on her back, she might be made more comfortable with a small pillow under her head and feet, a cushion or pillow under her knees, and a folded towel under her lumbar spine; this tends to lessen the strain on her back (Figure 7-17).

Resting is sometimes difficult for a mother who has several small children. Her rest periods might be coordinated with their nap times, or she may plan for several periods of quiet activity during the day. During this time, she might sit with her feet elevated and read stories to them. They might spend time together in a room where the children can play safely, occupied with toys or television, while the mother rests. Women in a clinic or doctor's office can help each other by sharing their methods for providing for periods of rest.

Mood Swings

Inadequate sleep and rest may contribute to a woman's susceptability to mood swings. Furthermore a physiological basis for the emotional lability of pregnancy has been hypothesized by a number of researchers. Some reports note that a de-

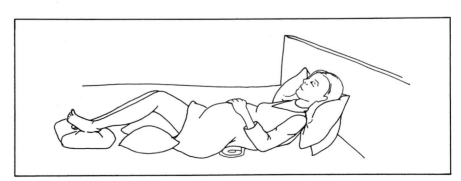

Figure 7-17. A comfortable position for relaxing during pregnancy.

crease in vitamin B_6 (pyridoxine) occurs as a result of increased levels of estrogen and progesterone. Adequate supplies of B_6 are necessary in the formation of catecholamines [3].

For some time researchers [15] have postulated a link between the affective disorders (depressions and elations) and changes in central nervous system catecholamine metabolism, particularly those leading to a decrease in norepinephrine. Treadway et al. [16] hypothesize that the decrease in norepinephrine levels in pregnancy and in the postpartum period may predispose the mother to affective disorders during these times.

Employment

More women than ever before are actively employed, for reasons of both self-satisfaction and economics. Generally there is no reason for them to stop during pregnancy, provided that they have no complications and provided that the nature of their work does not pose a threat to them or their babies. Certain safeguards are recommended: The pregnant woman should avoid severe physical strain, she should have adequate periods of rest, she should use good body mechanics, and she should avoid toxic substances, such as benzene and toluene, carbon monoxide, chlorinated hydrocarbons, lead and its compounds, mercury and its compounds, phorphorus, x-rays and radioactive substances, and turpentine. She might be further restricted by employment policies, although many of these are currently under review.

Traveling

Generally travel has no bad effect on pregnancy. Some airlines impose restrictions on pregnant women, and some require various degrees of information from her physician before she takes the trip. If she goes by car or bus, it is recommended that she stop at least every two hours to walk about, in order to enhance her circulation. Driving is not contraindicated, and although the use of seat belts is controversial, they may be buckled low over the abdomen. When the lap belt is used, the shoulder belt should also be used whenever possible. During the last trimester the woman should consider the distance she is traveling from home; if she should go into labor, it would be best for her to be delivered by the obstetrician who has been caring for her and in whom she has confidence.

Immunizations

Vaccinations with *live* viruses that can cross the placental barrier and be hazardous to the fetus are generally to be avoided during pregnancy. Therefore, it is important that a woman receive her immunizations prior to pregnancy (or have a pregnancy test done before being immunized if there is the possibility that she may be pregnant). In addition, women who are vaccinated with live viruses should be advised to use a contraceptive during the subsequent two or three months.

The Advisory Committee on Immunization Practices of the Public Health Service and the Committee on Infectious Diseases of the American Academy of Pediatrics have reported on various vaccinations [14]. *Smallpox* virus has the potential for infecting the fetus at any time during pregnancy, although it rarely does so. Therefore, if at all possible this vaccination should be postponed until after pregnancy. If the risk of exposure to *yellow fever* is great, a pregnant woman may receive its live virus vaccine. The live virus vaccines for *mumps* and *measles* should never be given to a pregnant woman. The vaccine for *rubella* has a definite potential for infecting the fetus and placenta; it, too, is never given during pregnancy. If there is danger of *cholera* infection, pregnant women should receive the killed bacterial vaccine, since its adverse maternal or fetal effects are not well documented. Pregnancy is not a contraindication to the use of Salk polio vaccine or rabies vaccine. Generally considered safe for administration during pregnancy are vaccines against influenza, epidemic typhus, and typhoid; tetanus and diphtheria toxoids; and tuberculin and histoplasmin tests.

Medications

The best policy for a pregnant woman is to take as few medications during her pregnancy as possible, since it is not known what effect many drugs have on fetal growth and development. Before any drug is given, its advantages must outweigh the factor of such unknown risks (as well as any known fetal risks) (Table 7-5).

Smoking and Drinking

Many obstetricians recommend that cigarette-smoking be avoided or decreased during pregnancy. Studies have shown that mothers who smoke bear smaller infants than do nonsmokers, particularly if they smoke more than one pack of cigarettes a day [2, 11]; presumably the nicotine crosses the placental barrier. The overall neonatal mortality and the incidence of prematurity, fetal abnormalities, and stillbirths do not seem to be higher, however.

Alcohol does cross the placental barrier. Its use in moderation has not been shown to produce abnormal changes in the mother or the fetus or to affect the course of pregnancy. The prenatal and postnatal underdevelopment of the fetus seen in cases of chronic alcoholism is thought to be related to accompanying malnutrition or alcohol toxicity. Some cases of malformations of the heart, face, head, and extremeties have also been associated with it. The caloric content of alcohol is usually high, which may be a consideration when mothers are "calorie-conscious." The sodium content of beer may be relevant when dietary sodium must be restricted.

Sexual Activity

There is no evidence to indicate that the pregnant woman with no unusual complications should not engage in intercourse or masturbation to orgasm until late in the third trimester or even until the time of labor, depending on the couple's needs. This is a subject that is frequently neglected by health professionals who counsel pregnant couples; they may assume that the sexual adjustments that become necessary with pregnancy occur as a matter of course and therefore need no discussion. Such an assumption does a great disservice to the woman and her partner.

Table 7-5. Fetotoxic Drugs

Maternal Medication	Possible Fetal or Neonatal Effect
Antidiabetic agents	
Chlorpropamide	Increased incidence of intrauterine fetal death
Antithyroid drugs	
Thiouracil, inorganic iodides	Goiter, mental retardation
Antibiotics	
Erythromycin	Hepatic injury
Streptomycin	Nerve deafness
Sulfonamides	Kernicterus
Tetracyclines	Hemolysis, hepatotoxicity, inhibition of skeletal growth, discolored teeth
Hormones	
Androgens, progestogens, estrogens	Advanced bone age, masculinization (applies to androgens and some progestogens)
Diuretics	
Thiazides	Bone marrow suppression
Analgesics, narcotics	
Salicylates (excessive)	Neonatal bleeding
Heroin, morphine	Neonatal death or convulsions, tremors
Sedatives, tranquilizers	
Meprobamate	Retarded development
Phenothiazines	Hyperbilirubinemia
Phenobarbital (excessive)	Neonatal bleeding
Barbiturates	Neonatal depression
Vitamins	
Vitamin D	Cardiac malformations
Vitamin K (excessive)	Hyperbilirubinemia
Antineoplastic agents	Multiple anomalies / Abortion
Anticoagulant drugs	
Coumarins	Fetal death or hemorrhage
Antieclamptic drugs	
Magnesium sulfate	Flaccidity, lethargy, neonatal depression

Source: S. G. Babson et al. *Management of High-Risk Pregnancy and Intensive Care of the Neonate* (3rd ed.). St. Louis: Mosby, 1971.

Masters and Johnson [10] have detailed some of the physiological changes that relate to the pregnant woman's response for which she can be prepared. Breast tenderness during advanced sexual tension, which may be severe in the first trimester, tends to decrease in the second and third trimesters. Increased pelvic vascularity and chronic engorgement contribute to high levels of sexual tension in the last half of pregnancy; the woman's sexual drives may become more intense at this time. Vaginal lubrication is greatly increased. Orgasms may be very strong.

Patterns of sexual activity are likely to change throughout pregnancy due to physical discomfort, loss of interest, fatigue, fear of injury to the baby, or, toward term, difficulty in finding a compatible position. Mutual masturbation or oral-genital techniques may be used more frequently, and alternative positions for intercourse may be attempted. The side-by-side position (with the couple either face to face or the man facing the woman's back) is less exhausting, avoids deep penetration, and puts less pressure on the woman than other positions do. She may find the female superior position uncomfortable, and this disadvantage may outweigh the advantage of being able to control the depth of penetration. Vice versa, the sitting position often results in deep penetration, which may be uncomfortable or harmful for the woman.

Whatever position or technique the couple chooses, they should take sensible precautions against excessive abdominal pressure, deep penile penetration, and infection. There is little reason to prohibit vaginal intercourse at any time during pregnancy, provided that the woman does not have a history of spontaneous abortion or premature labor. In addition, she should not have a ripe cervix, ruptured membranes, pain, spotting, or bleeding. Since strong uterine contractions occur with orgasmic response, both from intercourse and masturbation, couples should be cautioned that orgasm may initiate labor contractions if the woman is within three weeks of term. Whether or not premature labor can be attributed to orgasmic response remains controversial [10].

REFERENCES

1. Basu, H. K., and Jeffcoate, N.   Local fibrinolytic activity in the pregnant uterus. *American Journal of Obstetrics and Gynecology* 107:1188, 1970.
2. Buncher, C.   Cigarette smoking and duration of pregnancy. *American Journal of Obstetrics and Gynecology* 103:942, 1969.
3. Butterworth, C. E., Jr.   Interactions of nutrients with oral contraceptives and other drugs. *Journal of the American Dietetic Association* 62:510, 1973.
4. Hytten, F., and Leitch, I.   *The Physiology of Human Pregnancy*. Oxford: Blackwell Scientific, 1971.
5. Krieg, A., and Henry, J. B.   Pregnancy tests. *Postgraduate Medicine* 42:48, 1967.
6. Laidlaw, J. C., Ruse, J. L., and Gornall, A. G.   The influence of estrogen and progesterone on aldosterone secretion. *Journal of Clinical Endocrinology* 22:161, 1962.
7. Landau, R. L., Plotz, E. J., and Lugibihl, K.   Effect of pregnancy on the metabolic influence of administered progesterone. *Journal of Clinical Endocrinology* 20:1561, 1960.
8. Llewellyn-Jones, D.   *Fundamentals of Obstetrics and Gynaecology,* Vol. 1. London: Faber and Faber, 1971.
9. Luce, G. G., and Segal, J.   *Sleep*. New York: Coward-McCann, 1966.
10. Masters, W. H., and Johnson, V. E.   *Human Sexual Response*. Boston: Little, Brown, 1966.
11. Mulcahy, R., and Knaggs, J.   Effects of age, parity, and cigarette smoking on outcome of pregnancy. *American Journal of Obstetrics and Gynecology* 101:884, 1968.
12. Physicians seek reason for clay eating. *Journal of the American Medical Association* 201:26, 1967.
13. Radioreceptor assay of human chorionic gonadotropin: Detection of early pregnancy. *Science* 184:793, 1974.
14. Safety of immunizing agents in pregnancy. *Medical Letter on Drugs and Therapeutics* 12:23, 1970.
15. Schildkraut, J.   The catecholamine hypothesis of affective disorders: A review of supporting evidence. *American Journal of Psychiatry* 122:509, 1965.
16. Treadway, C. R., Kane, F., Jarrahi-Zadeh, A., and Lipton, M.   A psychoendocrine study of pregnancy and the puerperium. *American Journal of Psychiatry* 125:1380, 1969.
17. Ueland, K., Novy, M. J., Peterson, E. N., and Metcalfe, J.   Maternal cardiovascular dynamics. *American Journal of Obstetrics and Gynecology* 104:856, 1969.

FURTHER READING

Applebaum, R. M.   The modern management of successful breast feeding. *Pediatric Clinics of North America* 17:203, 1970.

Broadribb, V., and Corliss, C.   *Maternal-Child Nursing.* Philadelphia: Lippincott, 1973.

Clausen, J., Flook, M., Ford, B., Green, M., and Popiel, E.   *Maternity Nursing Today.* New York: McGraw-Hill, 1973.

Fitzpatrick, E., Reeder, S., and Mastroianni, L.   *Maternity Nursing.* Philadelphia: Lippincott, 1971.

Greenhill, J. P., and Friedman, E. A.   *Biological Principles and Modern Practice of Obstetrics.* Philadelphia: W. B. Saunders, 1974.

Hellman, L. M., and Pritchard, J. A.   *Williams Obstetrics.* New York: Appleton-Century-Crofts, 1971.

Lerch, C.   *Maternity Nursing.* St. Louis: Mosby, 1970.

Page, E., Villee, C., and Villee, D.   *Human Reproduction* (2nd ed.) Philadelphia: Saunders, 1976.

Philipp, E., Barnes, J., and Newton, M.   *Scientific Foundations of Obstetrics and Gynaecology.* Philadelphia: Davis, 1970.

Theuer, R.   Effect of oral contraceptive agents on vitamin and mineral needs: A review. *Journal of Reproductive Medicine* 8:13, 1972.

Treloar, A., Behn, B., and Cowan, D.   Analysis of gestational interval. *American Journal of Obstetrics and Gynecology* 99:34, 1967.

Wiedenbach, E.   *Family-Centered Maternity Nursing.* New York: Putnam, 1967.

Woods, N.   *Human Sexuality in Health and Illness.* St. Louis: Mosby, 1975.

Ziegel, E., and Van Blarcom, C.   *Obstetric Nursing.* New York: Macmillan, 1972.

Chapter 8 Nutritional Needs During Childbearing

METABOLIC CHANGES IN PREGNANCY

Certain aspects of the maternal physiological changes related to pregnancy have not been discussed, namely the differences in the metabolism of essential elements such as water, carbohydrates, lipids, and protein, as well as those other substances that relate to the nutrition of the pregnant or lactating woman. It is unfortunate that our knowledge and understanding of the metabolic changes during pregnancy are incomplete. However some of the adjustments in carbohydrate and insulin metabolism have been documented; for instance, fasting blood sugar values are lower in pregnancy. Insulin responds differently to a glucose load, a phenomenon that is observed throughout pregnancy but is more obvious in the later stages of pregnancy. While insulin seems to have a normal effect on blood glucose in early pregnancy, in late pregnancy the large extra quantities of insulin that are released do not have a corresponding extra effect on blood glucose levels [9]. This same reaction has been noted in both men and nonpregnant women who have received large doses of progesterone [10]. Progesterone and estrogen may play a part in promoting a state of insulin resistance. During pregnancy there is also increased resistance to injected insulin, since the fall in blood sugar it produces is not as great as that in the nonpregnant woman.

The source of insulin antagonism in pregnancy has not been specifically defined, but there are a number of speculations [9]. It may be that insulin, like thyroxin and many other hormones, might be more protein-bound. The growth hormone-like characteristics of human placental lactogen (HPL) include insulin antagonism. The elevated levels of serum corticosteroids in pregnancy might also be expected to antagonize insulin, probably by accelerating its destruction in the liver. Another contributing factor may be the increased levels of fatty acids; their high levels in late pregnancy may result from increased lipolysis due to HPL. It has been suggested that the mechanism of insulin antagonism by HPL and by growth hormone may be through higher levels of serum fatty acids. Insulin is also thought to be destroyed by a placental enzyme reaction.

Increased amounts of circulating insulin and low blood glucose may be responsible in part for the increased appetite and food intake during pregnancy. Increased insulin action might explain the amount of fat storage that takes place. It may also be that the fainting episodes that are common at the beginning of pregnancy are hypoglycemic rather than vasovagal in nature [9]. The increasing need for more insulin in later pregnancy to counteract increasing insulin metabolism puts additional stress on the pancreas. It is not surprising that the woman whose pancreas has little natural reserve may not be able to produce enough insulin, resulting in the development of gestational diabetes.

Plasma lipids are generally high in pregnancy, and the level tends to rise throughout its course. This may be a reflection of increased fatty-acid synthesis, possibly by the liver. There is extensive storage of fat in adipose tissue. Progesterone may act to reset a lipostat in the hypothalamus during pregnancy. Following delivery this mechanism probably returns to its nonpregnant level and the woman loses much of her added fat.

In most normal pregnancies, there is a positive sodium balance. As previously mentioned, this results from the increased glomerular filtration rate as well as the presence of large amounts of progesterone secreted by the placenta. Progesterone slows absorption of filtered sodium through the renal tubules. Through the renin-angiotensin-aldosterone pathway, aldosterone is released as part of a compensatory mechanism to counterbalance the salt-losing tendency of progesterone. With the resulting sodium reabsorption that occurs in the kidneys, a positive sodium balance results. To maintain fluid balance and proper osmosis, extra water is retained in the maternal tissues and contributes to the woman's weight gain during pregnancy [15].

It is still not known how the levels of most nutrients are controlled during pregnancy. Most of the nutrients that have been measured are found to exist at a lower concentration in the pregnant woman than in the nonpregnant woman. Dietary deficiency or failure of absorption is probably not responsible for most of the low levels, although many of them can be artificially raised by large dietary supplements [9]. Excretion by the kidney probably plays only a small role. One possible reason for the reduced levels of many nutrients is a resetting of different homeostatic mechanisms. It may also be that the lowering of nutrient levels in the maternal blood produces a balance that favors transfer to the fetus rather than the maternal tissues.

The basal metabolic rate is increased during pregnancy for many reasons: increase in muscle mass of the uterus, breast growth, fetal mass and placenta, and increased cardiac and respiratory loads. The total increase is about 20–25 percent over the nonpregnant state; it requires about 300 additional calories daily to meet these increased energy and nutrient demands. The current emphasis in obstetrical practice has been placed on the mother's intake of ample calories during her pregnancy, which represents a swing from previous stringent restriction of maternal weight gain. The goal of the previous restriction was presumably to produce a baby of low birth weight for easy delivery and to reduce the incidence of preeclampsia. Now it is recognized that maternal weight restriction and nutritional inadequacy may indeed contribute to a high perinatal mortality in the United States through fetal growth retardation, hypertensive disorders, abruptio placentae, and premature delivery [15, 16].

The exact nutritional requirements of the pregnant woman and her fetus have not been established. Very few women in the United States suffer from severe malnutrition, but many will begin a pregnancy with inadequate nutritional reserves. The increased demands of pregnancy deplete her nutrient stores, and deficiencies soon become evident. Even with treatment it may take months for the mother to feel recovered.

Table 8-1. Analysis of Weight Gain in Pregnancy (in Grams)

Part of Body	10 Weeks	20 Weeks	30 Weeks	40 Weeks
Fetus	5	300	1500	3400
Placenta	20	170	430	650
Amniotic fluid	30	350	750	800
Uterus	140	320	600	970
Breasts	45	180	360	405
Blood	100	600	1300	1250
Extracellular extravascular fluid	0	30	80	1680
Depot fat	310	2050	3480	3345

Source: F. Hytten, and I. Leitch. *The Physiology of Human Pregnancy.* London: Blackwell Scientific, 1971.

NUTRITIONAL NEEDS DURING PREGNANCY

The total weight gain expected during pregnancy in women with unrestricted balanced diets averages 11–13 kilograms (24–28 pounds), most of which can be accounted for by the products of pregnancy and by maternal physiological changes (Table 8-1). The weight gain is minimal in the first trimester; over the second and third trimesters it occurs at a rate of about 0.2–0.5 kilograms (0.5–1 pound) per week. During the second trimester about 60 percent of the weight gain occurs in the woman, while during the third trimester the fetus accounts for 60 percent of the weight gain [17]. Restrictive weight control or reduction is not advised during pregnancy because of the likelihood that it will result in nutritional deficiencies for the woman and fetus.

The nutritional needs of the pregnant woman mainly depend on a well-balanced diet, with nutrients from each of the basic four food groups. It must be remembered that the woman's general health at the time of her infant's conception is a result of dietary habits that have been established throughout her lifetime; thus, it is her prepregnancy nutrition that may be most important of all (Table 8-2).

Table 8-2. Recommended Daily Dietary Allowances of Some Selected Nutrients for Pregnancy and Lactation[a]

Nutrients	Nonpregnant 15–18 yr, 54 kg (119 lb)	Nonpregnant 25 yr, 58 kg (128 lb)	Pregnancy 15–18 yr	Pregnancy 25 yr	Pregnancy Added Need	Lactation 15–18 yr	Lactation 25 yr	Lactation Added Need
Calories	2100	2000	2400	2300	300	2600	2500	500
Protein (gm)	48	46	78	76	30	68	66	20
Calcium (mg)	1200	800	1600	1200	400	1600	1200	400
Iron (mg)	18	18	18+	18+		18	18	
Vitamin A (IU)	4000	4000	5000	5000	1000	6000	6000	2000
Thiamine (mg)	1.1	1.0	1.4	1.3	0.3	1.4	1.3	0.3
Riboflavin (mg)	1.4	1.2	1.7	1.5	0.3	1.9	1.7	0.5
Niacin (mg)	14	13	16	15	2.0	18	17	4.0
Ascorbic acid (mg)	45	45	60	60	15	60	60	15
Vitamin D (IU)	400		400	400		400	400	

[a]Two specific nonpregnant groups were chosen as samples: 15- to 18-year-old, 119 lb group and 25-year-old, 128 lb group.
Source: Research Council, National Academy of Sciences. *Recommended Dietary Allowances.* Washington, D.C., 1973.

Protein

As part of her 300 extra daily calories, the pregnant woman should have an additional daily allowance of 30 grams of protein. The nitrogen composition of fetal tissue rises from 0.9 grams at conception to 55.9 grams at term. In addition, 17 grams of nitrogen is stored in the placenta, 1 gram in amniotic fluid, 17 grams in maternal breast tissue, and 40 grams in the uterus. There are maternal reserves of 200–350 grams of nitrogen, stored to protect the woman against losses during labor and delivery and to prepare her for lactation. Increased blood volume and blood constituents, especially hemoglobin and plasma protein, contribute to the woman's need for increased intake of protein. Complete protein foods include milk, eggs, cheese, fish, and meat; legumes, nuts, and whole grains are additional protein sources.

Minerals

Calcium and iron are the minerals that receive special attention during pregnancy. In general, intake of calcium should be increased by 400 milligrams daily, to a total of 1.2 grams daily. Calcium stores of the woman increase from 4 grams at the middle of pregnancy to 30 grams at term. Fetal stores increase from 1 gram at the middle of pregnancy to 23 grams at term. Calcium is necessary for rapid mineralization of fetal skeletal tissue as well as formation of fetal tooth buds. Dairy products are an excellent source of calcium; other sources are whole or enriched cereal grain and green or leafy vegetables. Some women, in their zeal to meet their calcium needs, will drink too much milk, disturbing their calcium-phosphorus ratio, which may result in leg cramping. They might be reminded that 3–4 cups of milk or equivalent dairy products would be sufficient to meet their needs.

Iron supplements after meals are usually recommended to increase the woman's normal daily intake of 18 milligrams of iron. The total iron requirement of pregnancy is approximately 1000 milligrams: 300 milligrams for the increase in total red cell volume, 300 milligrams for the fetus, 70 milligrams for the placenta, and 500 milligrams or more in blood loss at delivery and post partum. Some iron is saved (about 150 milligrams), since during pregnancy no iron is lost through menstruation. Most iron demands occur in the second half of pregnancy, during which time the fetus stores a three- to four-month's supply in its liver. For this reason, the National Research Council (NRC) has recommended that pregnant women receive 30–60 milligrams of ferrous iron as a daily supplement during the second and third trimesters. The needs of the fetus are always met, even if at the mother's expense. In order to compensate for this acute demand during the last half of pregnancy, maternal uptake of iron from her gastrointestinal tract may be increased eight to ten times, and her iron-binding capacity is greatly increased [7]. Food sources rich in iron include liver, other meats, dried fruit and beans, green vegetables, eggs, and enriched cereals.

Vitamins

Increased amounts of vitamins A, B, C, and D are usually recommended for the pregnant woman. The NRC recommends a daily increase of 1000 IU of vitamin A during the last half of pregnancy. Good food sources of vitamin A include liver, egg yolk, butter or fortified margarine, dark green and yellow vegetables, and fruits.

During pregnancy the need for the B vitamins is great, since these vitamins are an important part of the increased metabolism associated with pregnancy. Folic acid is particularly important, and a daily supplement of 0.2–0.4 milligrams is recommended by the NRC if the diet is not adequate. Most of the increases in the other B vitamins will be supplied by a well-balanced diet.

The NRC has recommended a daily increase of 15 milligrams of vitamin C for the pregnant woman. Besides functioning in the formation of connective tissue and vascular systems, vitamin C also enhances the absorption of iron, which is necessary for the increased hemoglobin mass. Good food sources of vitamin C include citrus fruits, melon, berries, tomatoes, leafy greens, and cabbage.

It is very important that the pregnant woman receive an adequate amount of vitamin D, since it is necessary for the proper function of calcium and phosphorus in the growth of fetal skeletal tissue. Her diet should provide at least 400 IU of vitamin D daily; sometimes supplements are ordered by the physician. Vitamin D is abundant in fortified milk and margarine, butter, egg yolk, and liver.

NEEDS DURING LACTATION

During lactation, there are additional nutritional requirements. The pregnant woman needs to add 500 calories to her nonpregnant diet, an increase of 200 calories over her diet during pregnancy. This increase, which may be 500–1000 calories more than the usual adult requirement, provides calories for both milk content and milk production. The average daily milk production is 800–850 milliliters, with a caloric value of 500–600 calories; the energy consumed in producing that amount of milk uses another 200–400 calories.

The lactating woman has protein needs of 20 grams more than the nonpregnant allowance (a decrease of 10 grams from the protein needs during pregnancy); the amount of calcium, iron, and vitamin C needed is the same as during pregnancy. She will need an increase of about 2000 IU of vitamin A over her nonpregnant daily intake as well as increased amounts of the B vitamins. To ensure adequate milk production, the mother should be certain to increase her own intake of all fluids (water as well as other beverages).

There are many common beliefs about the relationship of various foods to breast milk. These include the belief that beer improves lactation and that some foods, such as cabbage, onions, and chocolate, pass through breast milk and give the infant gastrointestinal symptoms. There is no basis in fact for either of these assumptions. It cannot be denied, however, that beer would certainly add to the woman's daily fluid and caloric intake [21].

SPECIAL CONSIDERATIONS

While all pregnant or newly delivered women should receive diet counseling, some women need particular attention directed to their nutritional needs. Women who have a rapid succession of pregnancies often have depleted nutrient stores. Those who have a low prepregnancy weight for their height may experience an increased incidence of hypertensive disorders and prematurity. Women who have very limited weight gains during pregnancy may deliver low birth weight infants. Overweight pregnant women often have diets high in fat and carbohydrate and low in protein, minerals, and vitamins. Women with low incomes or those whose religious or philosophical beliefs limit their diet to certain foods should have their intakes assessed. Pregnant girls who are biologically immature form another group needing special guidance [6].

Teenage girls have been cited as having the poorest dietary habits of any age group. Their diets have been reported to be inadequate in calories, protein, iron, calcium, and vitamins A and C [11, 18]. This is especially detrimental for girls under 17 years of age, because their growth and development has not been completed. When a pregnancy is superimposed on her own biological nutritional demands, the pregnant adolescent is competing with the fetus for essential nutrients. Additionally, those girls who mature rapidly and reach menarche early are at a time of peak velocity of adolescent growth, yet their skeletal maturation is less advanced [19], which means that their pelvic capacity has not yet reached adult size. The resulting neonatal, postnatal, and infant mortality rates in young mothers are much higher than those for the population in general. The younger the mother, the greater the increase in infant mortality is likely to be. In addition to increased mortality, teenage mothers have many more low birth weight babies.

CURRENT RESEARCH

While there have been studies noting the effects of poor nutrition on fetal development in man, the majority of the findings in this area have been reported from animal research. Applying these results to human development has to be seriously questioned; animals have higher metabolic rates than humans, and the products of conception in animals form a larger proportion of the total weight of the animal. The birth weight of a litter may represent 75 percent of the mother's weight in experimental animals, while a human infant may represent only 6 percent of a woman's total weight. Inadequate diets in experimental animals have reduced birth weights 20–25 percent, while in women, where severe starvation has been present, birth weights have been reduced only 5–10 percent of the usual weights [13]. Experimental animals are often from inbred strains that represent better control of genetic variables, a factor almost impossible to control in human studies.

Animal studies have shown that maternal malnutrition has degenerative effects on the fetal and newborn central nervous system. The brains of these animals had a reduced total number of cells, decreased cell size, and decreased enzymatic content and activity [3]. Fetal lung tissue showed decreased cell multiplication and cell size and a reduction in total weight of the lung.

There have been additional reports that maternal nutritional deprivation (especially protein and caloric deprivation) adversely affects cognitive, emotional, and neurological development. Animals of malnourished mothers have shown abnormalities in activity level, response to stimuli, and ability to learn tasks, as well as the brain changes already noted [16]. The earlier and more prolonged the period of deprivation, the more profound and irreversible the changes have been.

Human studies have reported similar results. In humans, the peak period of brain growth is in prenatal life, but cell division in some regions of the brain continues through the first year of life. It has been postulated that during these critical periods of cellular proliferation, nutritional deprivation of the fetus and young infant could result in permanent cellular changes in the composition of the adult brain. Post-mortum examination of malnourished infants showed a 15 percent reduction in the number of brain cells if the malnutrition occurred after birth in infants with a normal birth weight. The reduction was 60 percent if the malnutrition occurred prenatally (in which case the infants had low birth weights) [12].

Reports from many parts of the world have shown a close association between poor maternal nutrition and high fetal and infant mortality. A child born to a severely malnourished mother may almost catch up to the normal for his age in physical growth, when given an adequate diet in later years. It is believed, however, that the nervous system impairment occurring during the critical period of development may be irreversible and may leave the individual with permanently damaged intellectual functioning [14].

Burke and co-workers [4], reporting on a study involving over 200 mothers, noted that adequate nutrition and adequate protein, in particular, related positively to infant birth weight, length, and the overall condition of infants during the first two weeks of life. Ebbs and associates [8] reported an increased incidence of complications (miscarriages, prematurity, and fetal mortality) in a group of mothers with poor diets as compared with another group of mothers whose poor diets had been supplemented. When Balfour [2] supplemented the poor diets of one group with a milk product and additional vitamins and minerals, the fetal and neonatal mortality was significantly lower than that of the group whose poor diets were not supplemented. Cameron and Graham [5], after giving diet supervision to a group of pregnant women, found reductions in prematurity and fetal mortality rates over the control group. Smith [20] reported that when mothers were adequately nourished prior to a period of nutritional deprivation (calories less than 1000, protein less than 40 grams), there appeared to be slight, if any, effect on fetal weight if the undernutrition occurred prior to the sixth month of gestation.

CULTURAL IMPORTANCE OF FOOD

Most people eat for reasons other than physical sustenance. Eating has many meanings that are intimately tied up with an individual's whole way of life. Food habits, like other forms of human behavior, are the result of many personal, social, psychological, and cultural influences. The meaning and importance they have for the pregnant woman must be kept in mind before nurses or other health workers give diet counseling. The objective is not to change the dietary pattern so that it resembles that of the person doing the counseling but rather to assess the woman's needs and supplement her diet with needed foods acceptable to her. Emphasis should be placed on the desirable features of her diet and on methods of food preparation that preserve food values. Unfamiliar foods and methods of preparation must be assessed before changes are recommended.

Culture develops as a means of interpreting common life experiences and evolves over a long period of time, partially as a result of adaptation to the environment. Attempts to change these long-standing cultural habits by someone not familiar with them may be upsetting. Food habits, some of the oldest and most entrenched aspects of culture, exert a deep influence on people's behavior, as noted by Williams [21]. The cultural background determines what will be eaten and when and how it will be eaten. Items considered to be good food in one culture may be viewed with disgust and believed to cause illness in other cultures. In America milk is considered a basic food, while in some other cultures it is rejected and viewed as an animal mucous discharge. In some cultures, such as the Greek culture, bread is the main focus of the meal, with the other foods planned around it. In other cultures, meat serves this purpose. Foods eaten for one meal may be rejected for another: In the western part of the United States, ham, eggs, and fried potatoes are popular for breakfast; in the South grits are popular; and in New England pie is a favorite.

Food is a method of teaching and transmitting many aspects of one's culture. Thanksgiving traditionally involves a turkey; picnic foods are eaten on the Fourth of July. Traditional foods are associated with religious holidays. Food may also serve as the main expression of sympathy, sorrow, or support for a family. Cultures that value change lead families or individuals to seek constant variety in diets; because people may want to feel that they are geared for action, they may seek quick-cooking convenience foods [21].

Food is symbolic of sociability, warmth, and friendly gathering. Eating together binds a group or family and builds closeness and solidarity. Special foods closely associated with family sentiments form the most lasting habits throughout life, and when eaten in adulthood trigger a flood of childhood memories. Foods may be accepted because they are viewed as having high status or rejected because they carry low prestige.

Religious practices also dictate food habits. Pork is not eaten by Moslems; meat is restricted by Seventh-Day Adventists. Strict Hindus or Buddhists eat no meat, while liberal Hindus may eat no beef.

The dietary patterns of American Jews depend on the degree of orthodoxy they practice. Pork in all forms is prohibited by Orthodox Jews; beef, lamb, goat, and venison are allowed, as are chicken, turkey, goose, pheasant, and duck. All poultry and meat must be freshly slaughtered according to ritual and soaked in salted water (koshered) to remove all traces of blood. Fish must have scales and fins; thus all shellfish are excluded [21]. Eggs, fruits, vegetables, and grain are eaten without restrictions. Milk or milk products and meat are never combined at the same meal, or even cooked in the same utensils. The Jewish diet generally includes much fish, poultry (especially chicken), noodles, rye and whole grain breads, rich pastries and cakes, and stewed and canned fruits.

Food habits may also vary according to one's ethnic group. Mexican-Americans use many varieties of beans, rice, potatoes, peas, and some vegetables [1]. Chili pepper is popular and is supposed to bring good health. Little meat or milk is used;

however, some calcium is provided by tortillas made from ground whole corn soaked in lime water.

The Puerto Rican diet also does not include much milk. Rice and beans are foods used daily. Salt codfish, chicken, pork, and beef are favorites, as are tomatoes, peppers, onions, and seasonings added to dried peas and beans. Fruits such as bananas and oranges are commonly used.

Italian-Americans use a variety of pastas with various cheeses and sauces, and bread remains an essential part of the meal. Southern Italians use much fish and highly seasoned foods, while their Northern counterparts use more meat and root vegetables. Eggs, cheese, tomatoes, green vegetables, and fruits are used liberally [1].

The diet of those of Middle Eastern extraction has grains (such as wheat or rice) as the major source of calories. Eggs, butter, and cheese are used liberally; lamb is the favorite meat. Sour milk preparations, such as yogurt, are used commonly, and sweet milk is seldom used.

The Chinese diet includes meat, fish, eggs, rice, and a large variety of vegetables. The amount of meat eaten is small, although pork is very popular. Fish is used commonly. Grains provide the main source of calories.

Western European and Scandinavian diets include a wide variety of meats, fish, vegetables, fruits, cheese, and grains. Central European diets derive much of the total calories from grains and potatoes. Pork and pork products, cabbage, root vegetables, eggs, fresh milk, sour cream, yogurt, and cheeses are used widely.

Most black Americans have incorporated to some degree dietary patterns of the South. Grits, rice, and potatoes provide the main source of carbohydrate. Dried peas and beans, fried fish, poultry, pork, game, greens, corn, and fruit are commonly eaten. Milk, milk products, and cheeses are not used extensively. These dietary patterns, like those previously mentioned, are generalizations and much individual variation can be expected. Black Americans born and raised in the North, for example, may have very few of the eating habits of their Southern counterparts. Evaluating these variations is essential in assessing dietary patterns prior to giving any dietary counseling.

REFERENCES

1. Anderson, L., Dibble, M., Mitchell, H., and Rynbergen, H. *Nutrition in Nursing*. Philadelphia: Lippincott, 1972.
2. Balfour, M. Supplementary feeding in pregnancy. *Lancet* 1:208, 1944.
3. Brasel, J. A., and Winick, M. Maternal nutrition and prenatal growth. *Archives of Diseases of Childhood* 47:479, 1972.
4. Burke, B., Beal, V., Kirkwood, S., and Stuart, H. The influence of nutrition during pregnancy upon the condition of the infant at birth. *Journal of Nutrition* 26:569, 1943.
5. Cameron, C. and Graham, S. Antenatal diet and its influence on stillbirth and prematurity. *Glasgow Medical Journal* 23:1, 1944.
6. Cross, A., and Walsh, H. Prenatal diet counseling. *Journal of Reproductive Medicine* 7:265, 1971.
7. Desforges, J. Anemia complicating pregnancy. *Journal of Reproductive Medicine* 10:111, 1973.
8. Ebbs, J., Tisdall, F., and Scott, W. The influence of the prenatal diet on the mother and child. *Milbank Memorial Fund Quarterly* 20:35, 1942.
9. Hytten, F E., and Leitch, I. *The Physiology of Human Pregnancy*. Philadelphia: Davis, 1971.

10. Kalkoff, R. D., Jacobson, M., and Lemper, D. Progesterone, pregnancy, and the augmented plasma insulin response. *Journal of Clinical Endocrinology* 31:24, 1970.
11. King, J. C., Cohenour, S. H., Calloway, D. H., and Jacobson, H. N. Assessment of nutritional status of teenage pregnant girls. *American Journal of Clinical Nutrition* 25:916, 1972.
12. Korones, S., Lancaster, J., and Roberts, F. *High-Risk Newborn Infants.* St. Louis: Mosby, 1972.
13. Langer, A., Haing, C., and Harrigan, J. Impact of maternal nutritional deficiency on the fetus. *Journal of the Medical Society of New Jersey* 71:194, 1974.
14. Manocha, S. Malnutrition—its impact on prenatal and postnatal life of the baby. *Journal of Reproductive Medicine* 10:41, 1973.
15. Oakes, G., Chez, R., and Morelli, I. Diet in pregnancy: Meddling with the normal or preventing toxemia. *American Journal of Nursing* 75:1135, 1975.
16. Osofsky, H. Relationships between nutrition during pregnancy and subsequent infant and child development. *Obstetrical and Gynecological Survey* 30:227, 1975.
17. Pitkin, R., Kaminetzky, H., Newton, M., and Pritchard, J. Maternal nutrition: A selective review of clinical topics. *Obstetrics and Gynecology* 40:773, 1972.
18. Seiler, J. A., and Fox, II. M. Adolescent pregnancy: Association of dietary and obstetric factors. *Home Economics Research Journal* 1:188, 1973.
19. Shank, R. A chink in our armor. *Nutrition Today* 5:2, Summer 1970.
20. Smith, C. Prenatal and neonatal nutrition: Bordon Award Address. *Pediatrics* 30:145, 1962.
21. Williams, S. R. *Nutrition and Diet Therapy.* St. Louis: Mosby, 1973.

FURTHER READING

Ademoware, A., Coury, N., and Kime, J. Relationships of maternal nutrition and weight gain to newborn birthweight. *Obstetrics and Gynecology* 39:460, 1972.
Duggin, G. G., Lyneham, R. C., Dale, N., Evans, R. A., and Tiller, D. J. Calcium balance in pregnancy. *Lancet* 2:926, 1974.
Moghissi, K., Churchill, J., and Kurrie, D. Relationship of maternal amino acids and proteins to fetal growth and mental development. *American Journal of Obstetrics and Gynecology* 123:398, 1975.
Thompson, M., Morse, E., and Merrow, S. Nutrient intake of pregnant women receiving vitamin mineral supplements. *Journal of the American Dietetic Association* 64:382, 1974.
Van de Mark, M., and Wright, A. Hemoglobin and folate levels of pregnant teenagers. *Journal of the American Dietetic Association* 61:511, 1972.
Watney, P. J. M., and Rudd, B. T. Calcium metabolism in pregnancy and in the newborn. *Journal of Obstetrics and Gynecology of the British Commonwealth* 81:210, 1974.
Williams, S. R. *Essentials of Nutrition and Diet Therapy.* St. Louis: Mosby, 1974.

Chapter 9 Education for Childbirth

COMMUNICATION

Communication skills enable the nurse to have a better perception of the needs of individuals and families. Meaningful, goal-directed communication requires conscious effort on the professional's part. Since communication is the core of interaction between people, it must be effective for adequate teaching and learning to occur.

Effective communication is dependent on a number of elements, perhaps the most important of which is the ability to listen. The nurse must listen with a "third ear." More than hearing the words other individuals say, she must hear what they are actually trying to say. Additionally, the nurse should not concentrate entirely on verbal communication, since she may miss much of the real message if she hears only this. Nonverbal communication has long been considered a more reliable expression of true feelings, since there is less conscious control over nonverbal behavior. Listening is enhanced by staying close to the individual, being in a comfortable position, perhaps being seated to signify available time, giving that individual full attention, and remaining silent except to indicate interest and support.

Another essential element in effective communication is the nurse's ability to focus on other individuals, keeping her own needs and desires separate. The nurse must have access to the couple's frame of reference, taking into account their perception of their situation and their feelings, concerns, and desires before the nurse can act or even assess the situation with any degree of validity.

Communication must also be appropriate. Replies should fit the circumstance, be relevant, and be matched to the initial statement. The communication should be efficient, using the couple's language or using simple words, not medical jargon. The couple should also be given time to receive and evaluate the message and to respond. Feedback is another critical element in effective communication; it helps to clarify the information and to alter the original message. However, nonverbal feedback should not be interpreted without verbal validation.

There are many variables both conscious and unconscious that play a part in the communication process. They include intelligence, surroundings, emotions, interests, physical perceptual ability, and differences in the interpretation of words. Differences in personalities of the communicators and prejudicial attitudes can play a role in either facilitating or blocking the communication process.

Knowledge of the subject being addressed and past experience are two additional factors that have an impact on communication. It is often assumed, for example, that mothers who have had previous pregnancies know more about childbearing than they do. The authors are reminded of a woman who, after delivering her third child, was bothered by drainage from her navel. She believed that the baby's umbilical cord had been directly connected to her own umbilicus and that the baby's cord had not been tied tightly enough, accounting for the leakage. On the other hand, multiparous women can be an untapped source of practical information for nurses.

The frequency of previous communication with the individual can be a favorable variable. This supports the need for nurses to get to know their patients and talk with them as often as possible. Some clinics make special efforts to have couples meet with the same personnel at each visit, so that a more meaningful relationship can be established.

The cultural background of the nurse can assert itself silently. The nurse may violate the couple's morals and values if she imposes her own likes and dislikes on the couple. The nurse must avoid the trap of deciding what they need on the basis of her own experiences and values. Likewise, stereotyping results in a mind-set that hinders nurses from responding to the uniqueness of others. Many nurses believe that all primigravidas have long labors. The authors remember one primigravida who had a two-hour labor being verbally chastized by the staff for not coming to the hospital as soon as labor had begun. Even though this is exactly what she had done, she could find no one to believe her.

Service or ward patients are often stereotyped as knowing less than private patients, an orientation that has often resulted in their withholding information from the professional staff. Such patients may be resistant to ideas of staff members while the patients assess whether they are accepted or rejected. This is most often a test of staff stereotypes and prejudices.

TEACHING

Effective communication forms the basis for effective teaching. The first step in teaching is to develop objectives. What is to be accomplished by the teaching? The objectives or goals developed must be realistic; they should be developed and defined so that they can be used to evaluate teaching when it is completed. For example, it would be difficult to evaluate the objective "to teach individuals about pregnancy." A more specific objective, "to identify common discomforts of pregnancy and helpful relief measures during the first trimester," is easier to evaluate in relation to the group's learning.

In developing objectives for childbirth education, the nurse must assess the population to be taught. What is it they want to learn? What are the cultural background and the socioeconomic and educational levels of the group? Are there commonly held folk beliefs about pregnancy in the community that the nurse must address? If so, are some of the beliefs based in fact, so that the nurse may reinforce these while slowly calling attention to the fallacy of others? Are the objectives being developed consistent with the philosophy of the agency or institution?

Other members of the health team must also be consulted in developing the objectives. Teaching will remain an isolated phenomenon rather than an integral part of care if that teaching is done by one or two people without involving other personnel who will be caring for the family. By meeting with other health care workers, the nurse may learn much more about the population to be taught, in addition to finding possible resource people to help with the teaching. The nurse should also advertise that teaching classes will begin shortly and should make the other team members feel that they have a part in the development of the classes. The nutritionist can provide invaluable information on the dietary patterns of the population. The social worker can provide a cultural, socioeconomic, and age profile of the group, in addition to knowing community agencies and resources available to the group. Nurses in the antepartum clinic, delivery room, and postpartum and nursery units can provide information on topics that need to be taught; because of their contribution the nurses are more willing to reinforce the teaching and to help in its evaluation.

After developing the objectives, the nurse must focus on some basic principles of the learning-teaching process. The learning must be active, that is, the individuals must be involved in the process. If the discussion focuses on common discomforts of pregnancy, the nurse might begin by asking members of the group what discomforts they have experienced, and then each should be discussed, rather than presenting a prearranged lecture on that subject. Discomforts that do not come up in discussion can be addressed at the end.

A second basic principle of teaching is that the learning must be meaningful. The nurse as teacher must address "where the learner is now," that is, the learner's current life situation. She must show the individual that the learning has a purpose and will facilitate more intelligent adjustments in the future. Teaching a woman to increase the iron in her diet, for example, should focus on the effects it will have on her and the baby. Her current dietary habits, including cultural and socioeconomic factors, and her individual likes and dislikes must be explored. The changes in her diet must have meaning for her before she will follow through. This illustrates a third principle the nurse must always remember: Learners are different and have different capacities, goals, interests, attitudes, life experiences, and perceptions, as well as different educational and cultural backgrounds. All of these factors must be considered in order to make the learning meaningful.

Another principle the nurse as teacher must remember is that the learner must be motivated. Most childbearing families are well motivated to learn about the process. They want the pregnancy to result in a healthy baby and a good experience for each of them. The learner must also be physically and mentally ready to learn. Timing is important: The exhausted mother in the active stage of labor is hardly ready to learn about child care. The nurse should remember that the more an individual accepts the goal, the more meaningful and effective the learning will be. The woman who cannot accept the fact that she is pregnant will learn little until that conflict is resolved.

As a teacher, the nurse must make the learner feel comfortable. This can be accomplished by controlling the environment so that physical comfort is possible and by avoiding direct questions that may threaten the individual within the group. Periods of stress, anxiety, or pain will interfere with learning. The nurse should remember that learning feeds on success. The woman who contributes something to the discussion should be recognized for her contribution. The learner should be helped to identify and apply previous learning. Likewise, the learning that has taken place should be reinforced, which can be done by the nursing staff in the clinic, labor and delivery rooms, and postpartum and nursery units, even though they may not have been directly involved in the initial teaching. It is important that a record of the teaching plan be made, so that it can accompany the mother's chart as she enters the other units.

The method of presentation depends on the material being presented and the group being taught. This may be a well-educated group that learns best through written materials and group discussion, or it may be a group that normally reads little but watches a great deal of television and learns best through audiovisual materials (such as large charts or posters, slides, movies, or videotapes). Teaching psychomotor skills, such as bathing and dressing infants, may best be learned through demonstrations. Teaching nutrition may best be done by having a room where a group of women eat lunch together and discuss dietary patterns. Some institutions are now making videotapes about topics such as child care, bathing the baby, and postpartum exercises; these videotapes can be viewed at any time in the woman's room during her hospital stay. Whatever method is used, the woman or couple must be actively drawn into the situation in order for effective learning to take place.

GROUP TEACHING

Most often, childbirth education is carried out through group teaching (Figure 9-1). The advantages of group teaching are that it saves time for those teaching, individ-

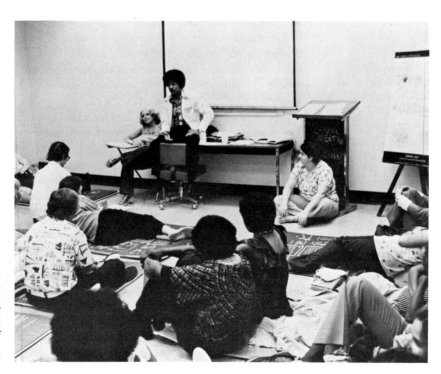

Figure 9-1. Physician and nurses participate in childbirth preparation class. Their relaxed manner puts the group at ease. (Courtesy of Pennsylvania Hospital, Philadelphia, Pa.)

uals within the group may become aware of common problems, and the questions raised may be questions that less vocal members would hesitate to raise. There is also a mutual sharing of ideas and experiences.

Prior to the first group session, the objectives and plan are developed. The setting should be clean and bright, with the chairs in a circle so each person can be seen and heard. During the first session the nurse should introduce all of the people and try to learn their names. The purpose of the sessions should be discussed from the nurse's perspective, and the expectations of the group should be elicited.

If discussion is the method chosen, it should begin with general, nonthreatening questions so that individuals will respond and gain confidence in answering and speaking in front of the group (learning feeds on success). The questions should be directed toward the group, so that no individual feels "put on the spot." This approach will maximize spontaneity and make members feel more secure (individuals must be secure for learning to take place). Members should be encouraged to talk about their particular experiences (learning must be meaningful to them). As the group begins talking, the nurse's role changes from an active participant to an active listener (learning should be active). The nurse's role now may be to keep the group's discussion on the original topic, to correct misinformation or misunderstanding, to encourage all to participate, making sure the quiet individuals have a chance to express their views, and to summarize the important points.

The teaching process is not complete without evaluation, which provides the teacher with some degree of satisfaction and direction for changes and improvements. The nurse may evaluate the effectiveness of the teaching directly by observing changes in the woman's or family's behavior. The evaluation may also be made through discussions with the women and their families. A written evaluation form may be used after a class or a group of classes. During class, nonverbal communication, such as facial expressions of anxiety, confusion, or boredom, can be validated by the nurse's questions; this provides for reassessment and redirection. Statistics may also provide some indication of effectiveness. If women in the community had been coming to receive their initial prenatal care during the later months of pregnancy and now are doing so earlier, the educational process may be a factor; this assumption can be validated by discussion with them.

CHILDBIRTH EDUCATION

Organized childbirth education has been a relatively recent development. The great scientific advances of the nineteenth and early twentieth centuries brought about a change of location for childbirth—from the home to the hospital; this change was accompanied by a change in attitude toward the birth process itself. Formerly, birth was associated with the company of family and friends and with normal health, despite the dangers. However, in the modern era birth seems more associated with the hospital, the doctor, and illness, despite the increased safety.

In 1932 in England, Grantly Dick-Read [2] began to speak and write in opposition to much of the medical intervention in childbirth, such as the use of forceps and anesthesia. He formulated a philosophy on which he then based a method of natural delivery. Dick-Read proposed that, through the ages, fear and anxiety were introduced by society into pregnancy and childbirth. Negative experiences related by family members and friends were reinforced by scenes in literature and motion pictures.

Dick-Read wrote that fear and anticipation of pain arouse natural protective tensions in the body, both psychic and muscular. Unfortunately, these muscle tensions tend to oppose dilatation of the birth canal during labor and make the outlet rigid. This resistance causes pain by exciting nerve endings in the uterus that respond to excessive tension. Thus, a process that Dick-Read referred to as the fear-tension-pain syndrome is set in motion. To break the circular reaction, Dick-Read advocated overcoming fear, eliminating anxiety and tension, and replacing them with calmness and relaxation.

To this end, Dick-Read held antepartal courses in education for childbirth, aimed at eliminating fear and overcoming ignorance. He also devised a series of physical and respiratory relaxation exercises aimed at reducing mental and physical tensions. The physical exercises were largely influenced by Helen Heardman, a physiotherapist in England. These exercises included tailor sitting, squatting, and the pelvic rock (Figure 9-2); their aim was to increase the elasticity of perineal muscles, mobilize the joints of the pelvis and back, and foster general improvement of circulation in the pelvic area.

Dick-Read's followers were taught to control their breathing by four respiratory exercises. These are integrated with different phases of labor to demonstrate to the woman how they will help her and to motivate her to practice them. The exercises included deep respiration for relaxation during the latent phase of the first stage of labor, more rapid respirations (25 per minute) for distraction during contractions in the active phase, breath-holding for pushing, and short panting respirations (40 per minute) at the time of delivery.

It is now recognized that excessive panting may result in improper alveolar ventilation. Some think that the respiratory alkalosis produced by hyperventilation may contribute to increased maternal suggestibility and some amnesia [1]. By disturbing

Figure 9-2. Pelvic rocking exercise to relieve back pain. The woman first allows her back to sag while holding her head up; then she lets her head drop and arches her back.

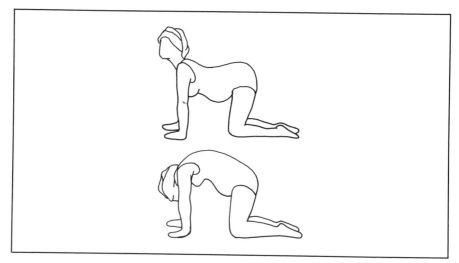

the acid-base balance, severe hyperventilation can be detrimental to the fetus [6].

Dick-Read advocated learning relaxation by concentrating on each part of the body separately, from the toes toward the head, contracting and then relaxing the muscles. He believed that the best way to support the mother in labor was based on the three Ps and the three Cs—patience, peacefulness, personal interest, confidence, concentrated observation, and cheerfulness. It was important that the woman never be left alone, since loneliness generated fear. If she had a consistent coach, particularly one who believed in the value of the method of preparation being used, the woman would be able to cope with her labor very well.

Dick-Read believed in showing the baby to the mother immediately after delivery so that she might fully experience the great moment of giving birth and a profound sense of achievement. Although Dick-Read's philosophy included the use of analgesics when necessary, the thrust of his writing emphasizes the avoidance of these "unnatural aids," as he called them.

Dick-Read's method was introduced to the United States under the direction of Dr. Thoms of Yale University. While the Western world was contemplating its merits, the Russians were applying a different approach based on pavlovian psychology, which was presented in 1950 at a World Congress of Gynecology held in Paris. A French obstetrician, Dr. Fernand Lamaze, became so interested that he later traveled to the Soviet Union to learn more about it. He and his colleague, Pierre Vellay, were responsible for popularizing this method of preparation of childbirth in the Western world.

According to the pavlovian philosophy, the degree of discomfort caused by uterine contractions is influenced by two important factors: (1) The actual physiologically transmitted discomfort (the strength of the pain signal to the brain) and (2) the behavioral response to this signal once it has been interpreted. The exercises taught by the Lamaze method are based on the theory that conditioned reflexes minimize the strength of the signal received in the brain and alter the behavioral response to whatever signal is received.

This method takes advantage of the fact that the brain can accept, integrate, interpret, and transmit only one set of signals at a time. If the strongest set of signals arriving at the brain comes from the uterus and is interpreted as a labor pain, the behavioral response is likely to be one of discomfort. If, however, at the time of the uterine contraction, a series of actions begins that requires for its successful execution stronger signals than those the uterus sends, then the uterine signals assume second place and the conscious perception of the uterine contraction diminishes markedly. The exercises of Lamaze (psychoprophylaxis) provide the strong stimuli necessary to take precedence over signals from uterine contractions. In addition, in this method the total preparation for childbirth involves learning what the process of having a baby entails, removing superstition and misinformation, and absorbing correct information. Such knowledge allows a woman to work effectively with her labor [5].

The Lamaze, or psychoprophylactic, method was popularized in the United States by the late Marjorie Karmel in her book, *Thank You, Dr. Lamaze* [4]. In 1960 interested laymen and health professionals founded the American Society for Psychoprophylaxis in Obstetrics (ASPO), which has been growing ever since. This is related, no doubt, to the satisfaction of the many mothers who have delivered using the Lamaze technique and their belief that others should have the opportunity to learn about the method.

Women who are educated by Lamaze method are instructed to time Braxton Hicks contractions during the last weeks of pregnancy and to do shallow fast breathing during the contractions. This establishes a relationship between these painless uterine contractions and the type of respiratory pattern to be used later during labor, thus building a favorable conditioned reflex that excludes the feeling of pain.

Pain-reducing procedures that are a part of the Lamaze training include slow breathing for the first part of labor, effleurage of the abdominal wall when active labor begins, pressure on the anterior-superior iliac spine to reduce abdominal pain, and pressure on the rhomboid triangle to reduce back pain when contractions are stronger. The mother must also be coached in muscle relaxation, best achieved in a half-sitting position with knees slightly flexed over a pillow. Carrying out all of these exercises in detail requires a great deal of concentration and a lot of encouragement from a good coach. Lamaze emphasized two periods when support is most needed by the woman in labor: When her cervix becomes completely dilated and when her perineum becomes completely distended.

Actually the Dick-Read and Lamaze methods of prepared childbirth are very similar in philosophy, techniques, and principles of management. Both depend on education to reduce apprehension and fear, to decrease anticipation of pain, and to decrease the pain sensation. Both methods offer respiratory exercises to achieve distraction and teach relaxation techniques to diminish pain.

The local groups of the International Childbirth Education Association (CEA) seem to advocate a less zealous approach than either Dick-Read or Lamaze, though they use the same general techniques. Although their philosophy does not lead parents to expect a "painless labor" nor one necessarily conducted without analgesia or anesthesia, they do emphasize the point that prepared parents usually require less medication. One of their aims is to foster in parents a sense of responsibility for their experience and provide them with ways in which they can participate in the birth of their baby. Affiliated with the LaLeche League International, they also try to help those mothers who wish to breast-feed to do so successfully for as long as they wish. To this end, through nursing mothers' groups, they offer information as well as practical suggestions and emotional support.

The Maternity Center Association in New York is another group that is active in promoting programs for childbirth education. An increasing number of such programs are developing throughout the United States.

Combinations of techniques are usually presented in childbirth education classes in this country. Generally the benefits enjoyed by the mother-participants could be enhanced if more involvement was encouraged for their "significant others" when labor and delivery are in progress. The presence of a support person other than the husband, such as a male friend, parent, relative, or other close friend, should be openly accepted by the maternity staff. Sometimes it is very threatening for hospital personnel to accept the fact that the woman is involved in what is happening to her and that she is actually exercising some control over it. Fortunately, the suspicion with which women who use "natural" childbirth techniques were viewed in the recent past has largely dissipated as preparation for childbirth has become more popular across the country.

The interpersonal relationships between the woman, her coach, and the attending nursing and medical staff form the foundation for the psychological analgesia that can result. It is dependent on the interplay of elements of suggestion, motivation, emotions, attention, and distraction. It is therefore important that all maternity personnel be aware of the basic principles of the method being used, so that they can offer reassurance and careful explanations of the sensations the mother is experiencing.

It is generally accepted that decreased apprehension, fear, and anxiety are of psychological and physiological value to the mother and to the progress of her labor. By whatever name, well-executed childbirth education programs will enable certain women to experience childbearing with deep emotional satisfaction. At the same time, it is recognized that being awake is not absolutely necessary, either for personal emotional growth or for the establishment of a warm mother-infant relationship, provided that parent-infant contact is initiated as soon as possible. Research [3] indicates that the more prepared women are for labor and delivery, the higher their level of awareness at delivery and their ability to cope successfully with it will be. This success is strongly associated with positive reactions to the infant and may also reflect the fact that individuals choosing childbirth education are already generally very interested and highly motivated to make the pregnancy experience as positive as possible.

A significant disadvantage is that the director of the educational program may insist on the importance of avoiding analgesic medications. When the woman feels that she must have some medication in order to continue, she is left to cope with her resulting guilt feelings. Research [1, 7] has indicated some controversy regarding differences in the effects of childbirth education methods and various forms of regional or general anesthesia on duration of labor, incidence of complications, blood loss, use of cesarean section, and postpartum complications. A compromise between prepared childbirth and the use of analgesics should not be neglected, as it is a worthwhile goal: The woman gets the benefit of both a well-planned educational program during her antepartal period and analgesia during labor if and when she needs it.

All of the childbirth techniques utilize principles of relaxation, which sometimes must be consciously achieved. The key to relaxation is correct basic posture and proper breathing; this is especially important during pregnancy, when body reserves are already taxed and fatigue readily accompanies increased tension. In labor, relaxation reduces muscular tension that may actually impede progress.

Controlled breathing provides one of the easiest ways to relax once correct posture is achieved. The exact rhythm is not as important as the comfort it provides. The Maternity Center Association advocates that a complete breath be used periodically during relaxation, followed by slow, quiet, easy respirations. With a complete breath (deep inspiration slowly exhaled under pressure) there is a more complete exchange of oxygen and carbon dioxide. Decreased muscular tension is accomplished when groups of muscles are systematically tightened and loosened. As a part of antepartal preparation, women are taught to contract their abdominal muscles and those of their pelvic floor.

Controlled breathing and relaxation techniques taught in classes sponsored by the Maternity Center are used during labor. During the first stage, deep breathing is done with a complete breath at the beginning and the end of each contraction. Approaching transition, the woman in labor uses modified deep breathing—a complete breath at the beginning and end, and quiet shallow throat breathing at the peak of each contraction. If she becomes dizzy or lightheaded, she is instructed to breathe more slowly. During transition she continues modified deep breathing, but blows out gently as she exhales on every third or fourth breath. In the second stage, pushing and panting are used as indicated.

The woman's partner (father of the child or other supportive person) provides her with practical assistance, close emotional support, and encouragement to go on. During early labor, he (or she) can encourage her to sleep and can provide information for the staff regarding how the woman is reacting to her labor and what she is finding distracting or helpful. He assists her to assume the positions she has practiced during labor, reminds her about her breathing patterns, times her contractions, and helps her to relax when he notices signs of tension (such as clenched fists, curled feet, or a wrinkled brow). If she has a backache, he can apply firm pressure during contractions. Effleurage brings relief for aching in her lower abdomen or thighs. He helps to keep her lips and mouth moistened with mouthwash, ice chips, or fruit-flavored candy drops. His firm coaching, assistance with pushing, and frequent reassurance provide valuable support for the woman. As long as the staff remains certain that she and the baby are safe, they should adopt an attitude of support but should not interfere with the relationship between the mother and her coaching partner. His involvement in her labor helps to make him an integral part of the birth process.

Until recently, many obstetricians and hospital administrators objected rather strongly to the father's presence in the delivery room. They were certain that he would probably contaminate the sterile drapes or that he might faint. Some even suggested that the experience might result in the man's impotence. Experience has indicated that their fears were groundless, and they are slowly changing their minds. However, the number of fathers in the delivery room remains small.

REFERENCES

1. Bonica, J. J. *Principles and Practice of Obstetric Analgesia and Anesthesia,* Vol. 1. Philadelphia: Davis, 1967.
2. Dick-Read, G. *Childbirth Without Fear.* New York: Harper & Row, 1953.
3. Doering, S., and Entwisle, D. Preparation during pregnancy and ability to cope with labor and delivery. *American Journal of Orthopsychiatry* 45:825, 1975.
4. Karmel, M. *Thank You, Dr. Lamaze.* Philadelphia: Lippincott, 1959.
5. Lamaze, F. *Painless Childbirth.* London: Burke, 1958.
6. Shnider, S. The Hyperventilation Controversy. In S. Shnider and F. Moya (Eds.), *The Anesthesiologist, Mother and Newborn.* Baltimore: Williams & Wilkins, 1974.
7. Zax, M., Sameroff, A., and Farnum, J. Childbirth education, maternal attitudes, and delivery. *American Journal of Obstetrics and Gynecology* 123:185, 1975.

FURTHER READING

Bing, E. *Adventure of Birth.* New York: Simon & Schuster, 1970.

Buxton, C. L. *Study of Psychophysical Methods for Relief of Childbirth Pain.* Philadelphia: Saunders, 1962.

Kitzinger, S. *Experience of Childbirth.* New York: Taplinger, 1972.

Preparation for Childbearing. New York: Maternity Center Association, 1972.

Vellay, P. *Childbirth Without Pain.* New York: Dutton, 1960.

Women's reactions toward childbirth. *Science News* 107:72, 1975.

Chapter 10 The Birth Process

ONSET OF LABOR

Labor consists of the regular, rhythmic contractions of the uterus, resulting in the birth of the infant and the delivery of the remaining products of conception. The mechanism responsible for the initiation of labor is unknown; theories that have been advanced include uterine stretch, oxytocin sensitivity, progesterone blocking, prostaglandin, and the fetal cortisol theory (which is currently receiving much research).

According to the uterine stretch theory, labor is initiated because the uterus functions as any other viscous organ. The more the uterine wall is stretched as pregnancy advances, the more irritable it becomes and the more easily it will contract. It is also theorized that as pregnancy advances, the intrauterine pressure increases, perhaps causing local ischemia and aging of the placenta, thus reducing the pregnancy stabilizing factors.

Proponents of the oxytocin theory note that as pregnancy advances, the uterus becomes more sensitive to oxytocin. The levels of endogenous oxytocin do not appear to be increased during the course of pregnancy, but concentrations in venous blood have been found to be elevated during labor [2]. One of the weaknesses of this theory is that pregnant women who have had hypophysectomies have a normal onset of labor. Recently research has shown that hormones previously believed to be produced in the pituitary may actually arise in the hypothalamus; this may be the case with oxytocin [9].

Prostaglandins have also been implicated as the initiators of labor, since they are able to induce abortion and labor. While they are present in amniotic fluid during labor, prostaglandins have not yet been detected in increased levels in the plasma of women before the onset of labor; however, decidual cells obtained immediately before labor have been shown to contain increased amounts of prostaglandins. Uterine contractions, according to one theory, are caused by prostaglandins released from the endometrial cells. This, in turn, may make the uterus more sensitive to oxytocin, increasing contractions and stressing the degenerating decidual cells further [15].

Progesterone has also been cited as a blocking agent. This theory holds that the estrogen effects that increase myometrial contractility are counteracted by the influence of progesterone in effecting hyperpolarization of the cell membrane, thereby blocking electrical conduction. The degenerative changes that take place in the placenta cause a withdrawal of the progesterone and its relaxant effects on the uterus [3].

One currently prominent theory is that the fetus at term produces increased levels of cortisol which inhibit progesterone production from the placenta. With an anencephalic fetus whose pituitary hypofunction causes adrenal hypofunction, labor may be delayed and pregnancy prolonged. Research in sheep shows that stimulation of the fetal adrenal gland can provoke premature labor. Recent research, however, suggests that elevated levels of cortisol found in fetal blood may be the result of labor, not the cause of it [20].

FACTORS AFFECTING LABOR

Pelvic Dimensions

The success of a woman's labor depends on a pelvis with adequate dimensions; normal size, shape, and presentation of the fetus; adequate uterine contractions; and psychological preparation and supportive care. Her pelvis should already have been evaluated for adequate dimensions prior to the beginning of labor (see Chapter 7), but reevaluation generally takes place upon admission to the hospital. In addition, the dimensions of the pelvis are capable of changing slightly during the process of labor [19].

Fetal Dimensions

The fetus is well prepared for labor during the last trimester. Its head is capable of changing its dimensions in order to accommodate itself to the woman's bony pelvis. While the skull bones of some fetuses are firmly ossified and capable of little change in shape, generally these bones remain relatively soft and able to change their shape and dimension. This is possible not only because the bones are soft but also because they are not united, remaining separated by membranous spaces known as *sutures*. The most important are the frontal (between the two frontal bones), the sagittal (between the two parietal bones), the coronal (between the frontal and parietal bones), and the lambdoid (between the back of the parietal bones and the margin of the occipital bone). With the exception of the temporal suture, these sutures can be felt by vaginal examination during labor (Figure 10-1).

Where two or more sutures meet, an irregular space is formed on the fetal head, known as a *fontanelle*. The two most important fontanelles are the anterior, a diamond-shaped area formed by a meeting of the sagittal and coronal sutures, and the posterior, a triangular area formed by a meeting of the sagittal and lambdoid sutures. Less important are the two temporal fontanelles formed by the junction of the lambdoid and temporal sutures, and the sagittal fontanelle, a space sometimes found midway between the anterior and posterior fontanelle. The sutures and fontanelles allow the fetal skull bones to overlap or override in order to pass through the woman's bony pelvis. This overlapping is known as molding and is the reason for elongation of the fetal head at birth.

During birth it is important not only that the fetal skull bones are able to override but also that the fetus' head passes through the birth canal with the smallest diameters presenting. When the head is fully flexed, the suboccipitobregmatic di-

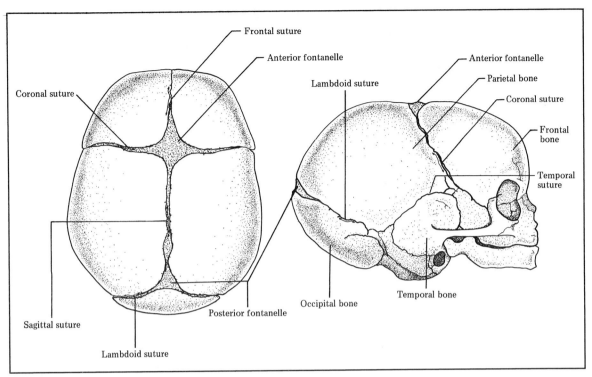

Figure 10-1. Fetal head bones, sutures, and fontanelles.

ameter enters the woman's pelvis (this diameter is measured from the middle of the large fontanelle to the undersurface of the occipital bone; it averages 9.5 centimeters, or 3.7 inches). As the fetal head assumes various extended positions, other diameters become important. With moderate extension the occipitofrontal diameter presents (this diameter extends from just above the root of the nose to the most prominent portion of the occipital bone; it averages 11.8 centimeters, or 4.6 inches). With marked extension the occipitomental diameter presents (this diameter extends from the chin to the most prominent portion of the occiput; it averages 13.5 centimeters, or 5.3 inches). Two additional measurements often evaluated during pregnancy or labor are the biparietal diameter (the greatest transverse diameter of the head, averaging 9.3 centimeters, or 3.6 inches) and the bitemporal diameter (the greatest distance between the two temporal sutures, averaging 8.0 centimeters, or 3.1 inches) (Figure 10-2).

Fetal Posture

During the last weeks before delivery, the fetus assumes a characteristic posture, or attitude, that is partially an attempt to accommodate itself to the space inside the uterus (Figure 10-3). Generally the fetus tries to conform to the shape of the uterine cavity by folding his extremities and bending his back. The head is sharply flexed, the chin almost resting upon the chest; the thighs are flexed over the abdomen; the legs are bent at the knee joints; and the arms are folded across the chest or are

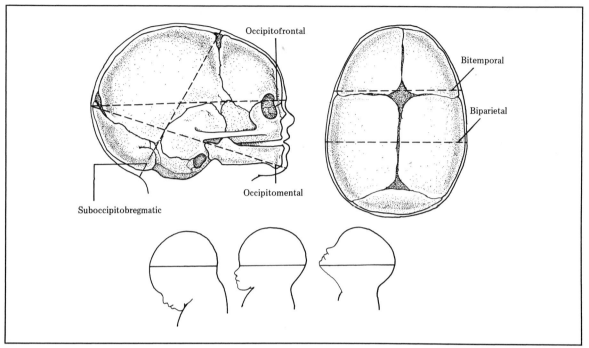

Occipitofrontal

Bitemporal

Biparietal

Suboccipitobregmatic

Occipitomental

Figure 10-2. Presenting diameters of the fetal head.

straight down at the sides. This whole posture is characteristically referred to as *fetal attitude* or *fetal habitus.*

Fetal Lie

The fetus also assumes a *lie,* (i.e., a comparison of its long axis to that of its mother) which can be either transverse or, more commonly, longitudinal (99 percent of fetuses at term). When the fetus assumes a longitudinal lie, either the head will present (cephalic presentation) and be felt on vaginal examination, or the buttocks or feet will present (breech presentation). In a transverse lie the shoulder will present. Whichever portion of the infant is deepest in the birth canal and is felt on vaginal examination is referred to as the presenting part; this determines the presentation of the fetus.

Fetal Presentation and Position

Cephalic presentations are classified according to the relation of the head of the fetus to the body. When the head is sharply flexed so that the chin rests on the thorax, the occipital area of the skull (vertex) is the presenting part (vertex presentation). Less commonly the head may be sharply extended, with the occiput in contact with the back; in this instance the face is felt on vaginal examination (face presentation). When the head is partially flexed, the large fontanelle is felt on vaginal examination (sincipital presentation), and when the head is partially extended, the brow can be felt upon vaginal examination (brow presentation) (Figure 10-4).

Figure 10-3. Fetal posture in utero in a vertex presentation.

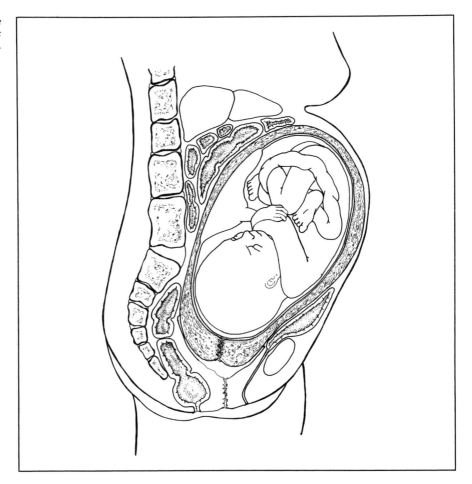

Breech presentations are classified according to the position of the thighs and legs of the fetus. When the thighs are flexed on the abdomen and the legs extended up onto the chest, the presentation is known as a single, or frank, breech. When the thighs of the fetus are flexed on the abdomen and the lower legs rest flexed on the thighs, the presentation is a full, or complete, breech. If one or both feet present first in the birth canal, the presentation is an incomplete breech of the type known as a single or double foot, or footling. Another form of incomplete breech presentation involves one or both knees presenting first (Figure 10-5).

With each presentation, a landmark has been designated on the presenting part to help identify the type of fetal presentation during vaginal examination. The landmark designated for identification on breech presentations is the sacrum; in vertex presentations, the occiput; in face presentations, the chin (mentum); in shoulder presentations, the scapula (acromium).

In addition to identifying the landmark, and thus the type of fetal presentation, it also becomes essential during the course of labor to identify the position of that landmark in relation to the right or left side of the maternal pelvis. The identifica-

Figure 10-4. Types of
cephalic presentation.
A. Vertex presentation.
B. Sincipital presentation.
C. Brow presentation.
D. Face presentation.

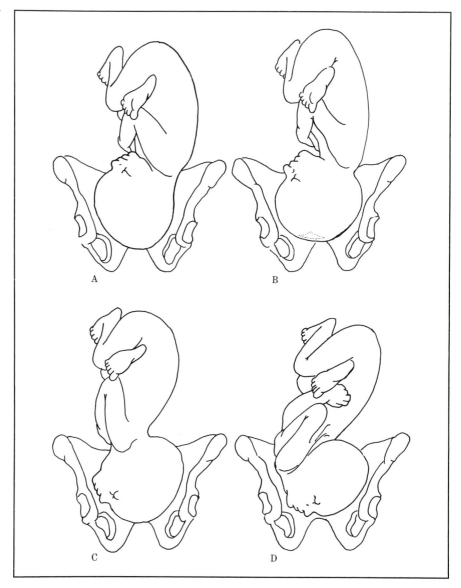

tion of this position enables the midwife or physician to ascertain the movements or rotation that will be necessary for the fetus to undergo prior to delivery.

The woman's pelvis is divided into four quadrants: a right and a left anterior quadrant and a right and a left posterior quadrant. A transverse position has also been designated as the position that divides the anterior and posterior portions of the pelvis.

In the vaginal examination the landmark is identified, and determination is made of the fetal position on the right or left side of the woman's pelvis and of its position in the anterior, transverse, or posterior portion of the woman's pelvis. For example,

*Figure 10-5. Breech
presentations. A. Full or
complete breech, with
thighs flexed on abdomen
and legs flexed on thighs.
B. Single or frank breech,
with legs extended over
anterior surface of body.
C. Incomplete or footling
breech; if both feet
present, as shown here,
this is known as a double
footling presentation.*

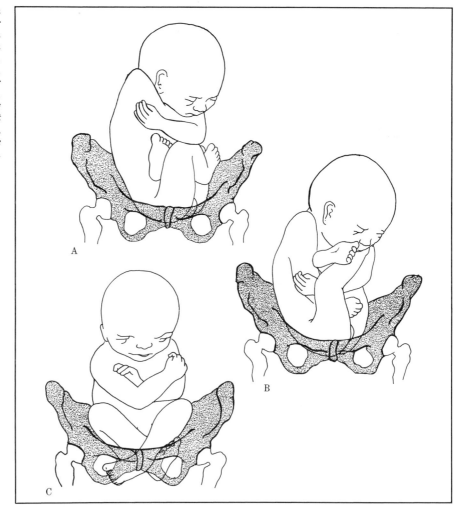

a vertex presentation with the fetus' occiput on the left side of the woman's pelvis and directed anteriorly would be designated as a left occipital anterior (LOA) position. Likewise, a breech presentation with the sacrum on the right side of the woman's pelvis and directed posteriorly would be designated as a right sacral posterior (RSP) position (Figure 10-6).

As term approaches, the incidence of vertex presentations is approximately 95 percent, breech 3.5 percent, face 0.5 percent, and shoulder 0.5 percent. About two-thirds of all vertex presentations are on the left side of the woman's pelvis and one-third on the right side. The fetal occiput is usually directed transversely. The incidence of breech presentations is much higher earlier in pregnancy; one study notes an incidence of 7.2 percent at 34 weeks [10]. As pregnancy advances, it is believed that the fetus takes advantage of the diminishing room within the uterus by positioning himself so that the bulkier buttocks and flexed legs are accommo-

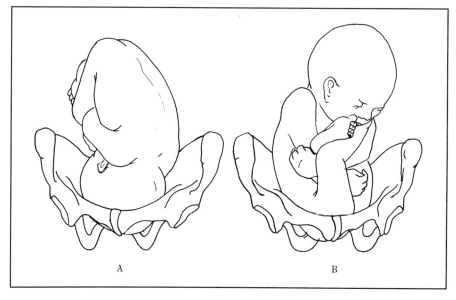

dated within the fundus. For the same reason, many fetuses with hydrocephalus are
born in breech presentations.

LEOPOLD'S MANEUVERS

The presentation and position of the fetus may be determined by abdominal palpation, auscultation, x-ray, ultrasonography, rectal examination, or vaginal examination. Determining fetal position by abdominal palpation is done by following the
four maneuvers suggested by Leopold and Sporlin. The woman should be on her
back with the examiner to her side, facing her head for the first three maneuvers and
facing her feet for the fourth (Figure 10-7).

The first maneuver is done by outlining the uterus with the fingertips, then gently
palpating the fundus to determine if the fetal head or breech occupies that portion
of the cavity. The head feels hard and round and is freely movable and ballottable,
while the breech feels large and nodular.

The second maneuver requires the examiner to outline the sides of the uterus
while applying gentle but deep pressure. On one side the back will be palpated as a
hard continuous structure, while the other side feels nodular, reflecting portions of
the fetal extremities. If the woman is obese or has excessive amniotic fluid, it is
suggested that the nurse apply deep pressure on one side of the abdomen while
palpating the other side; the procedure is then reversed.

In the third maneuver the nurse grasps the woman's abdomen above the symphysis pubis with one hand. If the fetal part grasped is movable, engagement has not
occurred; if engagement has occurred, the part gives the feeling of being fixed in the
pelvis. As in the first maneuver, the nurse should determine if the head or breech has
been grasped. If the head is the presenting part and the cephalic prominence (brow)
can be felt on the same side as the small parts, the head must be flexed and the
vertex presenting. If the cephalic prominence is felt on the same side as the back, the
head must be extended.

Figure 10-7. Leopold's maneuvers. A. First maneuver. B. Second maneuver. C. Third maneuver. D. Fourth maneuver.

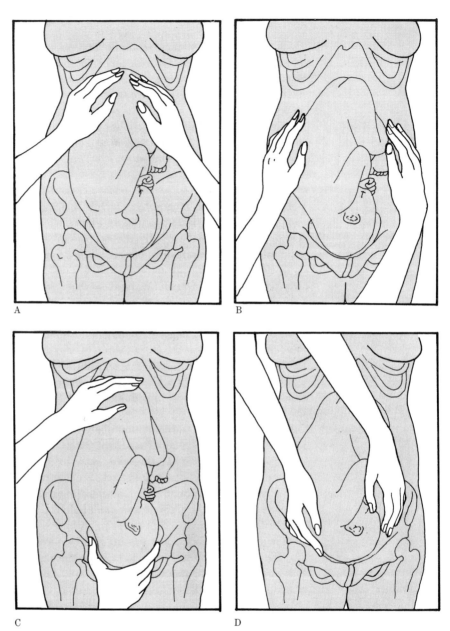

A

B

C

D

The fourth maneuver requires the nurse to face the woman's feet and palpate the lower portion of the uterus, sliding the fingers toward the birth canal. If the head is presenting, the fingers of one side will meet an obstruction (the cephalic prominence), while those on the other side will descend more deeply into the pelvis. Leopold's maneuvers are generally performed during the last few months of pregnancy or between labor contractions.

OTHER METHODS

Auscultation also aids in determining fetal position and presentation. In the later months of pregnancy and during labor, fetal heart sounds are best heard a short distance from the midline if the fetus is in an occipitoanterior position, since the heart sounds are heard best through the fetus' back. With the fetus presenting in an occipitotransverse position, the fetal heart sounds are heard lateral to the midline; in an occipitoposterior position they are found in the woman's flank. Generally in cephalic presentations the fetal heart sounds are best heard below the woman's umbilicus; in breech presentations they are best heard at or slightly above the woman's umbilicus.

The use of x-rays is sometimes needed to determine fetal position and presentation. However, ultrasonography, which is also used for this purpose, offers the advantage of locating fetal position and parts without hazards of x-ray radiation. (Other uses of ultrasonography in obstetrics include detection of early pregnancy, estimation of gestational age, identification of optimal sites for amniocentesis, localization of intrauterine contraceptive devices, and diagnosis of twin pregnancy, hydatidiform mole, intrauterine fetal death or growth retardation, placenta previa, fetal abnormalities, and ectopic pregnancy.)

Ultrasonography involves little preparation of the patient; the only requirement is that her bladder be full, since that will lift her uterus up and will provide a fluid-filled medium to aid in the transmission of sound. Oil or aqueous jelly is placed on the woman's abdomen so that the transducer can be moved back and forth with continuous airless contact between the transducer and her abdomen. The woman experiences no discomfort or problems, and usually will take an active interest in the whole procedure [5].

During labor when the cervix has dilated, fetal presentation and position can be identified on vaginal examination. Using a sterile glove, the examiner introduces the index and middle finger of either hand into the vagina. Upon palpation of the presenting part, the appropriate landmarks are identified. The sutures and fontanelles are found in a vertex presentation, the nose, mouth, and other portions of the face in a face presentation, and the sacrum and ischial tuberosities in a breech presentation. With a vertex presentation, passing the fingers behind the symphysis pubis and then in a sweeping movement passing them toward the sacrum has been suggested [10]. This movement causes them to cross the sagittal suture, which can then be followed to locate the fontanelles.

Uterine Contractions

Successful labor depends on adequate uterine contractions as well as appropriate pelvic size and position of the fetus. There are a number of characteristics that can be noted of uterine contractions during labor: The contractions are involuntary and are associated with some degree of discomfort. During the contractions of labor, the actively contracting upper portion of the uterus becomes thicker, while the lower uterine segment (isthmus and the cervix) becomes very thin. These changes divide

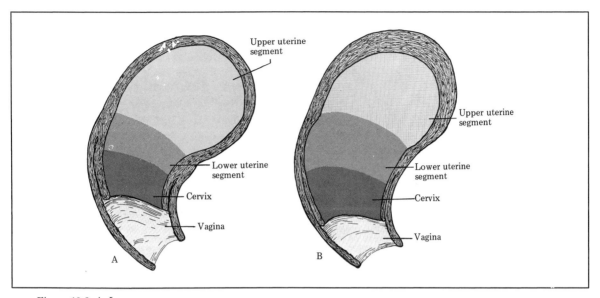

Figure 10-8. A. Lower uterine segment thick; upper uterine segment contracting. B. Later in labor. The upper uterine segment thickens, pushing the fetus downward. The lower uterine segment thins and relaxes, allowing the fetus to pass through that portion.

the uterus into two distinct zones, an upper portion, which is actively contracting, and a lower portion, which is passive.

At the completion of a contraction of the upper uterine segment, the cells of that segment do not resume their original length but become fixed at a shorter length. While this occurs in the upper segment, the lower uterine segment becomes stretched with each contraction. Upon completion of the contraction, the cells in the lower segment remain stretched and fixed at a longer length; this is called receptive or postural relaxation. As the cells become stretched, this portion of the uterus and cervix becomes thinner (Figure 10-8). If this phenomenon did not occur, the fetus would not be pushed further into the birth canal. The round ligaments also contract with each uterine contraction, elevating the fundus and aligning the fetus more directly with the curve of the birth canal.

MECHANISMS OF LABOR

If the woman's pelvis is of adequate size, the uterine contractions are adequate, and the size and position of the fetus are appropriate, the fetus will make adaptive movements enabling it to progress through the birth canal. The movements are caused by the involuntary uterine contractions during the first stage of labor, together with voluntary abdominal muscle contractions during the second stage. The positional and rotational changes of the fetus are also effected by the resistance offered by the woman's bony pelvis, cervix, and surrounding tissues of the birth canal. The events of engagement, descent, flexion, internal rotation, extension, external rotation, and expulsion do not occur separately, but rather overlap in time (Figure 10-9).

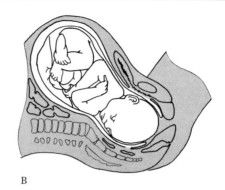

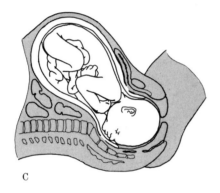

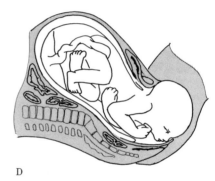

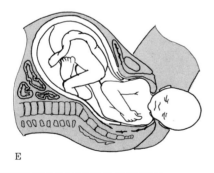

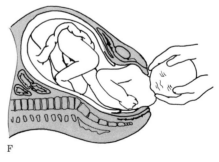

Figure 10-9. Labor and delivery. A. Cervical effacement complete; head flexed; descent begins. B. Descent continues; cervix dilating; internal rotation begins. C. Internal rotation complete. D. Extension. E. External rotation. F. Posterior shoulder delivered.

Engagement

When the fetal head enters the pelvic inlet, the biparietal diameter, which is the narrowest presenting diameter, will go through the narrowest diameter of the pelvis. The occiput will rotate to the widest portion of the pelvis. Since the widest diameter of the pelvic inlet is the transverse diameter, the fetal head most often enters the inlet in a transverse position. Engagement is often defined as having occurred when the biparietal diameter of the fetal head has passed through the pelvic inlet. Other clinicians prefer to define it as having occurred when the biparietal diameter has reached the level of the ischial spines. In primigravidas, the fetal head may sink into the pelvis enough during lightening to constitute engagement. In most multigravidas engagement occurs during labor.

Descent

Fetal descent occurs throughout labor and is essential for the rotational movements that must occur prior to birth. It is accomplished through the force of the uterine contractions on the amniotic fluid, or, after rupture of the membranes, on the portion of the fetus occupying the fundal area in the uterine cavity. During the second stage the efforts of the mother in bearing down increase intra-abdominal pressure and help effect expulsion of the fetus.

The degree of fetal descent may be described as floating, fixed, engaged in the midpelvis, or on the pelvic floor. Descent of the fetal presenting part is also described in relation to the ischial spines and is evaluated by stations. Station 0 is at the level of the ischial spines (engagement); stations -1, -2, -3, and -4 refer to 1, 2, 3, and 4 centimeters above the spines. When the presenting part is at station -4, the presenting part is floating. When the presenting part is 1, 2, 3, or 4 centimeters below the level of the spines, the station is referred to as $+1$, $+2$, $+3$, and $+4$. When the presenting part is at station $+4$, it is on the pelvic floor (Figure 10-10).

Flexion

Flexion is an important movement in the mechanism of labor, since it aids accommodation of the fetal head to the birth canal by effecting presentation of the smallest fetal head diameter, the suboccipitobregmatic diameter (9.5 centimeters). Pressure is exerted on the fetus by the uterine fundus; as the fetal head meets resistance from the lower uterine segment, cervix, or pelvic floor, it is tipped forward so that the chin lies close to the chest.

Internal Rotation

In accommodating to the birth canal, the fetal occiput rotates from its original position anteriorly toward the symphysis. This movement results from the shape of the fetal head, the amount of space available in the midpelvis, and the sling shape of the perineal muscles. The ischial spines project into the midpelvic cavity, causing

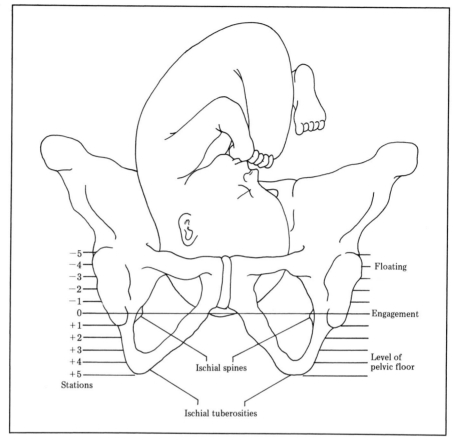

the anterior segment to be larger than the posterior and the anteroposterior diameter larger than the transverse. Since the occipital portion of the fetal head is larger than the frontal and sincipital areas, the occiput comes to occupy the anterior portion of the cavity. By doing this, the most flexible part of the fetal body, the nape of the neck, adapts to the curve of the birth canal.

Extension

As the fetal head descends further in the birth canal, it meets resistance from the perineal muscles and is forced into extension. The fetal head becomes visible at the vulvovaginal ring; its largest diameter is encircled (crowning), and it emerges from the vagina.

External Rotation

Following delivery of the head, the occiput rotates to the position it occupied prior to internal rotation. The anterior shoulder also rotates so that it comes to lie under the symphysis. When the shoulder rotation takes place, the occiput rotates further so that the head and shoulders return to their normal alignment.

Expulsion

Following delivery of the infant's head and internal rotation of the shoulders, the infant's anterior shoulder comes to rest beneath the symphysis pubis. The posterior shoulder is then delivered, followed quickly by the anterior shoulder, which slips from beneath the pubic arch. In some instances the anterior shoulder is delivered first. The remainder of the infant's body follows shortly.

THE WOMAN IN LABOR

Preliminary Events

Prior to the onset of labor, several events occur. In nulliparas, approximately two weeks before the onset of labor, the fetal head drops into the pelvic inlet, thus causing descent of the uterus. In multiparas, this phenomenon, known as *lightening,* generally occurs with the onset of labor. After lightening, the woman may experience more leg cramping and difficulty in walking as a result of increased pressure in the lower pelvic region. Urinary frequency also follows lightening, while breathing generally becomes easier.

As labor approaches and as the cervix begins to dilate and efface, the plug of mucus that filled the cervical canal during pregnancy is discharged along with a very small amount of blood from the surrounding capillaries. The discharge, referred to as *show* (or *bloody show*), usually precedes labor by a few hours or days. This discharge also commonly follows vaginal examination during the later weeks of pregnancy, and often there is an increase in the discharge following vaginal examination during labor. Occasionally, the membranes will rupture prior to the onset of labor.

False labor contractions, which may occur as early as three to four weeks prior to delivery, are an exaggeration of Braxton Hicks contractions, which occur during pregnancy. They can be differentiated from true labor contractions in a number of ways (Table 10-1).

Table 10-1. Differentiation of False Labor from True Labor Contractions

True Labor Contractions	False Labor Contractions
Result in progressive cervical dilatation and effacement	Do not result in progressive cervical dilatation and effacement
Occur at regular intervals	Occur at irregular intervals
Interval between contractions decreases	Interval between contractions remains the same or increases
Intensity increases	Intensity decreases or remains the same
Located mainly in back and abdomen	Located mainly in lower abdomen and groin
Generally intensified by walking	Generally unaffected by walking
Not affected by mild sedation	Generally relieved by mild sedation

Admission

The woman is generally advised to come to the hospital when her contractions are 5–10 minutes apart if she is a primigravida or when her contractions have established a regular pattern if she is a multigravida. Both primigravidas and multigravidas are also asked to notify the midwife or physician or to come to the hospital immediately if the membranes rupture, since the incidence of intrauterine infection rises significantly when membranes have been ruptured more than 24 hours.

When the couple or woman arrives at the hospital, the first action on the nurse's part should be to introduce herself. This establishes the initial tone of the interaction and communicates to the couple that someone acknowledges their identity. Initial impressions are generally long lasting, especially those established during times of stress.

Next it should be explained to the couple that it is necessary to find out how far the woman's labor has progressed, and that to do so, the nurse will be asking a number of questions, followed by a vaginal examination to see how much cervical dilatation has occurred. The nurse can begin by establishing whether or not this is the woman's first pregnancy. If not, she should be asked how long her last labor was and how long ago it was. How far apart are the woman's contractions, have her membranes ruptured, when did the contractions begin? Has she noticed any mucus or bloody discharge? If the woman reports ruptured membranes, this can be verified by placing a nitrazine-treated tape or swab in a pool of the fluid in her vagina. The presence of alkaline fluid will result in a positive test.

As the nurse begins asking the questions, she should observe the amount of discomfort the woman is experiencing. If she appears to be in obvious discomfort and is having contractions two or three minutes apart or if she shows any signs of wanting to bear down, it is essential that she be examined vaginally by the midwife or physician almost immediately.

If she is not in acute discomfort, the nurse should then take her vital signs, including temperature, blood pressure, pulse, respiration, and fetal heart sounds. The woman's blood pressure should be taken between contractions; during and immediately after a contraction, the blood pressure reading is higher. The fetal heart rate should also be taken between contractions and should be counted for a full minute; during a contraction and for 30 seconds thereafter, the rate may decrease [12].

In recording the woman's vital signs, the nurse also times the *duration, intensity,* and *interval* of the contractions. The duration of a contraction is timed from the beginning to the end of the contraction. The interval is measured from the beginning of one contraction to the beginning of the next. Each contraction has three phases: *increment, acme,* and *decrement.* Increment is the period of increasing intensity; acme, the period when the contraction is strongest; decrement, the period of decreasing intensity. The intensity of the contraction is measured by the nurse's ability to indent the uterus. When the nurse keeps her fingertips on the woman's fundus, a mild contraction feels like a tense muscle, a moderate contraction is more firm, and a strong contraction cannot be indented by pressure of the fingertips (it has been described as being as hard as wood).

The woman is examined vaginally by the nurse, midwife, or physician to determine the amount of cervical dilatation. Usually the woman will be admitted to the labor room or sent home on the basis of the extent of cervical dilatation and the evaluation of the woman's contractions.

If she is sent home, the woman or couple should be told that they were correct in coming to the hospital. This is usually a discouraging time and one that couples have commented on as having made them feel guilty and foolish. Knowing that this is a common feeling, the nurse can use this time to make them feel better about having come. They can be introduced to some of the staff members with the explanation that it would be good for them to meet, since they may be working together when the woman or the couple come the next time. The nurse might also take the opportunity to show them the inpatient unit if they have not seen it before. The nurse might also ask if they have traveled a distance to get to the hospital and suggest that they have a cup of coffee in the snack bar before going home. This enables them to discuss the events of the past few hours before driving in traffic.

If the woman is to be admitted to the labor room, some midwives or physicians will order that the woman be given an enema and/or have her pubic skin shaved. An enema may be ordered to evacuate the colon and thus provide more room in the pelvic cavity; a full colon is believed to impede the progress of labor. Also, feces from a full colon may be expelled during delivery and, if not wiped away, may contaminate the area unnecessarily. However, many women who have had an enema prior to delivery have more difficulty establishing regular bowel movements following delivery. If the woman's membranes have ruptured, enemas are generally contraindicated to prevent infection of the birth canal.

Some midwives and physicians feel that no pubic skin shave is needed; others call for a partial pubic shave (pubic hair removed from the top of the labia to the anus); others prefer all pubic hair removed. The pubic shave is justified as making episiotomy and its repair easier and aiding in keeping the perineum clean.

Following the initial admission procedures, the woman is admitted to a labor room. She and her partner should be oriented to the surroundings and introduced to the staff and the other women or couples who might be sharing the labor room.

The woman in true labor then begins progressing through the stages of labor. The first stage begins with the onset of true labor contractions and ends with full cervical dilatation; the second stage begins with full cervical dilatation and ends with the birth of the baby; and the third stage begins with birth of the baby and ends with the delivery of the placenta. The immediate postpartum period is sometimes referred to as the fourth stage of labor.

FETAL MONITORING IN LABOR

During the progress of labor, the condition of both mother and fetus is assessed very carefully. Electronic auscultation of the fetal heart is used as a means for assessing fetal condition. Recordings of fetal heart rate and uterine contractions can be obtained with internal or external monitors (Figure 10-11). Internal monitoring involves a silver electrode attached to the fetal scalp to transmit fetal heart signals and a catheter passed beyond the presenting part into the uterine cavity to record

Figure 10-11. A. Internal fetal monitoring. B. External fetal monitoring.

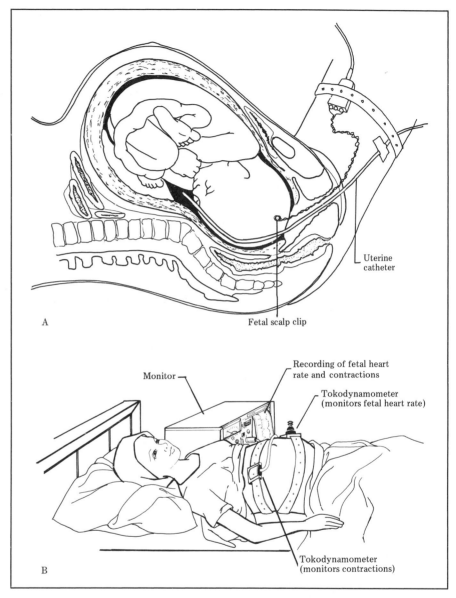

A

Uterine catheter

Fetal scalp clip

Monitor

Recording of fetal heart rate and contractions

Tokodynamometer (monitors fetal heart rate)

B

Tokodynamometer (monitors contractions)

the pressure of uterine contractions. External monitoring consists of external tokodynamometers strapped to the mother's abdomen to transmit fetal heart rate and uterine contractions. Internal monitoring is believed to yield more reliable information than external monitoring.

Originally, electronic monitoring of the fetal heart rate and uterine contractions was limited to women who were at risk of having a difficult labor or of fetal compromise. Currently, this monitoring is becoming routine for all women in labor in hospitals where the equipment is available. This method holds much promise for intervention in problems that would not even be detected by older monitoring methods using the fetoscope and abdominal palpation for uterine contractions.

Fetal heart rate patterns may undergo baseline changes or periodic changes. Baseline changes (tachycardia and bradycardia) occur when the woman is not in labor or between periodic changes. Periodic changes in the fetal heart rate (early, late, or variable decelerations) occur as a result of the uterine contraction.

Baseline Changes

A baseline fetal heart rate is obtained by taking the average rate over a tracing of several minutes. The normal fetal heart rate falls between 120 and 160 beats per minute. Fluctuations in the baseline rate are normal; the interaction between vagal and sympathetic tone causes variations of 3–10 percent of the baseline rate. Absence of this normal variability reflects immaturity of the autonomic nervous system as seen in the preterm infant, or the pharmacological vagal blocking action of drugs such as atropine; this condition is also seen late in the course of fetal hypoxia and is viewed as ominous. Fluctuations of more than 25 beats per minute may represent fetal overcompensation following recurrent late or variable deceleration and may be a forerunner of hypoxia.

Tachycardia (Figure 10-12, top tracing) ranges between 161 and 180 beats per minute (it is considered marked when it increases to more than 180). Baseline fetal heart rates that are higher than normal may result from immaturity of the fetal autonomic nervous system, maternal fever from amnionitis, maternal anemia, and minimal fetal hypoxia. Tachycardia associated with late or prolonged variable decelerations indicates fetal distress.

Bradycardia (Figure 10-12, bottom tracing) ranges between 100 and 119 beats per minute; it is considered marked when it falls below 100. Baseline fetal heart rates that are consistently low over a period of weeks are associated with congenital heart lesions. If, during labor, low fetal heart rates are also accompanied by marked fetal heart rate decelerations, the newborn will usually be depressed.

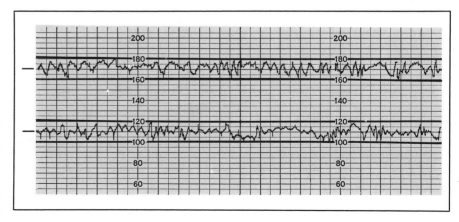

Figure 10-12. Baseline changes in fetal heart rate. Top tracing shows tachycardia (161–180 beats per minute). Bottom tracing shows bradycardia (100–119 beats per minute).

Periodic Changes

Approximately 30 percent of the time, the fetal heart rate responds to uterine contractions by decelerating. When the fetal heart rate begins to drop within 10 seconds after the onset of the contraction and returns to its baseline rate as the contraction ends, the response is called early deceleration, or Type I dip. The fetal heart rate during this deceleration is usually in the range of 100–140 beats per minute. The decrease is believed to be caused by compression of the head during the contraction. It is considered innocuous unless the decrease from the baseline rate is 45 beats per minute or more, in which case the physician should be notified. Early deceleration also can be elicited by digital pressure on the fetal head during vaginal examination or by the pressure of forceps during delivery. Since this pattern is mediated through the vagus, it will not be affected either by giving the mother oxygen or by changing her to a position lying on her side.

A late deceleration, or Type II dip, occurs when the fetal heart rate begins to drop 20 seconds or more after the beginning of the contraction, bottoms after the peak of the contraction, and returns to baseline after the end of the contraction. The fetal heart rate during this deceleration is usually in the range of 120–180 beats per minute but may go down to 80 on occasion. This pattern is found with impaired uteroplacental exchange and is considered ominous because it is related to fetal hypoxia. Each uterine contraction impedes uterine blood flow, imposing periodic stress on the fetus. Type II dips occur commonly with epidural anesthesia and oxytocin stimulation. It is not known whether this pattern reflects asphyxia to the central nervous system or if it reflects a direct effect on the fetal myocardium. The pattern is modified by the administration of oxygen, a change of maternal position so that she is lying on her left side, elevation of her legs, and increased intravenous fluids. Since patterns of late deceleration lasting for longer than 30 minutes are associated with fetal hypoxia, Hon [13] suggests that the labor should be terminated if the pattern persists this long after therapeutic measures are initiated. Since the range of heart rate in late deceleration (120–180) can be within the normal baseline range, this ominous sign easily can be missed with conventional monitoring using the fetoscope (Figure 10-13).

When the onset of decreased fetal heart rate varies in relationship to the onset of uterine contractions, these changes are known as variable decelerations. Variable decelerations are characterized by a rapid drop in fetal heart rate, followed by an interval of acute bradycardia, and then by a rapid return to the baseline. During these decreases the fetal heart rate is in the range of 60–160 beats per minute. The decrease (believed to be due to compression of the cord) is common during the final

Figure 10-13. Periodic changes in fetal heart rate. A. Early deceleration, or type I dip. B. Late deceleration, or type II dip. C. Variable deceleration, or type III dip.

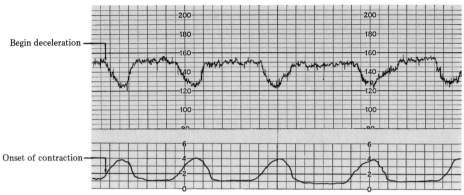

Begin deceleration

Onset of contraction

A

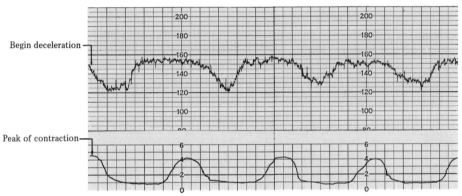

Begin deceleration

Peak of contraction

B

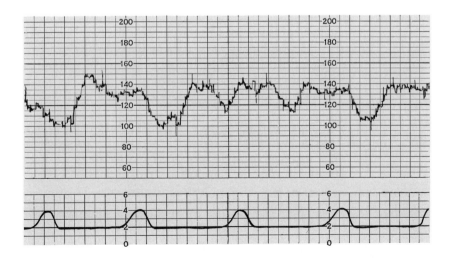

C

stages of labor as the fetus impinges on the cord during descent. A change in the woman's position may alter the pattern. Variable decelerations are thought to be innocuous unless prolonged, recurrent, or extreme in degree, (for example, if they persist for more than a minute or if the fetal heart rate drops below 60 beats per minute). In a well-compensated fetus, variable decelerations are followed by compensating reactive accelerations. A pattern of unrelenting, prolonged, variable, or late decelerations associated with an increased baseline fetal heart rate and decreased baseline variability suggests that fetal oxygenation is precarious and that operative delivery may be necessary.

Accelerations in response to uterine contractions are seen in fetuses with non-vertex presentations and immature central nervous systems or with maternal use of atropine-like drugs. In cases in which the fetus shows abnormal heart rate patterns, additional information can be obtained by means of scalp blood sampling, a technique that is especially helpful in the case of an infant who shows a pattern suggesting hypoxia and yet is delivered in good condition. When abnormal patterns are found, fetal acid-base status is evaluated. Under endoscopic visualization, the fetal scalp is cleaned, made hyperemic with ethyl chloride, coated with a silicone gel to promote formation of a blood globule, and incised with a stab blade; capillary blood is then collected. When placental function is limited, fetal asphyxia is revealed by increased carbon dioxide partial pressure and decreased oxygen pressure, pH, and base excess, all of which result in metabolic and respiratory acidosis. Reduced pH and reduced base excess reflect breakdown of glycogen to pyruvate and lactic acid by anaerobic pathways. Most authorities consider pH values of less than 7.20 to be critical [9]. While a single value may reflect maternal acidosis seen in prolonged labor, progressive decrease in *serial* pH determinations is an ominous sign.

Normal uterine contractions during the course of labor should show a regular pattern, with intervals of at least 2 minutes, durations of less than 90 seconds, and peak pressures of greater than 40 millimeters of mercury (Figures 10-14, 10-15). In the later phase of the first stage of labor (active labor), the amplitude approaches 75 millimeters of mercury. The contractions also should be well-rounded and symmetrical in appearance on the tracing produced by the monitor. Uterine contractions with intervals of more than 3 minutes and durations of less than 45 seconds may be associated with slow progress in labor.

In order to assure adequate uterine recordings, the tokodynamometer must be placed over the most contractile portion of the upper uterine segment. As labor progresses and the uterus descends, the tokodynamometer will need to be lowered also. Contractions that appear flat-topped may indicate that the belt is too tight, while contractions with sharp peaks may be the result of oxytocin infusion. With excessive oxytocin administration, a pattern of one large contraction followed by a smaller one may develop. A similar pattern may occur in persistent occiput posterior presentation.

THE FIRST STAGE OF LABOR

The first stage of labor is the longest of the three stages (Table 10-2) and is divided into three phases (Figure 10-16). During this stage the woman's cervix thins (efface-

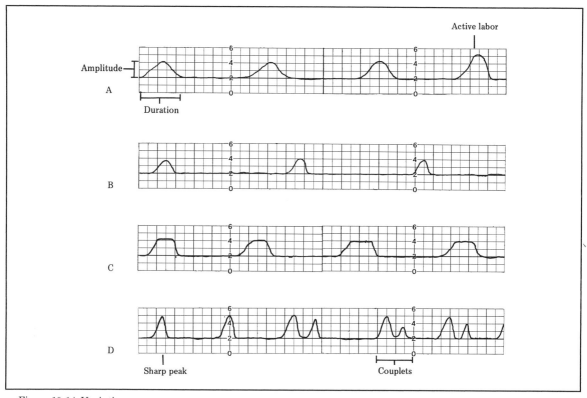

Figure 10-14. Variations in uterine contractions. A. Normal uterine contractions. B. Long intervals, short durations. C. Flat-topped contractions. D. Oxytocin contractions.

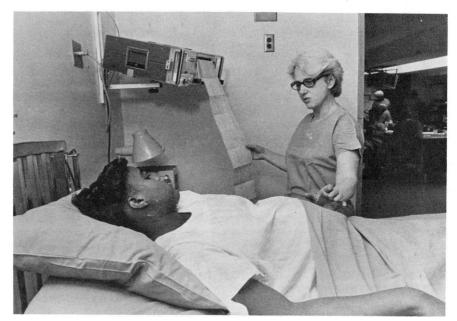

Figure 10-15. Midwife assessing the progress of the woman during labor. (Courtesy of Pennsylvania Hospital, Philadelphia, Pa.)

Table 10-2. Average Duration of Labor	Pregnancy	First Stage	Second Stage	Third Stage
	Primigravida	12½ hours	80 minutes	10 minutes
	Multigravida	7½ hours	30 minutes	10 minutes

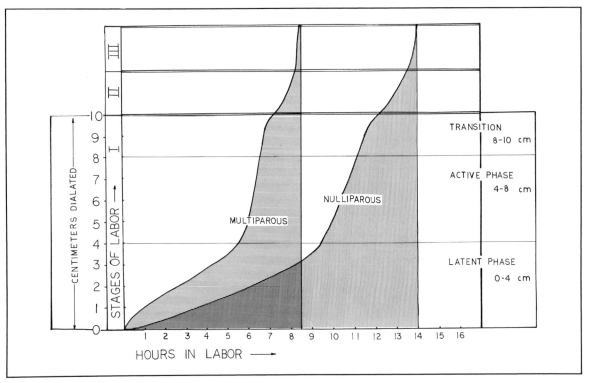

Figure 10-16. Time curves for normal labor in multiparous and nulliparous women.

ment). The cervical canal changes from a structure of approximately 2 centimeters in length to a circular orifice with paper-thin edges. During this process the muscular fibers around the internal os are pulled upward and incorporated into the lower uterine segment. In primigravidas effacement occurs prior to the beginning of cervical dilatation. In multigravidas the process occurs simultaneously with cervical dilatation (Figure 10-17).

The external cervical os progresses by dilatation from an opening a few millimeters in diameter to an opening large enough to allow birth of the fetus. When the cervical os has reached a diameter of 10 centimeters, it is referred to as being in the state of full or complete cervical dilatation. During the latent phase cervical dilatation progresses from 0 to approximately 4 centimeters.

Dilatation is accomplished by uterine pressure exerted on the amniotic sac (hydrostatic pressure) or, if the mother's membranes have ruptured, on the presenting part (fetal axis pressure). The amniotic sac or presenting part then serves as a wedge to effect cervical dilatation. As the cervix dilates, a reflex that further stimulates myometrial activity (Ferguson's reflex) [10] is activated.

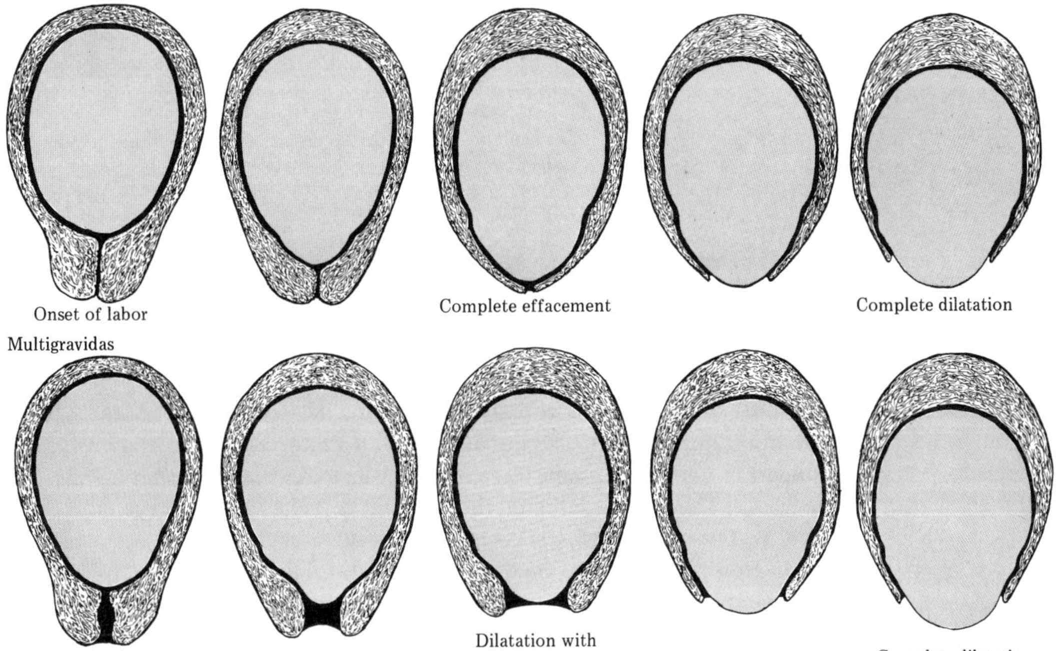

Primigravidas

Onset of labor   Complete effacement   Complete dilatation

Multigravidas

Onset of labor   Dilatation with   Complete dilatation
                          effacement

Figure 10-17. Dilatation and effacement in primigravidas and multigravidas. Primigravidas reach complete effacement prior to dilating. Multigravidas undergo effacement and dilatation simultaneously.

During the latent phase of the first stage of labor, the woman is generally comfortable. Her contractions are 20–40 seconds in duration and occur at intervals of 5–10 minutes. It is helpful for the nurse to suggest diversionary activity, perhaps watching television, reading, or a walk around the unit, provided the woman's membranes have not ruptured. If the woman's membranes have ruptured, she may still be allowed to walk around if the presenting part is far enough down in the pelvis that the umbilical cord cannot slip by and become wedged between the bony pelvis and the presenting part. At this time the nurse can also further assess the woman's feelings about the pregnancy and labor. If the woman or couple have attended classes in preparation for childbirth, this is a time when the nurse should ask them to describe and demonstrate the techniques they were taught; in this way the nurse can assess their understanding and performance of them. If the woman has not attended classes, the nurse can teach the types of breathing and pushing that will help the mother in the succeeding stages of labor (Table 10-3). During this time the nurse should also find out the expectations that the woman or couple have for their experience during the woman's hospital stay.

If the woman is accompanied by her husband (or by the baby's father, in the case of an unmarried woman) the nurse should assess their interaction and ability to work together. Whenever possible the nurse should assist him in helping the woman if he so wishes, teaching him techniques to increase his wife's comfort during labor. The couple should be allowed the privacy they need; when direct care is necessary,

Table 10-3. Breathing Techniques During Labor

Stage of Labor	Breathing Technique
Early First Stage	Relax, cleansing breath. Breathe deeply, slowly, rhythmically through contraction, then cleansing breath
Late First Stage	Assume comfortable position. Cleansing breath. Regular breathing to more shallow. With stronger contractions, accelerate breathing (very light throat breaths). Cleansing breath
Transition	Concentrate on breathing control. Cleansing breath. Breathe fairly deeply at beginning of contraction. Shallow breathing. Puff out on every third, fourth, or fifth breath if urge to push. Cleansing breath
Second Stage	Push toward vaginal opening as directed. Catch breath as needed. Relax pelvic floor. Go limp between contractions. Pant during contraction. Push gently as directed

Source: Modified from *Preparation for Childbearing,* published by Maternity Center Association, New York, 1972.

the nurse can do it without physically coming between them or breaking their eye contact (Figure 10-18). The nurse should also intervene when the husband needs support or a break, perhaps by saying that he looks tired and that he might like to get coffee. The nurse should tell the husband that she will stay with his wife until he returns. The husband, as well as the wife, needs support and encouragement during labor. He should feel that he has played a vital role in the birth of his child; when this is communicated, the family relationship is strengthened and his participation in child care is increased from the very start.

During the latent phase of the first stage of labor, many hospital routines allow the woman to have a clear liquid diet, since the maintenance of fluid and glucose levels aids in the effectiveness of uterine contractions. Since it is the early stage of

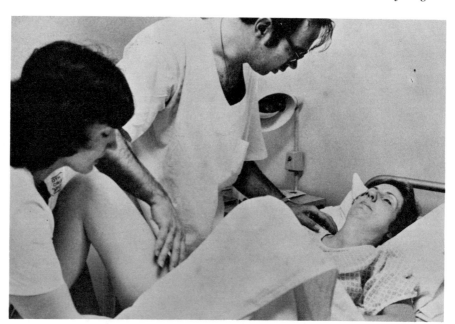

Figure 10-18. Midwife examines the woman but does not impose herself physically between the couple. (Courtesy of Booth Maternity Center, Philadelphia, Pa.)

labor, the stomach will be empty at the time of delivery, which eliminates the chance of aspiration of stomach contents. Some physicians prefer to give intravenous dextrose and water to maintain fluid and glucose levels during labor rather than allowing the woman to take anything by mouth. In either case, cracked ice is usually allowed by mouth and is appreciated by the woman during this period. The woman's fluid intake and urinary output should be monitored and recorded.

During the excitement of labor, especially when under the influence of analgesics, women often forget to void. A full bladder during labor can impede progress, cause pain, and lead to urinary retention after delivery. It is a good idea for the nurse to explain this to the mother and to remind her to void about every 2 hours during labor to avoid distention. The woman should also be reminded that perineal pads (sanitary napkins) are not worn during labor in order to prevent contamination of the vaginal area by fecal matter.

As part of the assessment during this period of labor, every hour the nurse monitors the woman's vital signs: blood pressure, pulse, and respiration, as well as contractions and fetal heart rate (which should range between 120 and 160 beats per minute). The blood pressure and fetal heart rate are taken between contractions because of the changes that occur during a contraction. The nurse should also listen occasionally to fetal heart rates during a contraction, to assess fetal response and heart rate changes during the stress of a contraction. The woman's temperature is usually checked every 4 hours during this phase unless a deviation is noted, in which case the temperature is taken more frequently; it is also checked more often when membranes have been ruptured for more than 12 hours.

With the beginning of the second or active phase (4–8 centimeters' dilatation) of the first stage of labor, the woman has completed one-half to two-thirds of the length of the first stage. This fact can be a source of real encouragement to the mother who has labored for so many hours with so little progress in terms of cervical dilatation. During the active phase, dilatation proceeds much more rapidly; the woman is usually more uncomfortable, because the intensity of the contractions has increased. Her contractions are now between 30 and 50 seconds in duration and are occurring at intervals of 2–5 minutes. The woman now needs continuous evaluation.

Her vital signs, including blood pressure, pulse, respiration, contractions, and fetal heart rate, are monitored from every 30 minutes in the beginning of this phase to every 15 minutes at its end. The nurse should always time the uterine contractions rather than relying on information from the woman, especially since the contraction begins about 10 seconds before there is any subjective feeling of discomfort. Occasionally, a woman will appear to be having strong, painful contractions when the contractions evaluated by the nurse do not coincide with the mother's reactions. Often the woman's anxiety level has greatly exaggerated her perception of the pain. Once the nurse is able to decrease the woman's anxiety through encouragement and comfort measures, the subjective pain tends to coincide more with the objective evaluation.

The fetus must also be carefully monitored. Bradycardia, an increase in fetal activity, and meconium-stained amniotic fluid in a vertex presentation may be signs of compromised fetal oxygenation and distress. If any of these occur, the physician should be notified and the fetus monitored very closely.

Fetal position can often be predicted by the location of the mother's discomfort and the position she assumes. When the woman complains of severe backache and is unable to lie on her back, the vertex may be in the posterior position. In this instance, the fetal heart tones are heard in her flank, and the contraction pattern may show a long contraction followed by one or two shorter ones. Chest (or costal) breathing may decrease the woman's discomfort [17].

If the woman is restless and rolls back and forth in the bed with equal discomfort in the back and front, the occiput may well be in a transverse position. In either the transverse or posterior position, vertex rotation may be speeded by having the woman lie on her side opposite the fetus' back. Lying on her side also keeps her uterus from compressing the inferior vena cava and permits better circulation.

When the fetus is in one of the anterior positions, the woman tends to lie on her back with the backrest elevated; the discomfort is generally concentrated over the symphysis and down into the groin area. The contractions are generally long and strong, but the woman may benefit by abdominal breathing. If the fetus is in a breech position, raising the backrest may make the woman more comfortable.

The nurse giving direct care or working through the woman's support person can use a number of comfort measures in helping the mother cope with labor. Since women react differently to labor, comfort measures helpful to some women may not be helpful to others. The nurse caring for a woman in labor must continually evaluate the woman's response to the measures being used; if one measure is not effective, another may be substituted.

Back pain may be relieved by applying pressure with the heel of the hand or some firm object such as a tennis ball to the small of the back (Figure 10-19). Some women get relief from a hot-water bottle applied to the back, while others find relief with an ice bag. Many women relieve the discomfort by lying on their side with the bed elevated or by doing pelvic rocking.

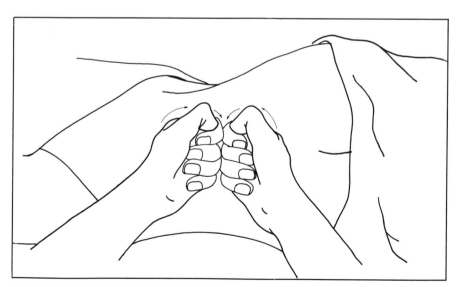

Figure 10-19. Applying sacral pressure.

Some women find that brushing their teeth or rinsing their mouths with mouthwash is very refreshing. Moistening the lips with a wet gauze pad or lemon and glycerine, sucking a piece of hard candy, or chewing gum are also helpful.

Another important comfort measure is to make sure the woman's perineum is clean and that she is resting on dry linens. She may also rest more comfortably if her feet are kept warm. A superficial circular stroking of the abdominal skin (effleurage) is comforting to some women.

Creating an environment that is conducive to rest is at least as important as the physical care the nurse can offer. The room should have soft lighting (keeping the overhead light on tends to make women more restless). Noise should be kept to a minimum. Women also find this period easier to cope with when someone is with them continuously.

Occasionally a woman becomes uncomfortable and cannot decide what will make her comfortable; at such times she needs direction. Often having her turn on her side, close her eyes, and try to rest between contractions while someone rubs her back is all that is needed. When this is done, many women are able to get considerable rest between contractions.

If the woman needs or requests analgesics she should receive them, provided that she is dilated approximately 4–5 centimeters if she is a primigravida, 4–6 centimeters if she is a multigravida. Analgesics given before this time can slow the progress of labor. Often a woman who requests analgesics early in labor can be made comfortable by other measures, and the amount of analgesic necessary can be decreased considerably. Whenever analgesics are administered, the woman's vital signs (including the fetal heart rate) should be checked just before administration. This will serve as a baseline should the woman or the fetus experience side effects from the analgesic.

The third phase (8–10 centimeters dilatation) of the first stage of labor is known as transition (deceleration phase); it is generally the most difficult of the phases of the first stage. The woman's contractions are between 50 and 60 seconds in duration, with an interval of approximately 2 minutes. Women need a great deal of encouragement and support at this point. They can be told that labor is almost over, since this stage usually averages 10 contractions or 20 minutes for multigravidas, and 20 contractions or 40 minutes for primigravidas [17].

The nurse may note that during the transition phase the woman automatically rests or sleeps between contractions; this is known as partial amnesia. During a contraction, pressure and massage to the sacral area helps, as does rapid shallow breathing. Since the woman perspires more now, she can be made more comfortable if her face and brow are wiped with a cool cloth.

During transition a number of signs and symptoms appear that should alert the nurse to the beginning of the second stage. These include an increase in bloody show, irritability, restlessness, and anxiety. Some women prefer not to be touched during this period. Women perspire much more at this stage and may develop hiccups or nausea and vomiting (a reflex sign of rapid cervical dilation). As the presenting part of the fetus descends, the woman will probably complain more of low back pain and pain in her upper thighs. Because of the pressure, she may experience involun-

Table 10-4. Assessment and Intervention During Labor and Delivery

Assessment	Intervention
Expectations for labor and delivery	Reinforce realistic expectations
Coping ability during labor	
Mother	Provide supportive measures
	Early labor: Use diversionary activities—walking, television, magazines; review breathing techniques; provide fluids and glucose
	Active phase: Work with woman or through her support person (nurse or other person remaining with woman); help with breathing techniques, back rub and sacral pressure for backache, mouth care, dry linens, change of position, adequate hydration, frequent voiding, analgesics when necessary, consistent encouragement, monitor vital signs; encourage rest between contractions, periods of privacy for the couple, quiet environment
Father	Encourage periodic breaks for the father or support person, recognition for his supporting role
Reaction to infant	Provide time and opportunity for parents to interact with each other and the infant; brief physical exam for infant, allowing close examination by parents—note normal newborn variations and unique features of their infant

tary leg shaking or involuntary bearing down. As the presenting part of the fetus reaches the perineal floor and presses on the rectum, the woman may complain of needing to have a bowel movement.

The membranes may rupture now if they have not ruptured before (while this may occur at any time in labor, it is most frequent during this period). When the membranes rupture, the fetal heart rate should be measured immediately, since on rare occasion the cord is washed down the canal with the fluid (prolapsed cord) and becomes wedged between the bony pelvis and the presenting part, compromising the fetal oxygen supply. The character and amount of amniotic fluid is also noted and recorded, since meconium-stained fluid may be a sign of fetal distress.

During this stage the nurse or supporting person should breathe with the woman during her contractions and apply sacral pressure and massage. Her perineum should be kept clean and the sheets or pads under her kept dry. She should be told that the end of labor is near, and she should be allowed to rest as much as possible between contractions (Table 10-4).

THE SECOND STAGE OF LABOR

The second stage of labor, which extends from full cervical dilatation to the birth of the infant, is a period that most women find less stressful than the first. Now the woman can increase the effectiveness of the uterine contractions by pushing.

At the beginning of a contraction the woman should lean forward, flex her legs on her abdomen, and grasp them just below the knee (Figure 10-20). She should take a

Figure 10-20. Woman in labor pushing with the coaching of her husband. (Courtesy of Booth Maternity Center, Philadelphia, Pa.)

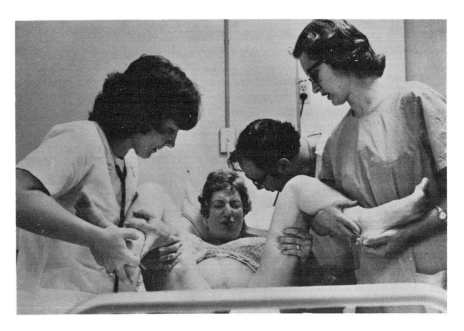

deep breath, blow it out, take another deep breath, hold it, and bear down using her abdominal muscles. The woman sustains her pushing while the nurse or support person counts to ten, then takes a second breath and continues pushing until the contraction is over. Maintaining eye contact with the woman during her pushing is usually helpful, as is a progress report on the amount of the baby's head that is visible. If she exhales while the contraction is still strong, she can take another deep breath and bear down again. The nurse continuously assesses the woman's ability to bear down with a contraction and, if improvement is necessary, the nurse can work with the woman directly or through her support person to improve her pushing. If fecal material is expelled during the bearing down, it should be removed at once and the perineal area kept clean. Between contractions the woman should close her eyes and rest. Fetal heart tones should be checked frequently, possibly after every other contraction. The woman's vital signs should continue to be checked approximately every 10 minutes.

The second stage is usually completed with an average of 20 contractions for a primigravida and 10 contractions for a multigravida. Since the second stage is short for a multigravida, she is generally transferred to the delivery room during the transition phase. In general, a primigravida is transferred when a portion of the fetal head approximately the size of a 50-cent piece can be seen at the perineum between contractions.

Once in the delivery room, the woman is positioned on the delivery table, with her legs placed in stirrups. Before being draped, her perineum is cleansed with an antiseptic solution. Prior to the crowning of the head, the midwife or physician may perform an episiotomy. This is an incision of the woman's perineal skin, vaginal mucosa, urogenital septum, constrictor cunni and transversus perinei muscles, fascia, and a few fibers of the puborectal portion of the levator ani muscle. An

Table 10-5. Lacerations of the Birth Canal

Degree of Laceration	Extent of Damage
First degree	Involvement of the fourchet, perineal skin, and mucous membrane of the vagina. No muscle involvement
Second degree	Involvement of perineal skin, vaginal mucous membrane, and muscles of the perineal body. No rectal sphincter involvement
Third degree	Involvement of perineal skin, vaginal mucous membrane, muscles of the perineal body, and rectal sphincter
Fourth degree	Sometimes used to designate involvement of the anterior rectal wall, in addition to the above areas

episiotomy enlarges the vaginal outlet, avoiding perineal tears (Table 10-5), which do not heal as well as repaired straight-edged incisions, and it allows the infant to be born with less effort. It also avoids prolonged and severe stretching of the muscles supporting the bladder and rectum, preventing later stress incontinence and vaginal prolapse. In addition, it decreases the duration of the second stage of labor, decreases pressure on the fetal head, which is especially important in delivery of premature infants, and makes application of forcep blades more accurate.

The incision may be made in the midline of the perineum (median episiotomy), or it may be made on an angle directed laterally away from the rectum on the right or left side of the mother's perineum (mediolateral episiotomy) (Figure 10-21). Usually infiltration with a local anesthetic precedes the incision, although some clinicians state that when the perineum is stretched, the pressure on the nerve endings at the

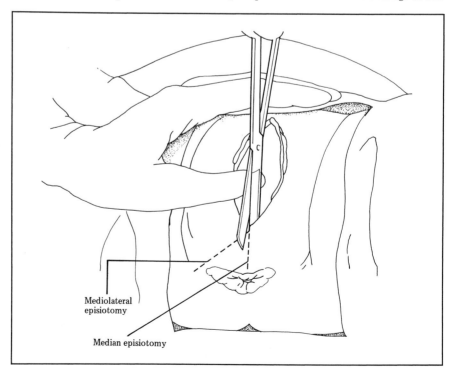

Mediolateral episiotomy

Median episiotomy

Figure 10-21. Sites for episiotomy incisions.

height of a contraction makes anesthesia unnecessary. Some mothers state otherwise!

The mediolateral episiotomy avoids the anal sphincter if further enlargement is necessary, but many women find it very uncomfortable during healing. The median episiotomy may necessitate further incision into the anal sphincter, but it is generally more comfortable for the woman during the healing process. Advocates of the latter method also state that it is easier to repair well and that it heals better with fewer complications.

After the head is delivered (Figure 10-22), blood and mucus are wiped from the infant's face, and his nose and mouth are suctioned, usually with bulb suction. Following delivery of the remainder of the infant's body, he is held below the level of

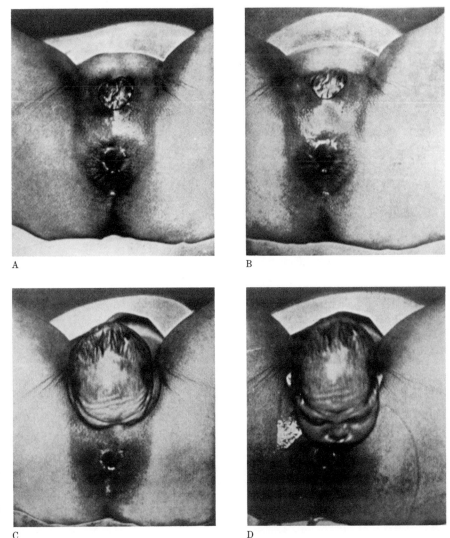

Figure 10-22. Birth of the infant's head. A. Head distends the perineum, anus flattens. B. Perineum much distended by the head, a process called crowning. C. Fetal head extended, perineum slipping back over the infant's face. D. Fetal head delivered, perineum retracted under chin. (From J. P. Greenhill and E. A. Friedman. Biological Principles and Modern Practice of Obstetrics. *Philadelphia: Saunders, 1974.)*

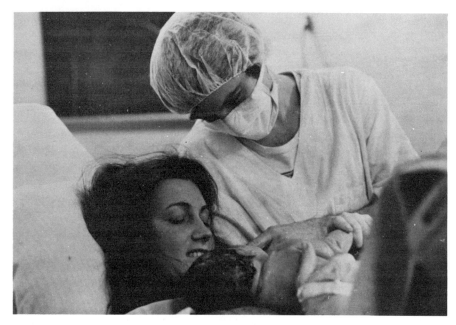

the mother's body, and his nose and mouth are suctioned further. His cord is clamped with two Kelly clamps and then cut between them. Some clinicians prefer to wait until the umbilical cord has stopped pulsating before it is clamped and cut; in this way the infant receives approximately 100 milliliters of additional blood from the placenta. Critics of this procedure argue that the infant does not need the additional blood and, in fact, becomes more likely to develop higher levels of bilirubin as the extra blood is broken down.

After the cord is clamped and the infant is breathing on his own, he is shown or given to his parents to hold briefly (Figure 10-23). In most hospitals the infant then receives routine newborn care.

NEWBORN CARE

It is extremely important that the newborn be kept dry and warm from the time of birth. Blood and amniotic fluid should be wiped off to prevent fluid evaporation from chilling the infant. The chilling can easily increase his metabolism and consequently his need for oxygen, which would cause him to use his readily available glucose and would induce an acidosis or aggravate the degree of metabolic acidosis already present. Metabolic acidosis in turn causes higher levels of bilirubin, since the binding of bilirubin to albumin is decreased.

Moore [18] stresses the amount of heat lost and notes that "a wet, small newborn loses up to 200 calories per kilogram per minute in the delivery room through evaporation, convection, and radiation. Realizing that an adult at full compensation generates only about 90 calories per kilogram per minute makes it easier to appreciate the severity of this heat loss." Wiping the infant dry cuts this heat loss in half.

Chilling also makes it more difficult for the infant's body temperature to increase and then stabilize after birth.

Although the newborn does not have the shivering mechanism of the adult for compensation, he does have brown fat, a source of heat that is unique to neonates. Deposits are found between the scapulas, around the neck and thorax, behind the sternum, and around the kidneys and adrenals. Brown fat is particularly rich in blood vessels and nerves and is believed to warm blood flowing through it, thus contributing to body heat. It is believed to hypertrophy after birth and then disappear several weeks later.

The newborn has a large body surface in comparison to his weight, which causes some of the difficulty of heat loss; because of this he experiences more heat loss than an adult. Perhaps to compensate in some degree, his extremities remain flexed immediately after birth, which decreases the exposed skin surface. While all of these factors contribute to heat loss in a normal newborn, in a low birth weight baby the problems are intensified. He has less subcutaneous fat to insulate him, a larger surface area in relation to his weight, a less flexed position, and smaller glycogen stores to be used when his metabolic rate increases. Therefore, it is especially important that he be dried and warmed immediately.

Once the infant is warm and dry, he receives an Apgar score, cord care, eye care, a vitamin K preparation, and an identification bracelet. He is also footprinted and assessed for gestational age.

Apgar Score

Apgar scoring of heart rate, respiratory effort, muscle tone, reflex irritability, and color is done at 1 minute and 5 minutes after birth (Table 10-6). The heart rate is generally regarded as the most important of the five items scored. It can be counted by using a stethoscope on the infant's chest wall, by feeling the pulsations in the cord, or by placing two fingers on the infant's left chest wall and counting for 30 seconds. A heart rate below 100 beats per minute is associated with asphyxia.

Respiratory effort is next to heart rate in importance, and a vigorous cry with regular respirations is given a score of 2. Muscle tone is scored according to the degree of flexion in the extremities. Normally the newborn keeps his extremities flexed, resisting extension; when the nurse extends a limb and then releases it, the

Table 10-6. Apgar Scoring

Sign	Score		
	0	1	2
Heart rate	Absent	Below 100	Over 100
Respiratory effort	Absent	Slow, irregular	Good, crying
Muscle tone	Flaccid	Some flexion of extremities	Active motion, flexed extremities
Reflex irritability	No response	Weak cry, facial grimace	Vigorous cry
Color	Pale, cyanotic	Pink body, extremities blue	Completely pink

healthy infant's response is to bring it back into a flexed position; this response merits a score of 2.

Reflex irritability is tested by flicking the sole of the infant's foot. If he responds by crying, he receives a score of 2, while a weak cry or change in facial expression merits a score of 1.

Color is evaluated according to the degree of cyanosis; if there is no cyanosis in the body or in the extremities, the infant receives a score of 2.

Infants who score between 0 and 3 are severely depressed, those scoring from 4 to 6 are moderately depressed, and those who score from 7 to 10 are free of immediate stress. Infants with low Apgar scores, particularly on a 5-minute test, have a significantly higher mortality and a higher incidence of neurological defects.

Cord Care

Routine cord care consists of tying off the cord 2 or 3 centimeters (approximately 1 inch) from the abdominal wall and then cutting it. The cord is tied with a rubber band, a cotton cord tie, or one of a variety of plastic clamps. The cord should be examined for the presence of three vessels—one large vein and two smaller arteries. Some hospital routines require that an antiseptic solution be applied over the cord stump.

Eye Care

The infant's eyes may become infected as his head passes through the vagina. Routine eye care is performed as prophylaxis against ophthalmia neonatorum, which causes a purulent inflammation of the conjuntiva and cornea. While the gonococcus is usually the organism responsible, pneumococcus, *Corynebacterium diphtheriae,* and other organisms can cause serious conjunctivitis.

Prophylaxis may be carried out according to modifications of Credé's method, which calls for the use of a silver nitrate solution in the eye. Generally two drops of a 1% silver nitrate solution are put in the conjunctival sac of the infant's eye. One minute later, sterile saline or water is used to flush out the eye. The irrigation should be directed so that the stream of irrigating fluid flows from the bridge of the nose and tear duct to the outer corner of the eye, serving to wash material away from the duct.

Some clinicians prefer to irrigate the eye before as well as after the instillation of the silver nitrate; in this way any blood or mucus is removed from the area. Others prefer not to irrigate the eyes at all, noting that the incidence of chemical conjunctivitis as a reaction to silver nitrate is no higher in infants who do not have their eyes irrigated after instillation of the silver nitrate. In some hospitals antibiotics such as penicillin or tetracycline are used for eye care instead of silver nitrate. However, this treatment carries with it the risk of the infant's developing a sensitivity to the antibiotic or the organisms' developing a resistance to it.

Greenberg and Vandow [8] questioned whether any single use of a drug in an infant's eye is really effective in preventing gonococcal ophthalmia; they reported the incidence of this infection with the use of a number of regimens. With no prophylaxis there were 25.5 cases per 100,000; using silver nitrate, 6.6; using saline, 7.4; using antibiotic ointments, 11.2; and using parenteral penicillin, no cases.

Vitamin K

As part of routine newborn care, 1 milligram of vitamin K is administered either in the delivery room or in the nursery, since the newborn is unable to manufacture vitamin K on his own due to inadequate intestinal flora immediately after birth. Vitamin K administration prevents decreases in plasma prothrombin levels and thus decreases hemorrhagic disease in the newborn.

Identification

Identification of the newborn is generally done by putting identification bracelets on both the mother and newborn and by footprinting the infant. The bracelets applied to the infant and mother should have matching identification numbers and note the mother's name, the infant's sex, and the date and time of birth. The bracelet put on the infant should be tight enough that it will not slip off in the nursery, but not tight enough to be constricting.

When taken properly, footprints can be a good source of identification [7]. The

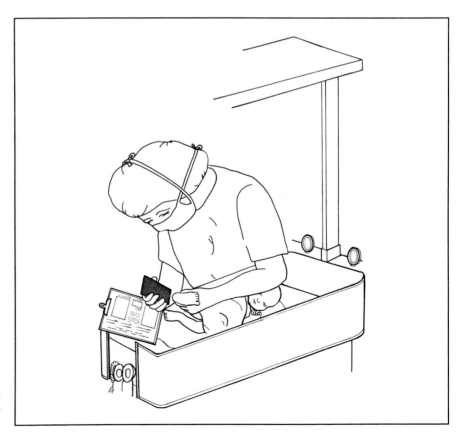

Figure 10-24. Footprinting the newborn (see text for details).

sole of the infant's foot should first be cleaned gently and dried (rigorous cleaning may well make the infant's skin peel). The sole is then pressed against the ink plate of the footprinter. The nurse should cradle the infant's foot between her thumb and index finger and place the infant's foot, heel first, on the footprint paper. By gently turning her wrist, the ball of the foot and the toes will be pressed between the paper and the back of her hand (Figure 10-24). The paper should be attached to a clipboard for stability and to provide a hard surface. The footprint should be checked to see if the ridges are distinct. The mother's thumbprints are also placed on the page.

Assessment

Immediately after birth the infant should be examined briefly to determine maturity and ascertain if there are any anomalies. The full-term infant will have sparse lanugo, cartilage present in his ears, formed nipples, creases over more than one-third of the soles of his feet, and relatively thick, smooth skin. The mature male infant will have rugae on his scrotal sac and descended testes, while the mature female infant will have labia majora that cover the labia minora. (For a more thorough assessment of gestational age see Chapter 17.) This postnatal assessment is important, since if the infant is preterm, postterm, or small for his gestational age, he is likely to experience a number of disturbances after birth.

Circulatory Changes

With the onset of respiration, a number of changes occur in the infant's circulatory system. Alveolar expansion at birth results in a decreased resistance in the pulmonary vessels, perhaps due to an increase in arterial Po_2, which causes a decrease in the right atrial pressure as the blood flows through the lungs. The increased blood flow from the lungs causes an increase in pressure in the left atrium, which in turn closes the foramen ovale. As the arterial Po_2 rises, the wall of the ductus arteriosus begins to constrict and close; it is usually obliterated by approximately two weeks of age, and most are sealed by two months [14]. The ductus venosus and umbilical arteries and vein become obliterated by two months of age.

If hypoxia occurs, the resistance in the pulmonary vessels increases and the blood flow through the lungs diminishes, changing pressures within the atria and opening the foramen ovale. The ductus arteriosus stops constricting and again shunts blood away from the lungs.

Occasionally an infant will be slow to breathe immediately after birth even though his heart rate is normal. This may happen as a result of undue pressure on the fetal head with a forceps delivery, abnormally long uterine contractions, or administration of large amounts of analgesia or anesthesia to the mother. Delay in respiration may also result from low maternal blood pressure or other factors that cause fetal distress. Often, rubbing the infant's skin when drying him and further suctioning of the upper airway [21] provide enough stimulation that he begins regular respirations and manages a lusty cry or two (Figure 10-25). He should also respond to a flick of the finger on the sole of his foot or gentle stroking of his back from his waist to his neck while he is held in the Trendelenburg position. If his respira-

Figure 10-25. Suctioning the newborn.

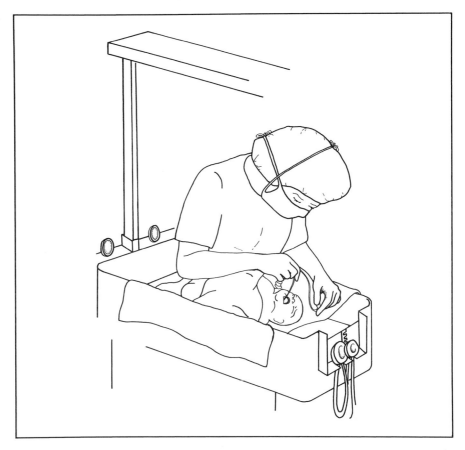

tions are still irregular, the infant will often respond after a very brief period of oxygen delivered via face mask.

Resuscitation of the Newborn

If after a minute the infant remains moderately depressed, appears limp and cyanotic, and has shallow, irregular, or gasping respirations, but maintains a heart rate above 100, he needs ventilatory assistance. A laryngoscope is passed, the airway cleared of any mucus or particles, and an airway inserted. Oxygen is then administered via a face mask attached to a hand-operated bag. The infant's chest should rise with each insufflation, and breath sounds should be heard in each lung. If the infant's respiration and color do not improve shortly, or if his heart rate drops below 100, endotracheal intubation is performed and he is given oxygen through a bag attached to the endotracheal tube.

If the heart beat remains depressed, external cardiac massage is started, using the index and middle finger over the left side of the infant's sternum (Figure 10-26). The heart is compressed at a rate of approximately 120 times per minute, and oxygen is administered by bag after every three cardiac compressions. The external massage is continued until the heart rate recovers.

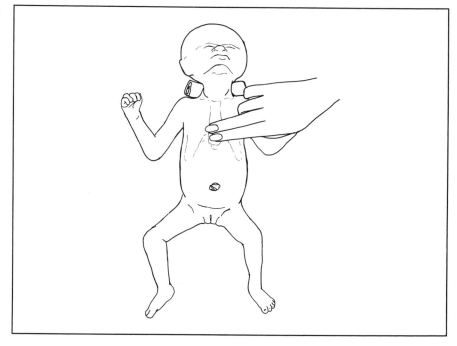

Prolonged hypoxia is accompanied by a metabolic acidosis, which is treated with administration of a 7.5% solution of sodium bicarbonate through the umbilical vein, provided that cardiac activity is adequate. When heart action is absent or depressed, the solution is infused into the infant's liver via the ductus venosus and remains there [14]. The infant also receives additional sugar, usually a solution of 10% dextrose. During resuscitation, the infant must be kept warm in order to ensure more rapid recovery.

Throughout the procedure, the nurse must consider the parents' feelings. When their infant fails to cry, their anxiety may be overwhelming. They must be told what is happening in a manner that does not increase their anxiety further, and they should be informed of any improvement as soon as it occurs. There is no better way of reassuring them and decreasing their anxiety than to allow them to see, touch, and hold the infant as soon as possible after his condition has stabilized. This can be done simply by moving the crib unit close to the delivery table and giving the parents some time with their infant. If the infant is transferred to the intensive care unit, the parents should be kept informed of his progress, and the father should be allowed to be with the infant as soon after transfer as possible.

THIRD STAGE OF LABOR

When the baby is born, the uterine cavity is obliterated. The uterus itself is almost a solid mass of muscle, with walls that are several centimeters thick; the fundus is usually just below the level of the umbilicus. With the decrease in size of the uterus, there is also less space available for placental attachment. To accommodate to the smaller area, the placenta first increases in thickness but is soon forced to fold on itself. The resulting tension causes the weakest layer of the decidua, the spongiosa, to break away, and the placenta begins to separate at that point. As a result of this continuing process, a hematoma forms between the separating placenta and the remaining decidua basalis; this hematoma may function in accelerating further separation. Usually placental separation occurs within a few minutes after delivery, 6–7 percent of the time within the first or second postpartum contractions.

After the separation of the placenta, the uterus becomes globular instead of discoid in shape. If the placenta remains in the uterus after separation, the fundus will rise up to or above the umbilicus or above the original position of the fundus. At the same time, a slight bulge appears just above the symphysis pubis, while the umbilical cord protrudes about 10–12 centimeters (4–5 inches) more than previously from the vulva. All of these signs indicate that the placenta has moved to the lower uterine segment or the upper part of the vagina. Because the formerly collapsed lower uterine segment becomes distended by the placenta, it mechanically lifts the tightly contracted body of the uterus to a higher level.

Studies have shown the periphery of the placenta to be the most adherent portion, so separation usually begins in a more central location. With central separation, the hematoma is thought to push the placenta toward the uterine cavity, where it becomes inverted; it descends, weighted with the hematoma. Surrounding membranes that are still attached to the decidua are dragged after it, and the shiny fetal surface of the placenta presents at the vulva. This type of placental presentation (Schultze's placenta) occurs over 70 percent of the time, usually accompanied by a gush of blood.

In the other method of separation (Duncan's placenta), the process begins at the periphery, with the result that blood collects between the membranes and the decidua and trickles from the vagina. The placenta descends to the vagina sideways, and the rough maternal surface appears first at the vulva. As can be surmised, with the continuous loss of blood in a Duncan separation, total blood loss may be greater. Fetal membranes usually remain in place until separation of the placenta is practically completed; they are then pulled off the uterine wall, partly by further contraction of the myometrium and partly by traction exerted by the separated placenta.

In some cases the placenta may be expelled by an increase in intra-abdominal pressure if the mother is coached to bear down. It is thought that this not only is less traumatic for her but also permits less fetal blood from the placenta to enter her circulation, which is particularly important in prevention of Rh sensitization. Unfortunately, women in the supine position can expel the placenta spontaneously only about 15–20 percent of the time. Since the figure is probably even lower when the woman has received anesthesia, artificial means of terminating the third stage of labor are generally necessary.

The usual method for delivering the placenta involves the midwife or obstetrician using manual pressure over the contracted fundus, thus using the uterus as a "piston" to expel the placenta, with the umbilical cord as a guide (Figure 10-27). If the placenta is not expelled quickly following separation, blood may be lost unnecessar-

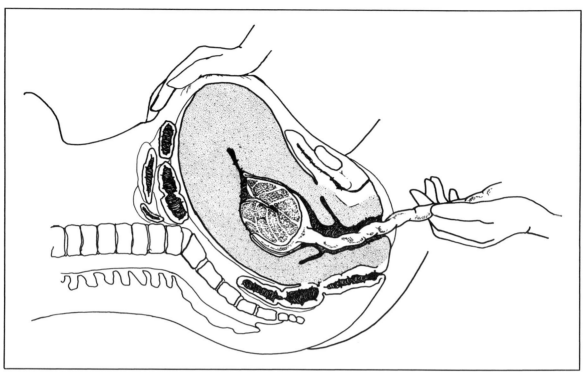

Figure 10-27. Expulsion of the placenta (see text for details).

ily. On the average, blood loss during and after vaginal delivery is around 600 milliliters. Nurses caring for a mother after delivery should be aware of what her estimated blood loss is so that they might assess its effect on the patient. Signs and symptoms of hypovolemic shock include pallor, tachypnea, air hunger, restlessness, euphoria, and vertigo.

Attempts to deliver the placenta prior to complete separation are not only futile but also dangerous, and excessive traction or pulling on the cord is never done, since part of the placenta may tear away and remain inside the uterus, predisposing the mother to hemorrhage and infection. However, manual removal of the placenta is sometimes necessary if bleeding is heavy and the placenta cannot be delivered otherwise.

The placenta is delivered carefully to prevent the membranes from being torn off and left inside the uterus; it is routinely examined for completeness and for the number of fetal vessels in the cord. As mentioned previously, retained placental fragments or membranes can easily cause postpartum hemorrhage by preventing adequate myometrial contraction.

THE FIRST POSTDELIVERY HOUR (Fourth Stage of Labor)

Sometimes the mother is extremely fatigued by the time she gets to the recovery room, so that care should be scheduled to allow for her maximum rest and to ensure privacy for the parents and their infant. If the baby has been transferred to the recovery room in the mother's or father's arms, the new family interaction has already been initiated.

If the parents have not had much opportunity to see their newborn while in the delivery room and if they desire it, time in the recovery room can be used to great advantage in helping them get acquainted. Since they may be apprehensive in handling their infant, the wise nurse stays with them, offering support, until they are comfortable. This also, of course, provides the nurse with an opportunity to make pertinent observations that can be passed on to other personnel who will care for the new family unit in succeeding days.

The first postdelivery hour, sometimes referred to as the fourth stage of labor, is a very critical period for the mother. It is the time that postpartum hemorrhage is most likely to occur as a result of uterine relaxation. After the baby and placenta are delivered, hemostasis is achieved at the placental site through vasoconstriction produced by the contraction of the myometrium. Oxytocin (Pitocin, Syntocinon), ergonovine (Ergotrate), and methylergonovine (Methergine) are used during the third and fourth stages of labor, principally to stimulate myometrial contractions and minimize blood loss. The tetanic effect of ergonovine is ideal for the prevention and control of postpartum hemorrhage, but it must be used carefully, since hypertension is a common side effect.

During the first postdelivery hour the mother is usually in the recovery room, where she can be closely monitored; her vital signs, the condition of the fundus, and lochia (vaginal discharge after delivery) are checked at least every 15 minutes. The fundus should remain firmly contracted, since even with slight relaxation it can quickly fill with blood and be unable to contract. If this occurs, the fundus should be massaged and the blood expelled.

In preparation for fundal massage the mother is asked to flex her legs and allow them to fall apart. The nurse palpates the mother's fundus by placing the side of one hand on top of and slightly cupped under the fundus while the other hand is placed over the symphysis pubis, exerting slight pressure (Figure 10-28). The fundus is usually felt in the midline, at or below the umbilicus. If it is boggy, it is rubbed lightly until it contracts firmly. It is important not to overmassage or overstimulate

Figure 10-28. Fundal massage (see text for details).

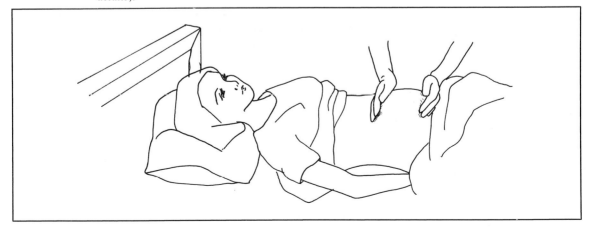

it, since the muscle may become fatigued and consequently relax. If blood has collected within the uterus, slight downward fundal pressure after the fundus is firm is usually all that is necessary to expel the blood.

In the recovery room mothers often are given intravenous fluids, commonly containing 10 units of oxytocin to promote uterine contraction. The intravenous fluids also result in rapid filling of the bladder, which may become distended and inhibit contractions by pushing the uterus high in the abdomen and displacing it to the right or left. A distended bladder may easily be seen and felt as a spongy, fluid-filled mass below the uterus and above the symphysis. If the mother has had block anesthesia that has not yet worn off, she may be totally unaware of the distention and may, in fact, be unable to void. In that case she will need to be catheterized (her voiding or catheterization is, of course, included in the nurse's notes).

The mother's perineum is inspected for swelling, or unusual tenderness when touched, or ecchymosis, all signs of a perineal or vaginal hematoma. The application of an ice bag may be ordered to lessen perineal edema and numb the area as anesthesia wears off. The mother's perineum is kept clean and dry, with regular changes of perineal pads and linen. Her lochia is routinely checked for color, amount, odor, and presence of clots. Since the discharge often pools under the mother's buttocks instead of collecting on the perineal pad, each examination should be a thorough one. If the lochia is excessive and the uterus is not remaining well contracted, or if there is a continuous bright red trickle, indicative of an unrepaired laceration, the mother should be placed on a pad count and her physician notified.

During the first hour after delivery the mother's vital signs should return to their prenatal base. Nurses should be particularly alert for an increase in the mother's temperature (dehydration, infection), an increase in blood pressure (preeclampsia), or an increase in pulse rate followed by a decrease in blood pressure (hemorrhage). It should be remembered that blood pressure and pulse rate usually do not show marked fluctuations in hemorrhage until after a large amount of blood has been lost and the circulatory system is unable to compensate for the decrease in volume.

Nursing care of the mother in the recovery room includes such measures to increase the mother's comfort as a clean gown, a cup of coffee or tea, ice water, or whatever she wishes to eat, if she is not nauseated. She may experience a postpartum chill and require an additional blanket, preferably already warmed. The cause of the postpartum chills is uncertain, but it may result from a nervous reaction, imbalance between external and internal body temperature due to muscular exertion, the sudden release of intra-abdominal pressure, or even infection.

Depending on the mother's condition, the recovery room can be a good place to educate the patient. The nurse may, for example, teach the mother how to palpate her own fundus and massage it until it is firm.

EMERGENCY CHILDBIRTH

Any nurse whose background includes an understanding of the essentials of adequate antepartal care, the conduct of labor and delivery, and the immediate care of the newborn should be able to apply that knowledge to situations outside of a prepared, organized environment. Some general principles are important in providing the mother and child with adequate protection and safety in an emergency delivery. The mother and baby should be considered as a unit, with the father involved as much as possible if he is present. Everything possible should be done to prevent infection, injury, and hemorrhage in the mother and baby. All necessary steps should be taken to ensure an adequate airway and the establishment of respiration in the newborn. For medical and legal purposes the time and location of birth should be recorded, as well as the names of the parents and any problems encountered.

Wherever the emergency delivery occurs, assessment of the general situation is the first priority. What is the condition of the mother and the fetus? How close is the delivery? How much time and what facilities exist for planning? Who will handle the delivery? Who will seek help? Who will prepare needed equipment? Very often the nurse is the most knowledgeable person present and is responsible for making the major decisions involved.

Whatever circumstances surround the delivery, basic medical asepsis is observed as much as possible. Since the baby is not born through an aseptic passage, no delivery is really sterile, but cleanliness remains an essential consideration. All care is directed toward maintaining physical and emotional reserves, interpreting progress to the mother and father, and providing rest, fluids, and support.

During the second stage of labor, the mother is constantly observed for signs of complications and exhaustion and is given encouragement as necessary. As the delivery becomes imminent, the nurse (after washing her hands) should wet the mother's perineum with a towel and liquid soap, if possible. As the baby's head crowns, the mother should be instructed to pant during her contractions, since this may give an additional 3–5 minutes for extra planning before the actual delivery. The woman's perineum is supported and protected with a clean towel (a sterile towel, if available, would be best). If there is no clean material, the birth canal and surrounding perineum is not touched, and the woman is instructed to keep her hands away from these areas.

Delivery of the Infant

Gentle pressure is applied against the baby's head as it emerges so that it is not delivered too rapidly; however, it is not held back. If the delivery attendant is unskilled, the head should be allowed to deliver spontaneously and should be supported as it emerges. If membranes are still present, they are removed. The umbilical cord is slipped over the baby's head if it is looped around his neck. Mucus and amniotic fluid are wiped from the infant's mouth and nose by stroking the nose downward and "milking" the throat with an upward movement on the neck and under the chin.

After the head is delivered, it usually turns spontaneously to one side or the other; occasionally it has to be gently rotated, in which case it should be turned in whichever direction it tends to go toward more easily. This motion will bring one shoulder anteriorly behind the symphysis pubis. With the baby's head in both her hands, the nurse can deliver the anterior shoulder by exerting gentle steady pressure down-ward. When the upper portion of the arm can be seen, the direction of traction should be reversed upward to deliver the posterior shoulder over the mother's peri-neum. This is done slowly and carefully, since there is no need to rush at this point.

As the baby's body is delivered, it is supported and then wrapped in a warm towel or clean cloth. After the parents have seen their newborn, the baby should be placed on the mother's abdomen with the head low so that the mucus will drain out. If he does not cry immediately, respiration will usually be stimulated by gently rubbing his back.

If proper equipment is available, the infant's umbilical cord is tied in two places after it has stopped pulsating. The ties should be made about 8 centimeters (3 inches) from the abdomen and 5 centimeters (2 inches) farther up; the cord should be cut between the ties if it can be done under aseptic conditions; otherwise it should not be cut, since the risk of infection is too great. In this case or if transportation is available, the cord and placenta are wrapped with the baby and are cut later when the baby and mother are in more favorable circumstances. No harm will result even in the extreme event that the cord is never cut, since the cord will dry naturally and fall off. Common household equipment can be sterilized to tie and cut the cord, including such items as wool, heavy cotton thread, or string and a kitchen knife, scissors, or a new razor blade.

Delivery of the Placenta

Following the baby's delivery, the mother is observed for signs of placental sepa-ration. Once this has occurred, the mother may be able to help push the placenta out. If not, gentle pressure on the contracted fundus toward the vaginal outlet will aid in placental delivery. Excessive traction is not exerted on the cord, since it may snap or a placental fragment may break off and be left in the uterus. The entire placenta can stay in the uterus for several hours without harm to the mother if she is monitored carefully for bleeding [4].

Once the placenta and membranes are delivered, they are examined thoroughly for completeness. If the mother's uterus is soft and bleeding, it is massaged to pro-mote contractions. Starting the baby on breast-feeding will stimulate the release of natural oxytocin to achieve the same effect. Using ice cubes or a heavy weight (for example, a book) just above the fundus or manual breast stimulation is also some-times recommended [4]. The mother is made as comfortable as possible, given nour-ishment (such as hot tea with honey, or salty broth), encouraged to void, and al-lowed to rest. If she is to be transferred to a medical facility, it would be better to give no fluids, since anesthesia may be necessary for repair of lacerations or for uterine exploration.

Care of the Newborn

Two important aspects of the routine care of the newborn are identification and warmth; also important are cleanliness (especially when dealing with the cord stump), gentle handling, and pertinent observations of the infant's condition.

Sometimes improvised methods of identification become necessary during wide-scale emergencies. The infant may be kept warm by wrapping him in lightweight blankets and placing him either next to his mother's skin (they can be wrapped together in the blankets) or in a warm place, such as in a box near an oven turned to a low heat.

The infant will also need food. Breast-feeding is preferable, but it should never be forced on the mother. A suitable formula can be prepared from powdered infant formula or dried skim milk. If there is no refrigeration, the formula should be made immediately prior to the feeding. Canned evaporated milk, diluted 1 part milk to 2 parts water, may also be used. If no bottles are available, milk may be placed in a teaspoon on the baby's lower lip or dropped on the inside of his cheek with a medicine dropper.

Other Situations of Emergency Childbirth

Emergency care of the pregnant woman may be necessary in her home, en route to the hospital, during local or national disasters, or even in the hospital itself. If the mother delivers precipitously in the hospital, there is usually an emergency delivery kit and sterile gloves in each labor room. The kit commonly includes two Kelly clamps, a plastic cord clamp, scissors, sterile towels, sponges, a bulb syringe, and a basin for the placenta. After the cord is cut, the baby and mother are usually transferred to the delivery room, where the placenta is delivered, the uterus is examined, and any lacerations are repaired. Care of the baby after an emergency delivery is the same as after a hospital delivery.

If the delivering mother is en route to the hospital in an automobile or taxi, she should be on the back seat with something under her buttocks (blanket, coat, skirt) to avoid contact with the seat, which has been used by many other people. When she reaches the hospital, usually she and the baby are taken directly to the delivery room. There the cord is cut, the placenta is removed, her uterus is explored, and any lacerations are repaired. The infant is usually taken to the isolation-observation nursery, where he can be closely watched for signs of trauma, fever, intracranial hemorrhage, or infection. Both mother and baby may be given prophylactic antibiotics.

If the mother in labor is at home and is on the floor, several thicknesses of heavy material (towels) should be placed under her buttocks to give a little more space for delivery of the baby's shoulders. If possible, she should be moved to a bed (or table) and positioned so she is lying crosswise with her buttocks slightly off the edge. She may place her hands under her thighs to support herself, or rest her feet on the backs of two chairs. If it is at all possible, the furnishings should be protected by newspapers, a plastic shower curtain or table cloth, towels, or old sheets.

In actual large scale disaster situations, principles of triage for obstetric patients will most likely be observed. Pregnant women who only need reassurance that their pregnancy is unthreatened and that they are not in active labor, in premature labor, or aborting are classified as requiring *minimal treatment*. Multiparas may be assigned duties in maternal areas and, with proper guidance, may be called on to assist in delivery or even to perform a delivery themselves. *Immediate treatment* is required for those mothers who are ready to deliver or who are actively aborting. Oxytocics may not be available, and unless hemorrhage is a major threat, no manipulation or instrumentation is even considered. Treatment may have to be *delayed* for women in active labor or with minor complications of pregnancy requiring nursing care; these women are allowed to progress until some spontaneous outcome is reached. *Expectant casualties* include those women in whom no normal spontaneous outcome can be expected (e.g., those requiring a cesarean section); treatment for these women will have to be deferred until more advanced obstetrical care is available.

For disasters and other emergency situations in which prior planning has been done, delivery kits are usually available. If there has been no time for planning, materials for meeting certain priorities of care should be gathered: for cleansing—liquid soap, alcohol, or vinegar; for adequate airway—bulb syringe, meat-basting syringe, a plastic straw, or rubber tubing of a small diameter; for padding and protection—newspapers, plastic bags, or old sheets and towels; for warmth—blankets, towels, clean sheets, shirts, or diapers; for a baby bed—a carton or box; for food—bottles and milk powder.

OBSTETRICAL ANALGESIA AND ANESTHESIA

Pain During Labor and Delivery

The pain of uterine contractions travels along afferent fibers via the posterior roots of the eleventh and twelfth thoracic nerves (sympathetic nervous system) to the spinal cord. Pain due to cervical dilatation and stretching of the birth canal travels via the roots of the second, third, and fourth sacral nerves (parasympathetic nervous system) to the spinal cord. Perineal pain is conducted via the pudendal nerve.

The exact mechanism that produces the pain of childbirth is a controversial issue. It is generally thought that the pain of the first stage of labor is primarily a result of cervical dilatation. This is corroborated by the fact that there is a definite interval of about 15–30 seconds after the onset of a contraction before pain is experienced. It takes this long for the amniotic fluid pressure to increase to 15 millimeters of mercury, the minimum pressure needed to distend the lower uterine segment and cervix, resulting in dilatation. (Pain is also felt when the cervix is dilated with an instrument or manually in pregnant or nonpregnant women [1]).

Pain is also probably caused by the contraction of the myometrium itself; the myometrium becomes ischemic or puts pressure on the nerve endings between the muscle fibers of the uterus. Perhaps the most severe pain of labor is produced by the distention of the pelvic outlet, vulva, and perineum, resulting in stretching (and possibly tearing) of the fascia, skin, and subcutaneous tissue of these structures. Other factors that contribute to the pain of childbirth include tension in the supporting uterine ligaments, pressure on the adnexa and peritoneum, and pressure on and stretching of the bladder, urethra, and rectum. Discomfort from these accessory structures is conveyed by sensory nerves associated with the ovarian plexus via the posterior roots of the tenth thoracic nerve.

The intensity of the pain depends on the intensity and duration of uterine contractions; the degree of cervical dilatation and how quickly it is reached; the degree of distention of the perineum; the patient's condition, age, pariety, and anxiety level; and the size of the infant and the birth canal. As a rule labor in the younger primigravida (under 30) is neither as long nor as painful as that in the older primigravida (35 or older), but it is longer than that of the multigravida [1].

During the first stage of labor, pain of contractions and cervical dilatation is referred to the lower abdominal wall and skin and to the soft tissue over the lower lumbar spine and upper sacrum. With more intense stimulation, the pain spreads to the upper thighs, midsacral area, and the umbilical region. During the second stage of labor, the pain is intense in the area of the vulva and perineum; however, during the third stage pain may again result from uterine contractions and from dilatation of the cervix by passage of the placenta.

Preparation for Anesthesia

The pregnant woman approaches anesthesia with the same fears as the person facing surgery; the most serious and most powerful fear, of course, is the fear of death. Fear of loss of consciousness and loss of control are closely related to each other. Also present are the fear of pain and fear of possible complications, such as paralysis due to spinal anesthesia. In addition, the mother may have heard about many unpleasant, if not terrifying, experiences from relatives and friends. There are also women who approach labor with the conviction that to request anything for relief of discomfort is an admission of failure. If it becomes necessary for them to be medicated, they often feel guilt or even depression following delivery.

Since it is known that pain, fear, and anxiety all cause a significant increase in the basal metabolic rate, reflex irritability, and oxygen demand [1], it becomes important to decrease each of these elements as much as possible. Fear and anxiety can be lessened with knowledge, so that parents who approach labor having attended childbirth education classes are usually able to cope with the situation more successfully. Unprepared women, on the other hand, tend to feel discomfort much more acutely and at an earlier phase of labor. In either case, the pattern of the woman's reactions depends not only on her present emotional state but also on her interpretation of pain in light of her past life experiences and the symbolic meaning of pain to her.

The analgesic techniques of childbirth education, psychoprophylaxis, and hypnosis are usually effective in the first stage of labor. Properly applied, each technique produces complete pain relief in 10–20 percent of laboring patients using that technique; these patients will require no anesthesia for delivery. In another 30–50 percent, pain will be decreased, and these women will need less medication than the unprepared patient. In the remainder of patients, the degree of pain does not seem to be affected [1].

Both prepared and unprepared patients in labor have certain needs, which they have identified for nurse researchers [16]. These needs include the relief of pain, the support of another human being, the assurance of their own safety and that of the baby, and the acceptance by those around them of their attitudes toward labor and their behavior during it. The nurse who supports and coaches parents through the process of labor develops a strong rapport with them and helps determine how well the parents are able to cope with the experience. Through her warmth and prompt response to requests, the nurse can make the parents feel that they are very important. This help is even more important when the laboring mother is solely dependent on the nurse for support.

Strong psychological support by the nurse can either make analgesia unnecessary for the patient in labor or greatly enhance its effects. In providing this support, the nurse reinforces whatever antepartal preparation the mother has had and reassures her that what she is experiencing is common and that medication is available if she needs it. A straightforward approach is used in explaining what is happening. Since mothers in labor are especially sensitive to their environment, they are very aware of the tone of voice, facial expression, disinterest, or false enthusiasm of those around them. They tend to interpret most of what they see and hear with reference to themselves. In spite of this fact, hospital staff members will sometimes have casual conversations among themselves within a patient's hearing, discussing other patients' conditions or laughing, with little realization that the mother may see herself as the topic of their discussion or laughter.

Because the mother is so open to suggestion during labor, she is likely to follow commands regarding breathing patterns, for example, even though she may say that it is impossible for her to do so. A nurse who is coaching a mother through labor can use this fact to great advantage; she should be careful to avoid anxiety-provoking terms like *pain,* using the more neutral term *contraction* instead.

Pain Relief in Labor and Delivery

In the middle 1800s anesthesia was used when Queen Victoria gave birth to Prince Leopold, and from that time the medical profession and lay public began to see it as having great potential in obstetrical practice. Research results in the past quarter century have added greatly to the knowledge and techniques of the relief of labor pain [1].

When considering analgesic and anesthetic needs, certain elements distinguish the woman in labor from the person facing surgery. There are actually two individuals to be cared for when the mother is in labor, and the respiratory center of the infant is highly vulnerable to sedative or analgesic or anesthetic drugs. The pregnant woman usually has little time to be prepared physically for anesthesia and often begins labor with some food in her stomach. Another difference is that some continuous methods of regional anesthesia permit the agent to be given throughout labor and thus over a longer period of time than most surgery lasts. Another very important consideration is that if the analgesia or anesthesia is begun too early in labor, it may stop progress entirely. The last major difference is that anesthesia is not an absolute necessity for labor and delivery, provided that the mother has no episiotomy to be repaired.

All methods of pain relief for the mother in labor and delivery have three essential criteria: fetal homeostasis, simplicity, and safety. Some methods of pain relief are associated with sustained or repeated maternal hypotension and thus reduce the Po_2 gradient across the placenta; under this type of stress, fetal homeostatic mechanisms become increasingly less competent. It is also known that potential complications increase in a direct relationship with the complexity of the method used for pain relief.

No completely safe and satisfactory method of analgesia and anesthesia has yet been developed in obstetrics. Probably the one that satisfies the three criteria best is proper psychological support throughout the antepartal period and during labor. This not only provides a natural sedative for the mother but also reduces her fears and anxieties. She tends to develop a feeling of confidence in her support person, the nurses, and the midwife or obstetrician. In this context, obstetrical anesthesia really begins with the first prenatal visit!

When the use of additional methods becomes necessary, as they do in the majority of women, usually they are not begun until there is evidence of progressive effacement and dilatation of the cervix. Usually the cervix is 4–5 centimeters dilated in the primigravida before medication is given and 4–6 centimeters dilated in the multigravida. Since labor may be prolonged if the medication is given too early, it is probably better if the mother receives it later [1].

The choice of technique depends on many factors, most important of which is the condition of the mother and the fetus. Has she eaten recently? Is she hypotensive or hypertensive? Is she dehydrated? Other significant variables include the stage of labor she is in, the rapidity of the progress she is making, and the expertise of the personnel who will administer her anesthesia. It should go without saying that the woman is never forced to accept a technique of analgesia or anesthesia against her wishes, barring very unusual circumstances.

Pain Relief During Labor

During the active phase of labor, the mother goes through two emotionally trying periods: (1) the end of the latent phase, when it seems as though she has labored so long and accomplished so little cervical dilatation, and (2) the more stressful time during transition, when the cervix is reaching full dilatation.

SEDATIVES AND ATARACTICS

Sometimes during labor, mothers are given sedative doses of barbiturates to produce a feeling of well-being and increased susceptibility to suggestion; however, sedatives do not produce analgesia. If they do not have the desired calming effect, occasionally a tranquilizer might be necessary.

For over 70 years scopolamine was used to potentiate the sedative effects of barbiturates and narcotics and to produce amnesia. Currently it is rarely used, since there are many better sedatives and tranquilizers available; in addition many mothers prefer to participate in their infant's birth and want to remember as many details of the event as possible.

NARCOTIC ANALGESICS

Narcotics are probably the most widely used analgesics for labor and the most simple to administer; they decrease fear and anxiety and promote physical relaxa-

Table 10-7.
Pharmacological Agents
Used in Labor

Drug	Maternal Side Effects	Effect on Labor	Placental Transmission	Effect on Newborn
Narcotics	Respiratory depression, bradycardia, orthostatic hypotension, nausea and vomiting, urinary retention	With optimum dose, none. If dose is excessive or given too early, slows progress of labor	Rapid	With proper use, mild depression; with excessive use, severe depression
Sedatives, hypnotics, and ataractics	Sleep, sedation, tranquilizing action, antiemetic; respiratory depression is dose dependent	With optimum dose, none; may enhance contractions. Excessive dose may slow labor	Rapid	Possible depression; may contribute to narcosis by potentiating narcotics
Anesthetic agents Pudendal block	If poor pain relief, apprehension and tachycardia	May eliminate urge to bear down	None	None, unless injected into maternal vessels; then results in fetal depression
Paracervical block	None	If given in latent phase, may arrest labor	Readily	Transient bradycardia
Epidural block	Hypotension, due to vasodilatation	Initial decrease in intensity of uterine contraction; urge to push interrupted	None	If maternal hypotension occurs, fetal distress results
Spinal block	Hypotension	Urge to push interrupted	None	If maternal hypotension occurs, fetal distress results

Source: Data from J. J. Bonica. *Principles and Practice of Obstetric Analgesia and Anesthesia,* Vols. 1, 2. Philadelphia: Davis, 1972.

tion and rest between contractions. However, they may slow the progress of labor if given before the active phase of labor and are specific depressants of neonatal respiration. The narcotic has its peak depressing effects on the fetus 2 hours after administration; to avoid the occurrence of that peak effect at the time of delivery (when the infant is under the most stress), the mother should be given the last injection 3 hours before the predictable time of delivery. She can also be given an injection if the delivery is expected in less than an hour [1]. Occasionally a narcotic and an ataractic will be administered together in the hope that the effect of the narcotic will be potentiated so that smaller doses may be used (Table 10-7).

REGIONAL ANALGESICS

The most common techniques used for regional analgesia during the first stage of labor are paracervical block, continuous caudal block, and continuous epidural block. Regional analgesia has many advantages: In contrast to narcotics it produces complete relief of pain, and it causes no maternal or neonatal depression, provided that there are no complications. If it is administered when the mother's labor is in the active phase, it does not impede the progress she is making. Continuous techniques can be extended for her delivery and may even be modified for cesarean section if necessary.

Regional analgesia permits the mother to remain awake during labor and delivery so that she can actively participate in the birth of her infant. Since regional anesthesia is a more complicated method than systemic drugs or inhalation agents, it requires greater skill to administer and the chance of failure (inadequate anesthesia) is greater. Complications can occur, notably maternal hypotension. Those techniques that produce perineal muscle paralysis (i.e., continuous epidural and caudal blocks) interfere with the mechanism of internal rotation and tend to increase the incidence of persistent posterior positions of the fetus [1].

Paracervical Block (Uterosacral Block).   In a paracervical block the anesthetic agent is placed along the base of the broad ligament and lateral walls of the lower uterine segment (Figure 10-29). It blocks the afferent sympathetic pathways (hypogastric plexus) as they pass through the uterovaginal plexus in the parametrium, relieving the pain of the first stage of labor but not the perineal pain of the second and third stages. Thus, it is not an anesthetic for delivery; at that point it is usually used in conjunction with a pudendal block. Analgesia occurs in 3–5 minutes and lasts 1–2 hours. The paracervical block may be repeated and seems to work best when given in the latter half of labor. It does not interrupt the mother's ability to push with her contractions.

Maternal complications with a paracervical block are rare, but there is a 10 percent incidence of transitory fetal bradycardia associated with its use. Although the cause is not certain, it is felt that the bradycardia may be the result of sudden absorption of the anesthetic, since the injection site is near the uterine artery [1].

Continuous Caudal and Lumbar Epidural Blocks.   Many patients who have had continuous regional analgesia during labor consider it the "ultimate" in pain relief. These techniques can be used on most mothers with normal uncomplicated labor; since they provide complete pain relief, they promote a feeling of calmness and well-being in the mother. Since she has to work less, her metabolism and oxygen consumption tend to decrease.

Both techniques may produce maternal hypotension, since they interrupt enough vasomotor segments to decrease peripheral resistance, venous return, and cardiac output. As this happens the mother's legs will become warm and may tingle. Even though the hypotension occurs less frequently and to a lesser degree than with a subarachnoid block, the mother should certainly have intravenous fluids running well before the procedure is started. Because it may take 15 or 20 minutes for hypotension to develop, the mother's blood pressure should be monitored very frequently (every 2 minutes) for 20 minutes after each injection. If the blood pressure is below 100 millimeters of mercury or decreased by 20 percent in a hypertensive patient, prompt treatment should be begun. In a normotensive woman, turning her to her left side (relieving pressure on the inferior vena cava) may be all that is necessary; however, it may be necessary to place her in the Trendelenburg position, increase the flow of intravenous fluids, and provide her with extra oxygen [1].

Both techniques, if begun too early in labor, may block Ferguson's reflex and

Figure 10-29. Paracervical
block (see text for details).

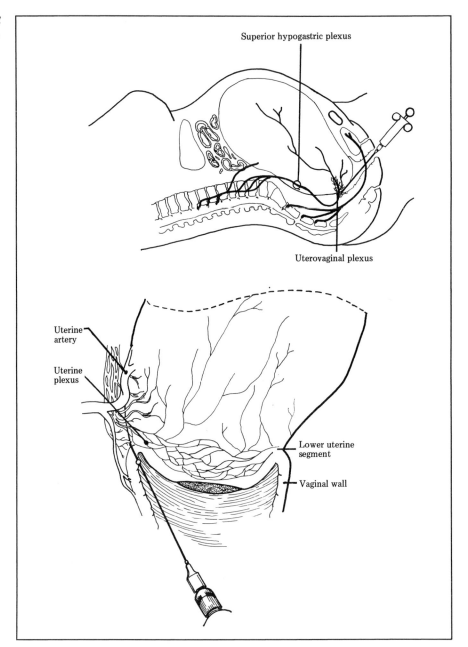

decrease uterine contractions. They may also relax the perineal muscular sling
enough to decrease the forces of internal rotation and may eliminate the mother's
urge to bear down during contractions in the second stage, in which case she will
need to be coached to do this. Both caudal and epidural blocks, when properly used
and when complications have not occurred, have no direct effect on the fetus and
cause no residual depression of the newborn.

In a continuous caudal block, the anesthetic is injected through a small catheter into the sacral canal (peridural space) via the sacral hiatus (Figure 10-30). In the sacral canal it anesthetizes a rich network of sacral nerves that emerge from the dural sac about 6–9 centimeters above.

In an epidural block the anesthetic is injected in the lumbar or lower thoracic peridural space (usually L4–L5), also through a small catheter (Figure 10-31). In both the caudal and epidural blocks the catheter remains in place throughout labor and the anesthetic agent is reinjected as necessary. The standard epidural block provides pain relief from T10 to S5 within 3–5 minutes. Compared with an epidural block, a caudal block requires more local anesthetic, the onset of pain relief is slower, and the chances of failure are greater. In addition, there is more risk of infection because the skin over the sacral hiatus is more difficult to keep clean than that over the lumbar region [1].

INHALATION ANALGESIA

If continuous regional analgesia is contraindicated for some reason, the mother may administer inhalation analgesia to herself as necessary. The most common agent used in this manner is trichloroethylene (Trilene); others include methoxyflurane and nitrous oxide.

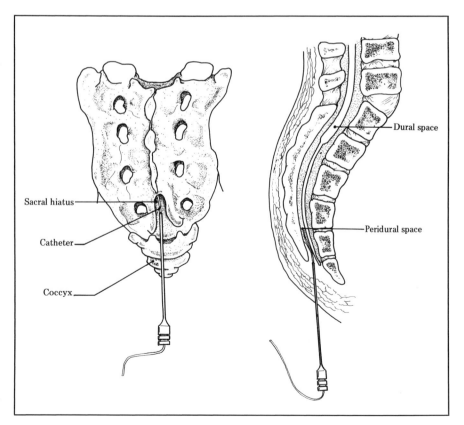

Figure 10-30. Continuous caudal block (see text for details).

Figure 10-30. Continuous caudal block (see text for details).

Figure 10-31. Epidural block (see text for details).

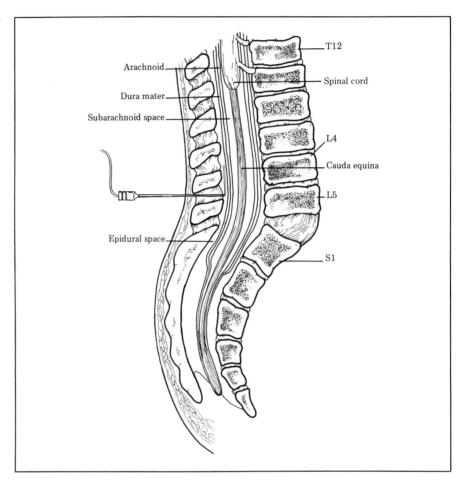

Arachnoid

Dura mater

Subarachnoid space

Epidural space

T12

Spinal cord

L4

Cauda equina

L5

S1

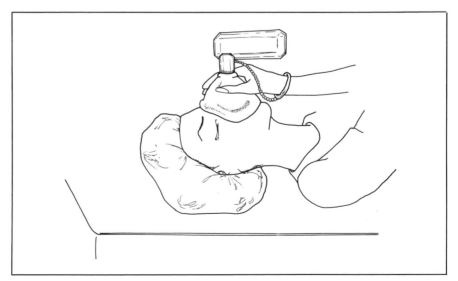

Figure 10-32. Use of the trichloroethylene mask (see text for details).

These agents are given by mask (Figure 10-32), and the woman is instructed in its proper use when she is in early labor. At the beginning of a contraction she applies it to her face, allowing no gaps for air to enter and dilute the anesthetic. She breathes deeply until the pain disappears, and then the mask is removed. A mechanism on the inhaler makes it possible to regulate the anesthetic concentration to produce analgesia without loss of consciousness.

Pain Relief During Delivery

PREPARATION FOR DELIVERY

In most cases primigravidas are moved to the delivery room when a portion of the infant's head can be seen between contractions; multigravidas are moved when they are in transition, or earlier if their labor is progressing rapidly. If the mother is unable to assist in her move to the delivery table because her legs are paralyzed, she should be supported and lifted gently, rather than transferred by grasping her shoulders and ankles. Anesthesia-induced paralysis in the lower extremities removes the protective action of muscles on joints. Consequently, if the woman is not handled carefully and if her back is stretched or twisted, she may suffer some tears of ligaments or muscle fibers that may later produce backache. Since sudden jarring apparently disturbs homeostatic mechanisms already stressed by block anesthesia, sharp movements may precipitate a hypotensive episode. During the transfer, the mother should not be made to sit up, since this too may cause orthostatic hypotension [1]. Needless to say, once she is on the delivery table, someone, preferably her nurse, should remain with her, monitoring vital signs and fetal heart tones and giving her constant support.

Women with caudal, epidural, pudendal, or subarachnoid blocks will not have the reflex urge to bear down during the second stage of labor. However, since these anesthetic techniques cause no weakness of the diaphragm and have little, if any, effect on abdominal muscles, the mother is still able to increase her intra-abdominal pressure effectively when she is properly coached and when she is informed of the beginning and end of each contraction.

When anesthesia is necessary for delivery, psychological support remains a very important adjunct to its successful administration. Constant reassurance, encouragement, and instruction from *one* person (usually the anesthesiologist at this point) will be most helpful and least confusing for the mother.

INHALATION ANESTHESIA

Inhalation anesthesia has the advantage of providing greater control of the depth and duration of anesthesia, a rapid smooth induction, and a quick recovery. Certain obstetrical problems, such as tetanic uterine contraction and Bandl's retraction ring, and procedures such as internal version can only be handled with transient deep inhalation anesthesia. On the other hand, a serious disadvantage is the danger of aspiration of stomach contents, which is one of the major reasons that the complications of obstetrical anesthesia rank fourth or fifth among the causes of maternal mortality. Consequently, inhalation anesthesia is contraindicated in women who have eaten recently, women who have acute respiratory infections or other respiratory diseases, and in women with severe diabetes, kidney or liver disease, or toxemia. It is also contraindicated when the infant is thought to be preterm. Another disadvantage of inhalation anesthesia is that it usually results in neonatal depression if given for longer than 5 minutes [1].

Nitrous oxide is a popular inhalation agent used for normal vaginal deliveries. Usually 40% nitrous oxide with 60% oxygen is satisfactory until the actual delivery, when 70% nitrous oxide with 30% oxygen produces adequate analgesia. Whatever the concentration, there must always be at least 20% oxygen in the combination. The main drawback of nitrous oxide is its lack of potency as a true anesthetic agent in concentrations that allow adequate fetal oxygenation.

Cyclopropane has a pleasant, rapid induction and recovery and can be used with high concentration of oxygen. A major disadvantage is its flammability and explosiveness; in addition, it can produce occasional cardiac arrythmias and has a tendency to cause fetal and maternal respiratory depression if deep anesthesia is required.

If trichloroethylene has been used during the first stage of labor, the mother is usually given a pudendal block to eliminate the perineal pain of the second stage. Trichloroethylene may then be continued throughout the delivery.

Ether is still considered useful by some, since it is inexpensive, easy to administer, and has a wide margin of safety. However, it does contribute to a high incidence of nausea and vomiting, and it also irritates the respiratory tract [1].

REGIONAL ANESTHESIA

The use of regional anesthesia for delivery generally produces no respiratory depression or other effects harmful to the mother and newborn. Since uterine tone is maintained, blood loss is usually less than with inhalation anesthesia. Since the mother is awake, the anesthesiologist is available to leave the mother and resuscitate the baby if necessary, and a pediatrician need not be present.

Subarachnoid Block (Spinal and Saddle). Subarachnoid block is thought to be the most widely used regional technique to produce terminal anesthesia for vaginal delivery. Its advantages include simplicity of induction and minimal side effects; the major disadvantages are maternal hypotension and postanesthetic headache. Usually this type of anesthesia is given to a primigravida when her baby's head is on the perineum; it is given to a multigravida at the beginning of the second stage of labor or when she is 8 centimeters dilated if her labor is progressing rapidly. The effects of the anesthesia usually last for about an hour [1].

In a low spinal block (saddle block) the agent is usually introduced into the cerebrospinal fluid in the subarachnoid space between L4 and L5. (Spinal blocks are usually introduced at the level of L3–L4—see Figure 10-33.) Generally a hyperbaric solution (specific gravity greater than spinal fluid) is injected into the woman's subarachnoid space while she remains in a sitting position, which enables the solution to gravitate to the lower part of the dural sac. She usually remains sitting for 1–3 minutes, depending on the amount of solution used, and then is placed flat on her back with two pillows under her head. Any change in intra-abdominal pressure during bearing down or any active effort to change position may cause a disturbance

Figure 10-33. Spinal block (see text for details).

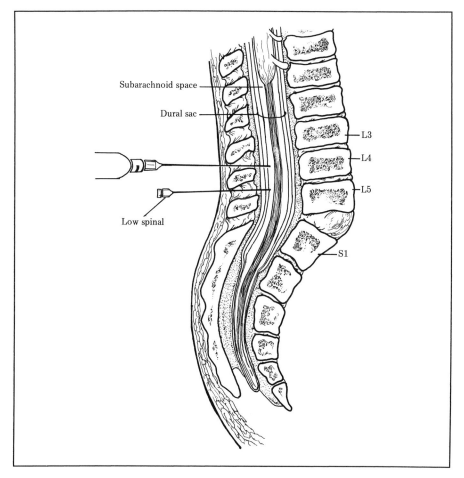

in cerebrospinal fluid pressure, enhancing the spread of the anesthetic solution. Because of this, the woman is instructed to remain as quiet as possible during the procedure. She can easily be reminded of this by the nurse, who should be supporting her in the correct position (Figure 10-34). The woman is also advised not to elevate her head for 6–8 hours (or as ordered) after delivery, to avoid a postspinal headache (see Chapter 11).

Extradural Blocks (*Caudal and Lumbar Epidural*).   Patients who have had continuous extradural blocks during labor receive a reinjection just before delivery, usually with a greater concentration of the drug. The dose is commonly administered with the patient in a sitting position ("sitting dose"), so that the effect of gravity results in adequate perineal anesthesia. This usually takes about 15 minutes to achieve and can permit a calm, unhurried, well-controlled delivery.

Pudendal Block.   A pudendal block provides relaxation and analgesia to the patient's perineum without disturbing uterine contractions or having harmful effects on the baby. However, it may eliminate the mother's urge to bear down. Since

*Figure 10-34. Sitting
position for spinal
anesthesia.*

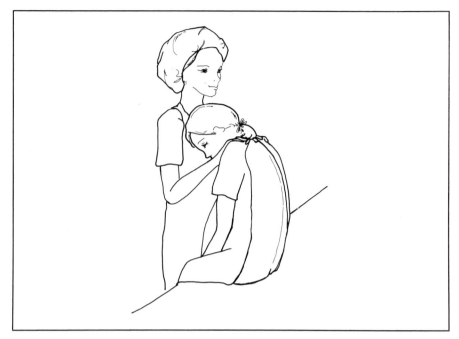

pudendal blocks are more difficult and time-consuming to give, they are followed by a higher incidence of failure (inadequate anesthesia) than subarachnoid blocks, and they provide no relief from the discomfort of contractions [1].

Each pudendal nerve is blocked in its position near the ischial spine (Figure 10-35). The transvaginal route provides less risk of infection and less discomfort than the transperineal approach. Transvaginal pudendal blocks must be done before the presenting part completely fills the vagina; otherwise the transperineal route becomes necessary.

If the block is improperly done, the inadequate pain relief will increase the woman's apprehension, anxiety, and fear. Possible maternal complications are hematoma formation and rectal puncture.

LOCAL ANESTHETICS

Absorption of the anesthetic, once it is injected into tissues, depends on the vascularity of the part and the solubility and concentration of the drug. Local anesthetics cause local vasomotor paralysis, thus increasing local blood flow and enhancing absorption. As a result, they are often administered with a vasoconstrictor (epinephrine), which prolongs the duration of action, increases the potency, and permits the use of smaller concentrations of the drug [1].

Local infiltration of the perineum for episiotomy repair has been used for many years. It is simple, effective, and practically free of maternal or fetal complications. It has no systemic effect on either the mother or the infant.

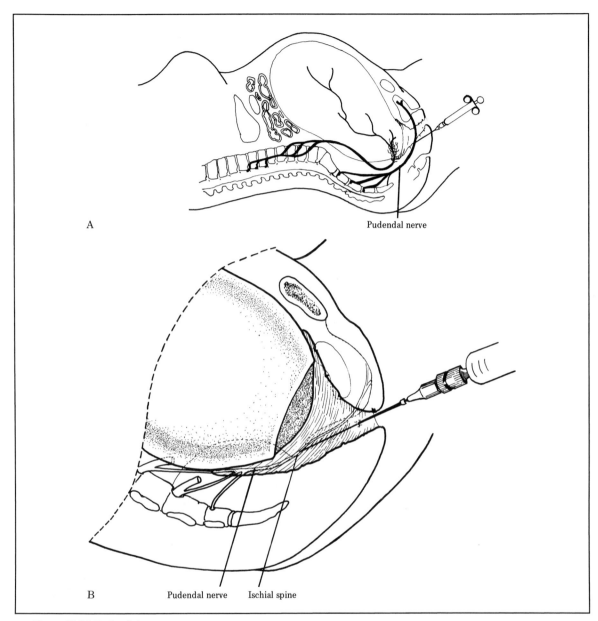

A

Pudendal nerve

B   Pudendal nerve   Ischial spine

Figure 10-35. Pudendal anesthesia administered by the transperineal route (A) or by the transvaginal route (B) (see text for details).

ABDOMINAL DECOMPRESSION

In the middle 1950s, abdominal decompression as a form of analgesia during labor was initiated by Heyns [11]; it entails the application of negative pressure around the abdomen of the mother in labor. A device is used to draw her abdominal wall anteriorly during a contraction in order to remove the resistance of the anterior and posterior abdominal wall muscles and allow free movement of her uterus. Theoretically this will shorten labor. The negative pressure is in the range of 35–77 milliliters of mercury, the higher levels being necessary for analgesia as the strength of contractions increases. After proper instruction, the mother is able to operate the apparatus herself with each contraction.

Sufficient analgesia is reported to occur in a high percentage of patients, with favorable effects on labor and the newborn. However, claims of shortened labor, improved fetal oxygenation, and prevention of fetal hypoxia have not been verified by objective studies. The method has not gained widespread favor [1].

HYPNOSIS

Hypnosis, one of the oldest medical arts, was first used to produce obstetrical pain relief in the 1830s. Isolated reports of its use in obstetrics were published between 1900 and 1940, and since that time interest in its use has grown. It has been accepted by both the American and British Medical Associations as an ethical part of medical practice.

Depending on the skill of the practitioner, about 40–50 percent of the patients who are prepared antepartally can be successfully hypnotized. While maintaining the active experience of childbirth, these patients show reduced levels of fear and apprehension. They are able to relax their perineal muscles effectively, resulting in less trauma to the birth canal, perineum, and fetal presenting part. It is reported that hypnosis shortens the first stage of labor in primigravidas by about 3 hours and by more than 2 hours in multigravidas [6]. Hypnosis precludes the risk of asphyxia in the newborn from chemical analgesics or anesthetics, although the use of post-hypnotic suggestion may cause maternal respiratory depression.

Childbirth under hypnosis can be a very gratifying emotional experience. In order for it to be successful, the mother must be willing to be hypnotized, and she must have the ability to concentrate, have average intelligence, be unafraid about hypnosis, and have absolute confidence in the practitioner. Hypnotic rapport can be transferred (during the first stage of labor) to other personnel who can, without previous training, induce and maintain the hypnotic state using a prearranged cue. However, it is necessary for the practitioner who has conditioned the patient to be present during the second stage of labor, and particularly during the actual delivery [1].

Many women who have been conditioned for childbirth are unable to remain relaxed in the distracting conditions of the hospital. It is helpful if they are placed in a quiet room and are spoken to as softly and as little as possible, avoiding any word that is suggestive of discomfort. Elements of surprise should be controlled as much as possible. If medication is necessary at any time, the amount given should be no more than enough to maintain the mother's relaxation.

REFERENCES

1. Bonica, J. J. *Principles and Practice of Obstetric Analgesia and Anesthesia,* Vols. 1, 2. Philadelphia: Davis, 1972.
2. Coch, J. A., Brovetto, J., Cabot, H. M., Fielitz, C. A., and Caldeyro-Barcia, R.   Oxytocin-

equivalent activity in the plasma of women in labor and during the puerperium. *American Journal of Obstetrics and Gynecology* 91:10, 1965.

3. Csapo, A. Function and regulation of the myometrium. *New York Academy of Medicine* 75:790, 1959.
4. Dickason, E., and Schult, M. O. *Maternal and Infant Care.* New York: McGraw-Hill, 1975.
5. Doust, B. D. The role of ultrasound in obstetrics and gynecology. *Hospital Practice* 8:143, 1973.
6. Flowers, C. E., Littlejohn, T. W., and Wells, H. B. Pharmacologic and hypnoid analgesia. *Obstetrics and Gynecology* 16:210, 1960.
7. Gleason, D. Footprinting for identification of infants. *Pediatrics* 44:302, 1969.
8. Greenberg, M., and Vandow, J. E. Ophthalmia neonatorum: Evaluation of different methods of prophylaxis in New York City. *American Journal of Public Health* 51:836, 1961.
9. Greenhill, J. P., and Friedman, E. A. *Biological Principles and Modern Practice of Obstetrics.* Philadelphia: Saunders, 1974.
10. Hellman, L. M., and Pritchard, J. P. *Williams Obstetrics.* New York: Appleton-Century-Crofts, 1971.
11. Heyns, O. S. Abdominal decompression of labour. *Journal of Obstetrics and Gynecology of the British Commonwealth* 66:220, 1959.
12. Hon, E. H. Electronic evaluation of fetal heart rates. *American Journal of Obstetrics and Gynecology* 83:333, 1962.
13. Hon, E. H. *An Introduction to Fetal Heart Rate Monitoring.* North Haven, Conn.: Corometrics Medical Systems, 1971.
14. Korones, S. B. *High Risk Newborn Infants.* St. Louis: Mosby, 1972.
15. Liggins, G. C. Fetal influences on myometrial contractility. *Clinical Obstetrics and Gynecology* 16:148, 1973.
16. Lesser, M., and Keane, V. *Nurse Patient Relationships in a Hospital Maternity Service.* St. Louis: Mosby, 1956.
17. *Mechanism of Normal Labor.* Columbus, Ohio: Ross Laboratories, 1970.
18. Moore, M. L. *The Newborn and the Nurse.* Philadelphia: Saunders, 1972.
19. Ohlsen, H. Moulding of the pelvis during labour. *Acta Radiologica: Diagnosis* (Stockholm) 14:417, 1973.
20. Pokoly, T. B. The role of cortisol in human parturition. *American Journal of Obstetrics and Gynecology* 117:549, 1973.
21. Roberts, J. Suctioning the newborn. *American Journal of Nursing* 73:63, 1973.

FURTHER READING

Brooten, D., and Miller, M. A. *The Frequency of Certain Signs and Symptoms Prior to Full Cervical Dilatation.* Unpublished M.S.N. thesis, University of Pennsylvania, 1970.

Drugging the baby too. *Science News* 106:348, November 30, 1974.

Fitzpatrick, E., Reeder, S., and Mastroianni, L. *Maternity Nursing.* Philadelphia: Lippincott, 1971.

Gross, H. N., and Posner, A. An evaluation of hypnosis for obstetric delivery. *American Journal of Obstetrics and Gynecology* 87:912, 1963.

Jolivet, A., Blancher, H., and Gantray, J. P. Blood cortisol variations during late pregnancy and labor. *American Journal of Obstetrics and Gynecology* 119:775, 1974.

Klaus, M. H., and Faneroff, A. *Care of the High Risk Neonate.* Philadelphia: Saunders, 1973.

Mahoney, R. F. *Emergency and Disaster Nursing.* New York: Macmillan, 1969.

Quilligan, E. J. Maternal factors influencing the onset of labor. *Clinical Obstetrics and Gynecology* 16:150, 1973.

Chapter 11 Normal Puerperium

UTERUS

In the immediate postdelivery period, the uterus becomes firm and globular, with its anterior and posterior walls in close apposition. Compared to its condition during pregnancy, it appears blanched because the contracted myometrium has markedly compressed the blood vessels of the uterus. During the following six-week period of involution (the puerperium), the uterus decreases in size, mainly because of the autolysis of cellular protein material, particularly actomyosin. As a result there is a tenfold decrease in the size of the hypertrophied myometrial cells, while the actual number of such cells decreases only slightly. The whole process leads to an increase in the nitrogen content of the urine for several days. Just after delivery, the uterus weighs about 1000 grams (2.2 pounds); one week after delivery it weighs 500 grams (1.1 pound); two weeks after delivery it weighs 350 grams (12 ounces); by the end of the sixth week the uterus has returned to its normal 50–70 grams (1.8–2.5 ounces).

The progress of uterine involution is measured daily by determining the height of the fundus, which can be done most accurately using the method described in Chapter 10. Following delivery and for the first two days thereafter, the fundus can be found usually about 12 centimeters (5 inches) above the symphysis pubis or around the level of the umbilicus. After that, it descends about 1 centimeter (0.4 inch) (or one fingerbreadth) a day, until by the tenth day it has descended into the cavity of the true pelvis and can no longer be palpated above the symphysis pubis (Figure 11-1).

After delivery of the placenta and during the postpartum period, uterine contractions continue but occur less frequently than they did during labor. Their pattern becomes incoordinate, a phenomenon that may be due to a decrease in the amount of oxytocin being secreted after delivery or to a decrease in uterine sensitivity to oxytocin stimulation, or both. The primipara's uterus tends to remain tonically contracted, so that she generally has fewer complaints of painful uterine contractions after delivery than a multipara. In about 75 percent of multiparas, the uterus contracts and relaxes at intervals, causing "afterpains" that may on occasion be severe enough to require analgesics. The release of natural oxytocin that accompanies breast-feeding may magnify the intensity of afterpains, as will the administration of oxytocics when they are indicated. In addition, blood clots or retained placental fragments will cause the uterus to contract more vigorously in an effort to expel them. Usually afterpains begin to decrease in intensity after 48 hours. Some mothers find that measures such as assuming a prone position, applying a hot-water bottle to the abdomen, voiding often and keeping the bladder empty, and drinking hot liquids help them to relax and provide some measure of relief.

Figure 11-1. Involution of the uterus during the puerperium.

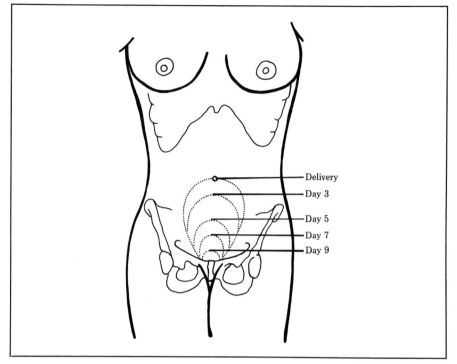

Since the pregnant uterus requires a more abundant blood supply than the nonpregnant one, a readjustment of its vasculature is necessary. Current theory suggests that the larger vessels become completely obliterated by hyaline changes and that new and smaller vessels develop in their place. Following delivery, the blood vessels and sinuses of the placental site rapidly become thrombosed. This area, which was originally the size of the palm of the hand, becomes progressively smaller and is replaced by new endometrium. No scar remains when the healing is complete.

The postdelivery decidua consists of the inner portion of the spongy decidual layer in varying thicknesses; within two days after delivery it has separated into two layers. The layer next to the myometrium contains the remnants of the uterine glands and is the source of new endometrium. During the first three weeks postpartum, the epithelium arising from proliferation of these glands covers the uterine cavity, with the exception of the placental site, which is usually covered by the sixth week. When this process is defective, late puerperal hemorrhage may occur. The other layer that lines the uterine cavity is infiltrated by leukocytes, becomes necrotic, and is cast off in the *lochia* (vaginal discharge) within five or six days after delivery.

The total amount of lochia after delivery is in the range of 150–400 milliliters. For the first two or three days, the red discharge (*lochia rubra*) contains bacteria, fatty epithelial cells, shreds of membrane, decidua, and blood. Later the amount of blood decreases and the discharge becomes paler or sometimes brownish (*lochia serosa*).

After the seventh to tenth day, the lochia becomes whitish or yellowish (*lochia alba*) because of the presence of leukocytes and serum. At about three weeks, the amount of lochia decreases; the flow finally stops when the placental site is healed completely. Lochia normally has the odor of fresh blood.

If the lochia remains red after two weeks, involution may be delayed or placental fragments may have been retained. If the lochia is excessive in amount, has an offensive odor, and contains solid particles, this may be a sign of bits of retained placenta and membranes. Infection should be considered if the lochia is scanty in amount and has an offensive odor. If the lochia is scanty but otherwise normal in characteristics, drainage may be poor, possibly because a small clot is obstructing the flow. Such an obstruction is usually associated with an elevation in temperature, which subsides when the obstruction is removed and good drainage is established.

Mothers should be told that ambulation usually increases drainage. Women may be needlessly alarmed by the different appearance of blood or an increased amount of blood in the lochia after they have returned home unless they realize that it may be a sign that their activity level has been too great. With increased rest periods, lochia will usually return to a normal color and amount; however, all lochial changes should be reported to the obstetrician.

Lochia may be more profuse in multiparas, and it may be greater when the mother is getting up for the first time. It is said to be less profuse in nursing mothers, although there may be a temporary increase in the amount of blood in the lochia while the infant nurses. In general, studies [1, 9] have indicated that routine administration of oxytocin other than in the immediate postdelivery period is unwarranted, since it does not decrease blood loss or hasten involution, and it probably adds to the discomfort of the mother by stimulating painful uterine contractions.

LIGAMENTS

The stretched uterine ligaments become shorter as they regain their tone. Until the ligaments, pelvic floor, and abdominal wall are restored to normal tonicity, the uterus is not supported well and may easily be displaced.

CERVIX AND VAGINA

Immediately after delivery the cervix and the lower uterine segment are flabby collapsed structures. During involution new cervical muscle fibers form and the cervical osses contract, so that by the end of the first 10 days the cervix and lower uterine segment are so narrow that it is difficult to introduce one finger into the external os. A finger will not pass through the internal os at all. The external os does not resume its prepregnant appearance, since lateral depressions from lacerations make it look more slitlike than circular.

After delivery the vagina decreases in size. The mucosal swelling disappears, tone increases, and rugae begin to reappear by the third week. It rarely returns to its nulliparous condition, however. What remains of the hymen are several tags of tissue, the *carunculae hymenales*. The external genitalia lose their fatty cushion and appear more flabby.

PERINEUM

The muscles and fascia of the pelvic floor have been overstretched during pregnancy and may have been torn or incised for an episiotomy during delivery. By the sixth postpartum week, their muscular function has returned to normal and there is little or no gaping of the introitus.

The perineum is observed daily for signs of proper healing, or evidence of infection, swelling, or hemorrhoids. Special care is taken to prevent infection and to prevent irritation of external genitalia from vaginal discharge. The mother is taught to do this for herself, but the nurse may choose to do perineal care once a day for the mother. This gives the nurse an excellent opportunity to observe the condition of the perineum while carefully noting the mother's facial expressions, which may indicate particularly sore spots. The nurse may also use this time for explaining the importance of doing the care correctly.

Perineal care may be done in a variety of ways. Cleansing solution may be poured over the perineum without separating the labia, to prevent the fluid from entering the vagina. The perineum is always cleaned from the vulva to the anal region, wiping with a downward stroke from front to back and using a clean tissue or clean side of the wipe for each stroke. The mother may be instructed to do her perineal care with her morning shower and after each voiding and bowel movement. She should also be instructed to wash her hands well before and after doing this.

Perineal pads (sanitary napkins) should be changed as often as necessary and after trips to the bathroom. The pad should be applied with a sanitary belt, sanitary panties, or pins in such a manner that it remains close to the body, not moving back and forth with the mother's activity, which would increase the likelihood of the transfer of organisms from the rectum to the vagina. On the other hand, the pad should not be applied so tightly as to cause discomfort.

Pads are applied and removed from *front* to *back*. They should be handled only on the side that will be away from the mother's body. The number of pads required in 24 hours varies according to the amount of lochial discharge; this number provides a means of estimating that quantity (if bleeding is heavy or excessive, a pad might be saturated every 30–60 minutes). If hemorrhage is suspected, patients are usually put on "pad counts" for a certain period of time.

A mother who had an episiotomy or lacerations at the time of delivery will experience varying degrees of perineal discomfort; a variety of measures may be taken to give her some relief. Sitz baths in warm water or a heat lamp directed at the perineum provides improved circulation and relaxation. She may be helped by witch-hazel compresses, analgesic sprays, sitting on rubber rings or pillows, or application of warm compresses or ice packs (ice in a rubber glove). Exercising perineal floor muscles not only improves circulation of blood in the area but also improves the muscle tone. The mother should be instructed to contract her gluteal muscles for 5 seconds and relax; contract gluteal muscles and press thighs together

Table 11-1. Assessment and Teaching During the Puerperium

Assessment	Observation	Possible Significance	Teaching Opportunities
Breasts			
Contour	Fullness, firmness, tenderness Tingling with or without pain Venous distention; warm skin; shiny skin; nodular	Milk may be coming in; possible engorgement; possible infection	Proper breast care; process of milk production; breast massage and expression; breast feeding and diet history and counseling; breast self-examination
Areolae	Soft, compressible, taut; presence of Montgomery's follicles	Areolar engorgement	
Nipples	Prominent, erect, flat, inverted, clean, caked, reddened, sore, fissured, cracked	Grasp of baby may be incorrect	Nipple eversion Proper nursing techniques
Colostrum or milk	Expressed, clear, bluish-white, cream-colored, yellow		
Brassiere	Proper fit and adequate support	Proper alignment of blood and lymph vessels; may prevent engorgement from becoming exaggerated and minimize discomfort	Importance of adequate support
Uterus	Firmness; position with regard to umbilicus and abdominal midline; afterpains; tenderness	Firmness shows proper involution; subinvolution possibly a result of infection retained placental fragments, atonia; incomplete bladder emptying; fibroids	Process of involution; uterine palpation; activity level after discharge and when to return to work
Bladder	Amount and frequency of voiding; distention; pain or burning on urination; flank tenderness	Normal postpartum diuresis; urinary retention; infection	Proper perineal care to prevent urinary tract infections; adequate fluid intake
Lochia	Amount and type; odor; presence of large clots	Normal involution; possible infection; retained placental fragments; obstructed flow	Changes in lochial appearance; when discharge should cease; proper application of perineal pad; resumption of menstrual periods; resumption of sexual relations; family planning
Perineum	Integrity of suture line; skin temperature and color; amount of discomfort; hemorrhoids	Normal healing; infection; inflammation; hematoma	Perineal care; sitz baths; suture removal; perineal tightening
Bowels	Constipation	Dehydration; inadequate roughage or fluid; discomfort; fear of rupturing episiotomy sutures	Diet history and counseling; assurance of strength of suture line
Abdominal wall	Diastasis	Poor muscle tone	Abdominal tightening; appropriate exercises
Homan's sign	Pain in calf upon flexion of foot with leg extended flat on bed	Possible thrombophlebitis	Inadvisability of leg massage and positions that impede circulation
Emotional status	Dependent, independent; elated, despondent; anorexic	Postpartum "blues," possibly more severe depression; inadequate support systems	"Listening ear"; assurance that mood swings are normal and temporary; referral to proper resource agencies in the community

for 7 seconds and relax; and contract gluteal muscles, press thighs together, and draw in the anus as though trying to stop a bowel movement for 10 seconds and relax slowly. If the gluteal muscles are held contracted during the process of sitting and moving in bed, this will keep the buttocks together, so that the mother sits on them rather than placing pressure on the suture line.

Sometimes the perineal body does not heal well. Scar formation may distort the base of the bladder and contribute to the development of stress urinary incontinence. Incontinence may also result from lack of good sphincter tone; the mother can improve and maintain this tone by periodically stopping urination midstream for a few seconds (Table 11-1).

ABDOMEN

Involution of abdominal muscles and fascia may require six to seven weeks. In some women the abdominal musculature never regains good tone, and the abdominal wall remains flabby and the skin loose. This is most likely to occur when pregnancies follow each other in rapid succession or when the abdomen has been excessively distended and the elastic fibers of the skin ruptured, such as in multiple pregnancies or patients with hydramnios.

The striae gravidarum fade to a silvery color; in other respects the abdominal wall generally resumes its normal appearance after six weeks. There may be marked separation or *diastasis* of the rectus muscles; if this occurs, that portion of the abdominal wall is formed just by peritoneum, thinned-out fascia, subcutaneous fat, and skin. If the mother is asked to raise her head and look toward her feet as she lies flat in bed, her diastasis will become accentuated (Figure 11-2). This provides an excellent opportunity to draw the mother's attention to the condition of her muscles and to interest her in exercises to improve their tone. One such exercise, which she may begin on the first postpartum day as she lies in bed, involves taking a deep breath, raising only her abdomen, and slowly exhaling. As she exhales, she

Figure 11-2. Postpartum diastasis.

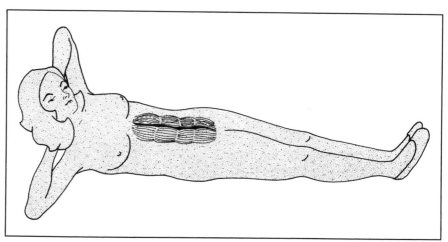

should pull her abdominal muscles in toward her back, hold them contracted for 5–10 seconds, and then relax. She may do this about five times daily.

Although it was formerly thought that an abdominal binder improved muscle tone and hastened involution, it is now known that it has neither effect. A girdle, which may make some women feel more comfortable, is not helpful in this respect either, since the abdominal musculature, not having been exercised, remains as lax as ever when the girdle is removed.

During involution when the abdominal muscles lack tone, they are unable to respond to noxious stimulation by spasm, as is normally the case. Consequently, abdominal rigidity is absent post partum in women who develop a visceral disease such as peritonitis.

SKIN

For the first few days post partum, a mother perspires profusely, especially at night. This normal reversal of the water retention of pregnancy may add to the increased thirst that is characteristic of the postpartum period. The diaphoresis gradually subsides and becomes normal by the end of a week. Since her perspiration sometimes has a strong odor, daily showers are important, not only for good hygiene but also for personal comfort. Because the perspiration is profuse at night, the mother might be advised to wear a hospital gown then and to save her fancy nightgowns for daytime wear.

The pigmentary changes that occur during pregnancy tend to regress during the postpartum period. However, some may never fade completely.

GASTROINTESTINAL SYSTEM

While some mothers may have a poor appetite for the first few days post partum, many more have voracious appetites and begin requesting food while they are still in the recovery room. This seems only natural considering the work of labor and delivery and the length of time without solid food. However, the time without solid food may lead to difficulty in having a spontaneous bowel movement.

Constipation may be a problem for other reasons also. The overstretched abdominal and perineal muscles are less effective in aiding defecation, and intestinal peristalsis is still decreased. Other sources of difficulty in having a bowel movement include perineal pain from an episiotomy, fear of rupturing the sutures, hemorrhoidal pain, and the cleansing enema that the mother may have had before delivery. Even if intravenous fluids have been given during labor, there may still be an imbalance between the fluids taken in and those lost during this period, which may leave intestinal contents drier than normal.

Prior to offering suggestions to alleviate constipation, it is helpful to determine the mother's normal bowel habits and what she usually does to relieve constipation. She may be helped by increasing her fluid intake, some of it perhaps in the form of prune juice, or by including fresh fruits and roughage in her diet. In addition, mothers who are ambulatory appear to have fewer problems with constipation. The relaxation that follows perineal tightening exercises (see page 256) may be of use when the mother is about to have a bowel movement.

If all else fails, a mild cathartic such as milk of magnesia may be ordered for the evening of the second day. If there has been no bowel movement by the morning of the third day, a small enema or a suppository may be ordered.

CARDIOVASCULAR-RESPIRATORY SYSTEM

In the immediate postpartum period, the blood volume remains high, reflecting the increased blood volume of pregnancy. Within a week it returns to normal, as does the leukocytosis, which has been accentuated during labor and immediately after delivery (the leukocytosis will be greater following long labors). During this same period, the plasma fibrinogen and sedimentation rate remain elevated. After labor and delivery the hemoglobin and hematocrit are also elevated as a result of hemoconcentration, but these values should return to normal levels within three to four days post partum, as the mother becomes more hydrated. If the hemoglobin and hematocrit are low, additional iron therapy, rest, and possibly transfusions may be necessary. Iron preparations are often routinely given in the postpartum period to compensate for blood loss during delivery and possible depletion of iron stores during pregnancy. In any case, dietary counseling is necessary, with emphasis on foods high in iron. It is a nursing responsibility to see that this is done.

As the blood volume decreases, women with superficial varicose veins may notice improvement. However, they should continue to wear elastic stockings and to avoid practices that would hinder circulation, since the deeper, larger veins may show less improvement.

The bradycardia sometimes found in the postpartum mother may be in the range of 60–70, but the heart rate may drop to 40 within two days after delivery (by the seventh to tenth day, the heart rate has returned to normal). This lowered heart rate is considered a good sign, whereas an elevated rate may indicate pain, nervousness, blood loss, infection, or cardiac disease. Although the cause is controversial [3], the low heart rate may result from a reduction in cardiac output without a reduction in stroke volume; therefore, the decrease in cardiac output is accomplished by a fall in heart rate [4].

TEMPERATURE

The mother's temperature, as well as pulse rate, is taken frequently in the postpartum period. In normal postpartum mothers, the temperature should not rise above 37.2° C (99.0° F). The transient rise often seen after labor usually falls to normal in 12 hours. While the criteria for febrile temperature elevations vary, that established by the U.S. Joint Committee on Maternal Welfare is generally accepted; they define morbidity as a temperature of 38.0° C (100.4° F) or higher in any two consecutive 24-hour periods during the first 10 days post partum, excluding the first 24 hours.

Temperature elevations appearing about the third postpartum day were once attributed to the milk coming in or "milk fever." Today it is believed that these elevations are probably due to genital infections, although extreme lymphatic and vascular engorgement may cause a temperature spike for a few hours. With even slight elevations, the temperature should be checked every 4 hours until it becomes normal for a minimum of two readings.

Temperature elevations after the first day post partum are usually due to endometritis or infections of the urinary tract. With both types of infection the mother may initially complain of chills and general discomfort.

Temperature elevations due to dehydration occur earlier after labor, generally within the first 24 hours after delivery. The mother is generally not aware of her elevated temperature even though she may have warm dry skin, flushed face, and dry mucous membranes. The mucous membrane between the gum and the cheek is one area that can easily be checked. While the mother's mouth may appear very dry, perhaps due to mouth-breathing, the area between the gum and the cheek will remain moist unless she is dehydrated. With increased fluid intake, the temperature usually returns to normal. Since the oral intake must be increased to as much as 3500 milliliters per day, it may have to be supplemented by intravenous fluids.

URINARY SYSTEM

Soon after delivery there may be an increase in urinary output, possibly because of increased muscular contractions of the kidney pelves and ureters and release of pressure on the ureters from the presenting part. Increased urinary output may also occur if the mother received intravenous fluid during labor or if she was unable to void because of pressure from the presenting part. Diuresis appearing in the first 48 hours post partum has also been attributed to the body's attempt to rid itself of the nitrogenous wastes that accumulate during labor [10] and to a fall in progesterone blood levels [7].

Voiding after delivery may be difficult. The bladder walls, trigone, and urethra may be edematous and hyperemic, with areas of bleeding in the submucosal layers. The bladder capacity post partum is increased, and the bladder may be less sensitive to fluid pressure as a result of trauma by the presenting part or due to the effects of anesthesia. The vulva may also be edematous, which contributes to the problem.

Mothers should void within the first 8 hours after delivery and should be checked carefully during this time for evidence of bladder distention. A full bladder may appear as a rounded area above the symphysis and may displace the uterus to one side, preventing it from remaining firmly contracted.

When the mother has a full bladder, she should be offered the bedpan and allowed to concentrate on voiding in private. If she is unable to void, getting her out of bed to the bathroom may be all that is needed. Other helpful measures might include turning on the faucet and having her listen to the sound of running water, pouring warm water over her vulva, and having her take a warm sitz bath. The relaxation following perineal tightening may be conducive to starting the flow of urine. When the mother does void, the amount of urine should measure over 100–150 milliliters.

Amounts less than this usually indicate incomplete emptying; the residual urine remaining in the bladder serves as a medium for the growth of organisms responsible for urinary tract infections.

If the mother is unable to void or if she voids in small amounts, she will need to be catheterized. Catheterization may be done after she voids small amounts to check the amount of residual urine remaining in the bladder. If there is more than 135 milliliters of residual urine, she should be catheterized after each voiding until the amount of residual urine is approximately 50–60 milliliters. As an alternative to frequent catheterizations, an indwelling catheter may be used for 24 hours, until the edema in the urethra, bladder base, and vulva have subsided. When the indwelling catheter is removed, a culture and sensitivity may be done from the catheter tip or bladder urine to check for possible contamination and infection. After the catheter has been removed, the mother is encouraged to drink fluids; she should void within the next 6–8 hours. When she does void, the nurse should record the time, the amount that she voids, any other significant characteristics of the urine, and the presence or absence of pain with voiding.

Within two to five days after delivery, another period of diuresis may occur as the extra fluids retained during pregnancy are excreted. Mothers may void up to 3000 milliliters per day, as compared to the 1000–1800 milliliters normally excreted. The urine may contain lactose secreted from the breasts as they begin milk production. In tests of the urine for glucose, the lactose will yield false positive results. Protein may also appear in the urine, as cells break down during the process of involution. This is usually gone by the third day, but may last for weeks in trace amounts. Acetone may also appear in the urine after prolonged or difficult labor, but usually disappears within the next three days. Within two to three weeks the dilatation of the kidneys and ureters is significantly decreased; however, complete return to normal size requires six to eight weeks.

BREASTS

Complex physiological changes occur in the breasts during the postpartum period. Estrogen, progesterone, and chorionic somatomammotropin have stimulated mammary growth during pregnancy; these hormones are withdrawn with the delivery of the placenta. The levels of progesterone and particularly estrogen decrease, removing their inhibitory effect on the activity of prolactin, the milk-producing hormone, and lactation begins. The beginning of lactation represents one of the major changes occurring during the postpartum period.

It will be recalled that the breasts are made up of 15–24 lobes arranged radially and separated from each other by fat. Each lobe includes several lobules; in each lobule there are smaller alveoli containing many acini cells. These specialized cells form a single layer of epithelium, beneath which lies a layer of connective tissue rich in capillaries. The epithelial layer produces the various constituents of milk. The lobules have ducts that join to form a single larger lactiferous duct for each lobe. These large ducts widen to form milk reservoirs behind the nipple; they narrow and open separately on its surface (Figure 11-3).

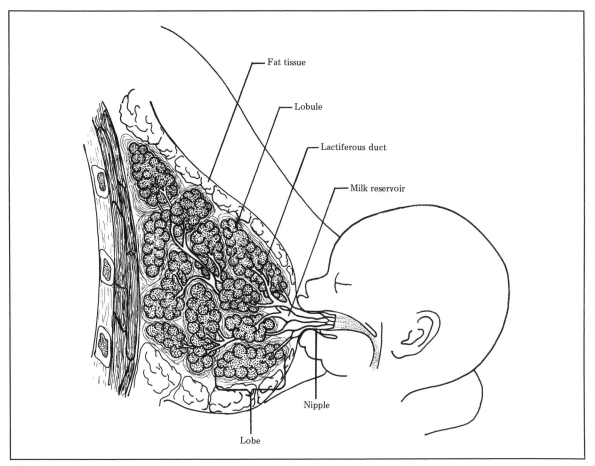

Figure 11-3. The lactating breast, with nursing infant.

There is little change in the condition of the breasts during the first two days post partum. While they do not contain milk, they do produce approximately 150–300 milliliters of colostrum per day. Colostrum, which often has a laxative effect on the newborn, is a yellowish fluid containing more minerals and protein (especially globulin) but less sugar and fat than mature milk. The production of mature milk generally begins on the third day post partum; however, if a newborn nurses within the hour after delivery and frequently thereafter, milk is produced in 24 hours. The breasts are producing only mature milk by the second week post partum.

The intensity and duration of lactation is believed to be dependent on the stimulus of nursing and on the regular withdrawal of milk as well as on the mother's state of mind, health, and nutrition. Through a complex neural mechanism, suckling by the infant not only promotes an adequate supply of milk by stimulating the anterior pituitary to secrete prolactin, but also has a beneficial effect on uterine involution by stimulating oxytocin release from the posterior pituitary.

Mothers who choose not to breast-feed may be given a lactation inhibitor while they are still in labor, immediately after delivery, or during their stay in the hos-

Table 11-2. Lactation Suppressants

Preparations	Administered	Side Effects
Synthetic estrogens		
Diethylstilbestrol	Begun first day after delivery given for five to seven days	Nausea, heavier lochial discharge, greater proportion of bright red blood.
Chlorotrianisene (TACE)	As above	As above
Methallenestril (Vallestril)	As above	As above
Estrogen-androgen combination		
Testosterone Enanthate and Estradiol Valerate (Deladumone OB)	During second stage of labor or immediately after delivery	Virilizing effects: hoarse voice, acne

pital. Estrogens that are given post partum to suppress lactation (Table 11-2) are thought to operate by blocking the peripheral action of prolactin (i.e. milk protein synthesis in the acini cells). It is known that the serum concentration of prolactin is high during pregnancy, but presumably its lactogenic action is prevented then by the elevated circulatory levels of estrogen and progesterone [2]. Some physicians prefer to give estrogen even to nursing mothers, with the intention of preventing engorgement. In India, folk medicine prescribes garlic for the newly lactating mother, since it contains plant estrogens and may prevent overfilling. Many authorities disagree with the practice of prescribing estrogens for nursing mothers, since there are insufficient data on the long-range effects of estrogens on the newborn.

If the mother is untreated and no effort is made to withdraw the milk after it "comes in," the pressure produced by milk remaining in the ducts and alveoli, as well as the pressure produced by the engorged blood vessels and lymphatics, results in the cessation of secretory activity. The engorgement subsides, usually within 24 hours, and lactation ceases. Nursing mothers may also experience engorgement when the milk initially comes in; engorgement may occur later if the breasts are not adequately emptied when the baby nurses.

Engorged breasts are typically hard, full, tender, shiny, and perhaps reddened. The mother may be made more comfortable with a well-fitting supportive brassiere or binder, applications of warm or cold compresses, or mild analgesics. In addition, the nursing mother may relieve some of the tension within her breasts by manually expressing her milk (Figure 11-4), which can be done by placing the fingers on the periphery of the breast and gradually massaging centrally toward the nipple. With this action the milk is worked down into the reservoirs from which it is expressed by massaging the areola. The mother places her thumb and forefinger at the areolar margin, pressing back in toward the chest and bringing the fingers together rhythmically, approximating the action of a baby's jaws. A lotion or ointment on the peripheral portion of the breast lubricates the skin and reduces friction. The manual expression of milk is more effective if warmth has been applied; for this

Figure 11-4. Manual expression of milk. 1. The mother massages her breast, starting from the periphery and working toward the nipple. 2. She then places her thumb and forefinger at the alveolar margin and presses in toward her chest. 3. She then brings her fingers together rhythmically.

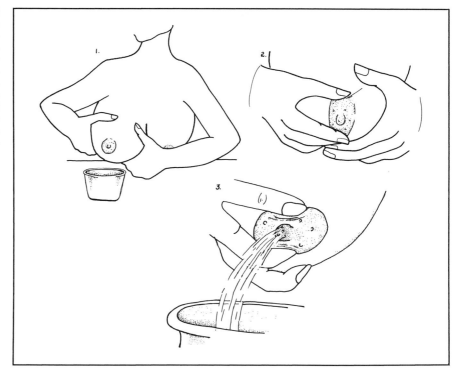

reason, many mothers express their milk during or after their shower. This procedure may be done several times each day if necessary. Many authorities discourage the use of a breast pump in the treatment of engorgement, since they feel that its forceful pull traumatizes the tissues.

Nipples usually require little extra attention in the postpartum period other than cleanliness and attention to fissures. Since dried milk may accumulate and irritate the nipples, the area should be cleaned before nursing with warm water and a soft cloth. Soap should not be used since it removes sebum, which keeps the nipple soft and protected against infection.

Cracked nipples may be caused by an incorrect grasp by the baby. The nipples should be examined under a good light to see whether there is actual cracking or the subepithelial petechiae that are precursors to cracking. Healing measures include exposure to air and light for 20 minutes following nursing. Feeding may need to be discontinued from the involved breast for 24–48 hours, then begun again for periods as short as 3–5 minutes. A healing ointment, such as A and D ointment, may be used. Nipple shields may be advised, although these may cause the mother's nipple to be drawn out considerably, which may delay healing or cause additional trauma.

Some mothers have trouble with leaking milk, which is common until about the sixth week. This problem diminishes as full nursing is established and the internal reservoirs have stretched enough to hold the milk. The mother may find that placing absorbant material, such as gauze pads or a portion of a perineal pad, inside her brassiere will prevent the milk from staining her clothing.

GENERAL CONSIDERATIONS

Ambulation

Prior to World War II, women remained in bed for 7–10 days after delivery. During the war, it was often necessary to evacuate the hospital wards in England, and postpartum women were forced to ambulate early; the results of this experience made earlier ambulation preferred. It improves lochial drainage, circulation (with fewer complications of embolism and thrombophlebitis), bowel and bladder functioning, and muscle tone. Mothers generally state that they feel better and stronger when they have been out of bed and walking about. It is now well accepted that mothers may ambulate in 8–12 hours or less after delivery.

As is the case for any patient allowed to ambulate for the first time, the mother should sit on the side of the bed for 5–10 minutes before getting up. Her feet should be placed flat on a chair rather than allowed to hang over the edge of the bed, in order to promote better circulation in her legs. Mothers should be strongly encouraged to wait for assistance before getting out of bed for the first time, since they often become dizzy or faint.

The mother may shower once she is ambulating, unless she has had a cesarean section or tubal ligation and the incisional area needs to be kept dry. Some physicians encourage sitz baths in the tub to relieve perineal discomfort; others allow full tub baths when the mother is discharged.

In some hospitals, mothers who have had spinal anesthesia are kept in a recumbant position for 8–12 hours to prevent postspinal headaches. It is believed these headaches are due to spinal fluid leakage through the puncture site in the dura, causing a decrease in spinal fluid pressure and subsequent traction on pain-sensitive structures within the cranial cavity (to prevent this, smaller gauge needles are now used in administering anesthesia). If postspinal headache does occur, the mother is encouraged to rest flat in bed and increase her daily fluid intake up to approximately 3500 milliliters. A tight abdominal binder may be applied to increase intra-abdominal venous pressure, thereby increasing cerebrospinal fluid pressure. Analgesics of varying strengths may be used, depending on the severity of the headache.

Weight Loss After Delivery

Once allowed out of bed, mothers invariably want to be weighed. Unfortunately, they are often disappointed to learn that they have not lost as much weight as they had hoped to lose. Approximately 5.4 kilograms (12 pounds) are lost after delivery of the baby and the placenta, and from fluid and blood loss. A further amount of approximately 2.3 kilograms (5 pounds) is lost during the postpartum period, due to fluid loss. By the end of the postpartum period, any weight above prepregnancy weight represents fat, or an increase in breast tissue in those mothers who are breast-feeding.

In discussing weight loss with the mother during this time, the nurse should mention the additional 2.3 kilograms (5 pounds) that the mother may expect to lose in the six weeks after delivery. Also it is an excellent time to discuss diet with her, reviewing her diet history, encouraging well-balanced meals, and discussing ways to safely lose additional weight if she wishes. It is also a good opportunity to point out to the mother the ways in which children mimic their parents' habits. By beginning now, she can encourage her children to develop good eating patterns by practicing them herself. (See Chapter 8 for nutritional needs of the postpartum mother.)

Fertility and Sexual Relations

New mothers are always interested in knowing when they will resume ovulation and normal menstruation. In women who are not breast-feeding, menstruation generally occurs in four to eight weeks. In nursing mothers, menstruation occurs between two and 18 months post partum, although it most commonly returns in four months. Many women experience a very heavy menstrual flow during their first period after delivery, and should be told beforehand that this often happens. The first menstrual period may be anovulatory. Research studies [5] on nursing mothers report that during lactation the ovaries fail to respond to gonadotropins. Others report that the high levels of prolactin produced by vigorous nursing of the infant inhibit pituitary gonadotropins.

For whatever cause, it appears that in the majority of women, lactation results in a temporary infertility. This is especially true in those nursing mothers who also experience amenorrhea during lactation. However, infertility during lactation does not occur in all women, and pregnancy is possible during this period. Nursing mothers should be made aware of this so that they may use contraception if they choose. Oral contraceptive agents should be avoided if possible, since the increased estrogen and progesterone tend to interfere with the peripheral action of prolactin, thus decreasing the supply of milk. This is particularly true in the early stages of lactation. The hormones from the pill are present in the mother's milk, but they are not thought to affect the baby, although there have been few long-range studies on this subject.

Nursing mothers should also realize that when the baby is given early supplementary bottle feedings or solid food, the decreased nursing stimulation will result in a decreased prolactin level. This will increase the mother's ability to conceive as she resumes menstruation and ovulation.

Couples are commonly concerned about the question of when they will be able to resume intercourse. Perineal and uterine wounds should be healed before intercourse is resumed. Masters and Johnson [8] report that this occurs within two to four weeks; most physicians, however, ask couples to abstain until the first postpartum check-up, when it can be determined if healing has taken place. If a couple is unable to wait this long, it is important that the man use a condom to prevent introduction of infectious organisms into the woman's genital tract.

Some couples report a change in sexual desire after childbirth [6], and Masters and Johnson [8] have found in a limited sample of women that their physiological responses were reduced in rapidity and intensity. By three months after delivery these responses were normal again; the mothers who were not nursing recovered faster than the nursing mothers. If sexual response is decreased in the postpartum period, some factors that may contribute to the problem include fatigue, pain, fear, vaginal discharge, poor health, and anxiety about another pregnancy.

Discharge from the Hospital

Most new mothers and babies are discharged from the hospital in five days; however, in some areas they may be discharged in three days or even 24 hours after delivery. The earlier discharge reflects the fact that healthy mothers and babies should not remain in institutions where they may contact organisms resistant to antibiotics. Earlier discharge also reduces the cost of hospitalization. With early discharge, home follow-up is recommended.

As a part of their teaching in preparation for discharge, mothers are encouraged to report any unusual signs or symptoms, such as heavy or foul-smelling lochia or bright bleeding, breast pain (which may indicate mastitis when it occurs around the ninth or tenth day), leg pain (which may indicate venous thrombosis), persistent headache, backache (which may indicate pyelitis), and an elevated temperature. Postpartum instruction also includes teaching the mother the technique and importance of breast self-examination monthly, as described in Chapter 7.

The mother is also asked to resume her normal activities gradually once she is discharged. She should rest for at least 30 minutes when she gets home and several times during the day. If possible, she should avoid climbing stairs, especially for the first three or four days after discharge. If this is not realistic, the mother should limit her stair climbing as much as possible. Most importantly, she should not overtire herself, and she should be told that most women find it difficult to resume normal household activities for at least two weeks. The nurse must do more than merely offer these suggestions to the mother, she must explore with the mother how she will cope with these limitations in a way that will be acceptable to her. Usually before the mother leaves the hospital, she is given an appointment to return to her doctor in four to six weeks for a postpartum check-up.

REFERENCES

1. Adams, H., and Flowers C. E.   Oral oxytocic drugs in the puerperium. *Obstetrics and Gynecology* 15:280, 1960.
2. Brun del Re, R., del Pozo, E., de Grandi, P., Friesen, H., Hinselmann, M., and Wyss, H. Prolactin inhibition and suppression of puerperal lactation by a Br-ergocryptine (CB154). *Obstetrics and Gynecology* 41:884, 1973.
3. Greenhill, J. P., and Friedman, E. A.   *Biological Principles and Modern Practice of Obstetrics.* Philadelphia: Saunders, 1974.
4. Hellman, L. M., and Pritchard, J. A.   *Williams Obstetrics.* New York: Appleton-Century-Crofts, 1971.
5. Keettel, W. C., and Bradbury, J. T.   Endocrine studies of lactation amenorrhea. *American Journal of Obstetrics and Gynecology* 82:995, 1961.
6. Landis, J. T., Poffenberger, T., and Poffenberger, S.   The effects of first pregnancy upon the sexual adjustment of 212 couples. *American Sociological Review* 15:767, 1950.
7. Llewellyn-Jones, D.   *Fundamentals of Obstetrics and Gynecology,* Vol. 1. London: Faber & Faber, 1971.
8. Masters, W. H., and Johnson, V. E.   *Human Sexual Response.* Boston: Little, Brown, 1966.
9. Newton, M., and Bradford, W. M.   Postpartal blood loss. *Obstetrics and Gynecology* 17:229, 1961.
10. Philipp, E.   *Obstetrics and Gynaecology.* London: Lewis, 1970.

FURTHER READING

Applebaum, R. M.   *Abreast of the Times*. Miami: Applebaum, 1969.

Boyarsky, S., and Goldenberg, J.   Detection of bladder distention by suprapubic percussion. *New York Journal of Medicine* 62:1804, 1962.

Broadribb, V., and Corliss, C.   *Maternal-Child Nursing*. Philadelphia: Lippincott, 1973.

Clausen, J., Flook, M., Ford, B., Green, M., and Popiel, E.   *Maternity Nursing Today*. New York: McGraw-Hill, 1973.

Dewhurst, C. J. (Ed.).   *Integrated Obstetrics and Gynaecology for Post Graduates*. Melbourne: Blackwell Scientific, 1972.

Fitzpatrick, E., Reeder, S., and Mastroianni, L.   *Maternity Nursing*. Philadelphia: Lippincott, 1971.

Guttmacher, A. F.   *Pregnancy, Birth and Family Planning*. New York: Viking, 1973.

Kilker, R., and Wilkerson, B.   8-Point postpartum assessment. *Nursing '73* 3:56, 1973.

Law, R. G., and Friedman, M.   *Midwifery*. London: Staples, 1972.

Lerch, C.   *Maternity Nursing*. St. Louis: Mosby, 1970.

Morley, G. W.   The important "Ten B's" of postpartum hospital care. *Hospital Topics* 44:107, 1966.

Sherman, J.   *On the Psychology of Women*. Springfield, Ill.: Thomas, 1971.

Taylor, E. S.   *Beck's Obstetrical Practice*. Baltimore: Williams & Wilkins, 1971.

Wiedenbach, E.   *Family Centered Maternity Nursing*. New York: Putnam, 1967.

Wilson-Clyne, D.   *A Concise Textbook for Midwives*. London: Faber & Faber, 1971.

Ziegel, E., and Van Blarcom, C.   *Obstetric Nursing*. New York: Macmillan, 1972.

Chapter 12 Adapting to Parenthood

Following the exhausting effort of labor and delivery, the mother faces the task of making many readjustments, physiological as well as psychological. During labor she has concentrated her energy on coping with that experience. The mother, as well as the father, faces the postpartum period with the work of realizing that the baby has actually been born, beginning the tasks of parenting, and assuming new roles.

TAKING-IN

Reva Rubin [7, 8, 9, 10, 11], one of the most widely quoted authors on the subject of maternal behavior in the postpartum period, has identified the specific phases through which the mother passes. The first, or taking-in phase, usually begins with a deep refreshing sleep following delivery. At first the mother may not perceive how exhausted she really is because of initial feelings of exhilaration brought about by giving birth or because of emotional tension generated by her feelings of anticlimax and emptiness caused by separation from the baby. It has been reported that the mother may have sleep hunger for several days if this initial sleep is interrupted. This should have bearing on how nursing care is planned in the immediate postpartum period.

Rubin describes the mother's behavior during this phase as passive and dependent. She accepts what she is given, tries to follow directions, and makes few decisions on her own. Almost all mothers wish to discuss what they recall of their labor and delivery. It is as if a reconstruction of their experience confirms the reality of the postdelivery period. Nurses can be very supportive listeners, and their interaction is even more meaningful to the mother if they have been with her during labor and delivery. Because of the importance of this reconstruction process, labor floor nurses should make a special effort to visit their patients post partum.

During the taking-in phase, sleep and food take on added physiological as well as psychological importance in the mother's life. She may often state that she is hungry and require extra snacks throughout the day to become satisfied. This is a good example of how food plays an important part in the asking for care and the giving of care. She may also express concern about the oral intake of her baby. It is important that nurses take time to listen to the mother and to satisfy her needs and concerns as much as possible, which will help to reinforce the mother's feeling that she and the baby are very important people.

The father, at this time, may find that he must assume the companionship and supportive roles for the family. At the same time he may also be experiencing conflicting feelings and may feel exhausted by the emotional strain of the baby's delivery. He may be concerned about the mother and about her passivity and dependency. If he realizes that this is to be expected, it will be easier for him to assume responsibilities for making decisions and for maintaining the routine of home and family, responsibilities that have been previously shared. He may receive adequate support from the nursing staff if they maintain open lines of communication with him, providing him with the information and assistance he needs to cope with the changing needs of his new family.

TAKING-HOLD

As the mother's inner resources become replenished during the first few days post partum, she begins to become impatient with her dependency. Rubin describes the *taking-hold* phase, during which the mother expresses concerns about the present, particularly regaining control over her own bodily functions. Her anxieties may be increased by doubts about her ability to care adequately for her new baby. Insignificant difficulties she has in handling him may become monumental reinforcements of the concerns she is beginning to feel. Special privileges that were hers alone during pregnancy must now be shared with the baby.

One mother [12] has written of her conflicting feelings during this time; her recollections of old childhood experiences and strange dreams, both pleasant and terrifying exemplify postpartum introspection. The feelings that she recalls disappeared within a week, as she met success in caring for her baby and became reinvolved with her career.

During the taking-hold phase, the mother becomes more involved with her baby, which facilitates both the development of maternal concern and the tasks of mothering. As she meets success in caring for her newborn, her concern extends to other family members at home and what their activities have been in her absence.

With early discharge of maternity patients, most of the period of transition to mothering occurs after the mother has gone home. From a teaching viewpoint, it is unfortunate that the stage of her maximal readiness for learning is found now, when nursing staff are not as immediately available to her. Therefore, the time the nurse spends with her in the hospital becomes even more valuable, since an accurate assessment of her needs paves the way for the health teaching, anticipatory guidance, and appropriate referral necessary for a smooth transition to motherhood.

It is not uncommon for mothers at some time during the postpartum period to experience frequent temporary mood swings and to feel very vulnerable. Many factors may contribute to this disequilibrium, including the hormonal changes of childbearing, ego regression accompanying increased dependency needs, and discomfort, fatigue, and exhaustion following labor and delivery. In addition, she may be overwhelmed by her responsibilities when she goes home or by those responsibilities inherent in her new role. Therefore it is important to build up the mother's confidence in herself. Such reassurance is rarely solicited by the mother but is gratefully accepted whenever it is offered, particularly in the case of primigravidas.

During this period, the mother may cry for no apparent reason, be irritable, or have a poor appetite or insomnia. These "postpartum blues" often appear about the third day after delivery. A mother may feel guilty about such unaccustomed behavior, especially when she can assign no reason to it; she needs to be reassured that it is normal and acceptable. More severe or prolonged depression is usually a sign of a more serious condition.

During the time of the mother's taking-hold, her anxieties may be increased if the father becomes, as Anderson et al. [1] note, "totally involved with the baby and does not evaluate and respond to the mother's feelings and reactions. . . . Proud and elated over the prospect of parenthood, he may not be sufficiently in tune with the unspoken doubts and questions the mother may have." His behavior may be reinforced by her mood swings and, at times, unpredictable behavior. Skillful nurse-parent interactions now should encourage the couple to share ideas and feelings, which strengthens the family bonds. Encouragement and praise, along with constant reinforcement and careful teaching, are essential components of the nursing care of the new family.

FATHER'S ROLE

In today's society, the new role of father may bring with it many conflicts. One of these conflicts may exist between the traditional role of father as breadwinner and head of the household, and a more recently accepted role in which parental authority is shifted to the mother, with fathers assuming some of the nurturant and affectional functions traditionally associated with mothering. With this shift toward greater homogeneity in parental roles, it is generally accepted that fathers may enjoy tender feelings toward their children, but many must still cope with the old concepts of masculine ruggedness and aggressiveness.

Hines [3] notes that "in an environment where the feelings of the father are allowed to be expressed without censure, without fear of embarrassment, and without anyone accusing him of being unmanly, the father does show evidence of deep feelings for his baby right after birth." Today more of these feelings are being openly expressed. A father's investment in the birth of his child is increased by not simply allowing but encouraging fathers to participate during the prenatal period and during labor and delivery, with the support of members of the health team. This participation may also increase his feelings of adequacy as a new father, a mate, and possibly a man; in addition, it reinforces his feelings that the children are also his responsibility, not simply that of the mother. Far too many health personnel, however, continue to focus on maternal-infant interactions, and support the father little, if at all, in his adaptation to parenting.

Encouraging the father to have physical contact with his newborn from the time of birth certainly aids in the transition to fathering (Figure 12-1). He, as well as the mother, should benefit from the support and guidance of the health team in adjusting to and caring for his newborn. In some families where the mother-infant relationship is inadequate, the father-child relationship serves as a balance to support the child.

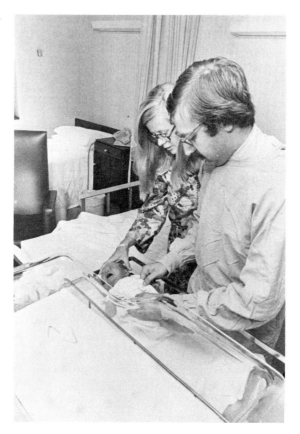

NEEDS CONCEPTUALIZED BY MOTHERS

Various studies have attempted to define the most pressing postpartum needs identified by the mothers themselves (Table 12-1). Lesser and Keane [5] outline three main physical needs expressed by mothers: sleep and rest, relief of discomfort, and bodily care. Emotional needs as identified by mothers in their study were more encompassing; these mothers wanted freedom from responsibility at home, freedom from anxiety, and a choice in whether or not they had to care for the baby initially. Lesser and Keane noted that the mothers' anxiety was relieved by the feeling or knowledge that their babies were in good hands and in good condition. They wanted to be allowed to examine their infants carefully to satisfy any questions they might have in this regard. They also wanted assurance that their own physical recovery was proceeding normally and expressed a desire for consistent information from the various staff members with whom they had contact. It is extremely important therefore to have a viable and consistently used system for record keeping and reporting, which makes it possible for mothers to receive consistent information.

The mother needs the nursing staff's acceptance of her dependency. Unfortunately the attitudes of staff members can easily convey the message that such

Table 12-1. Needs Verbalized by Postpartum Mothers

Need	Primiparas (11)	Multiparas (15)
More rest and sleep at home	9	4
More help in the home to allow more time for recovery	8	7
Help in planning baby care	9	2
Guidance in reestablishment of family relationships	4	9
Good meal planning for self and family	5	6
Knowledge regarding family planning	5	5

Source: Modified from E. Henning, G. Martoglio, M. Quita, J. Reinbrecht, and M. Strickland. A Dynamic Nursing Appraisal of the Puerperium. In N. Lytle (Ed.), *Maternal Health Nursing.* Dubuque, Iowa: Wm. C. Brown, 1967.

behavior is acceptable for only a short time and that after this period, since the mother is not "ill," she is expected to care for herself.

In the mother's transition from dependency to independence, the nurse is the primary person who helps her achieve this goal, by offering guidance as she resumes care for herself. Although many nurses automatically assume that multiparas do not need such help, this is not always the case. The security of the mother is best fostered by the noncritical nurse, one who stays by her side for a period of time and indicates her willingness to offer help. Again, whatever is being taught, it is imperative that the teaching be consistent; communication among staff members is essential.

Mothers who elect rooming-in are generally more successful in getting their needs satisfied [5], although the personality of the mother herself determines in part how well this occurs. The mother who verbalizes her questions is more likely to get them answered, but even she may be inhibited by an unfriendly or unwilling nurse. The nurse can be her chief source of gratification or denial, and the nurse is the key person responsible for whether or not the mother has a fulfilling postpartum hospital stay or one that reinforces her doubts, fears, and anxieties.

NEEDS CONCEPTUALIZED BY NURSES

Lesser and Keane [5] report that nurses generally recognize all the needs that the patients themselves reveal; however, their emphasis is different from that of the mothers. Many nurses believe that mothers have very little need for physical care and that they are an independent, happy group. They identify their chief function as teaching the mother care of herself and of the baby. They rarely mention the mother's need for a period of dependence and do not emphasize their possible role in meeting these dependency needs.

The degree to which nurses can successfully achieve this goal depends on their view of the postpartum needs of the mother. If nurses view her as an independent person with few needs other than physical ones, this lack of perspective provides a barrier to her effective care. There is another barrier inherent in this view. If nurses do not feel needed, their jobs may become routine, and their dissatisfaction leads them to seek gratification in ways other than direct patient contact. It is little wonder, then, that the mother feels that the nurses are not interested in her.

Another barrier may be found in the traditional separation of mothers and babies, with different nursing staffs caring for each. Nurses caring for the baby usually have limited contact with the mother, and that contact is only when the baby is being fed. This may not be sufficient time for the mother's questions to be answered or for her to receive enough information about her baby's progress. One remedy, of course, is to make additional visits to the mothers between feedings. The postpartum nurse tends to be concerned mainly with the mother's physical needs. The two nursing staffs often do not have common goals. Dual reports, given at change of shift, may ensure that the care of mother and baby is better coordinated. Another idea might be joint classes given by both staffs for groups of mothers, although some mothers may still need more individualized attention.

Nurses may create their own barriers by stereotyping groups of patients, by lacking insight to recognize the need that underlies a more superficial request, or by being unable to sympathize with the attitudes or goals of the mother.

Another barrier to effective care arises when nurses are pressed for time; the nurses then consider only those needs they judge to be essential, giving cursory attention to human relationships and needs for teaching and emotional support. Discharge instructions may be left for the last few hectic moments before the mother leaves the hospital.

PARENTING TASKS

Nurses may provide crucial support to parents as they assume their new roles and establish initial relationships with their newborn (Table 12-2). One of the parents' first tasks is recognizing the separate identity of their baby and establishing his individuality [7], a process which begins with their initial inspection of him after delivery. This is the time when parents first notice his specific features, and make such comments as "He has his mother's eyes" or "his father's chin." This association with others illustrates their initial problem in seeing him as a separate individual, with characteristics of his own. At the first opportunity, parents should be allowed to unwrap the baby and do a more thorough inspection. Nurses may use this occasion to explain some of the variations in newborns that may seem unusual to the parents, such as the cord stump, milia, and molding of the head. Now is a good time to observe relationships between the parents, and between them and their infant, for clues about family interaction and cohesiveness (Figure 12-2).

At this time parents are confronted with the reality of their newborn and they must reconcile this with their fantasies of the child they had expected, who may have been of the opposite sex. Sex is probably the major basis for the initial identification process [7]. It can have a strong influence on parents' reactions to the baby, on their handling of him, and on their emotional response of acceptance or rejection. If the differences between the characteristics of the idealized child and the real child are never really resolved in the parents' minds, the effects on their rela-

Table 12-2. Family Interactions with Newborn

Assessment	Intervention
Parents' interactions	
Are the parents interacting comfortably with each other?	Provide an environment in which parents can openly express feelings. Acknowledge that becoming parents requires new roles and responsibilities and that this adjustment often takes time
Parent-infant interactions	
Are the parents comfortable holding him?	Encourage and support both parents in holding him
Are the parents familiar with newborn care?	Teach both parents bathing, feeding, dressing, general hygiene of the newborn, how to cope with his behavior; have them care for their baby before discharge to increase their expertise and confidence in caring for him
Do the parents refer to him by name; make eye contact with him; talk to him?	Provide a role model by talking to the baby, making eye contact and calling him by name; explain the importance of this interaction
Do they refer to features that make him unique?	Encourage both parents to examine the baby closely, and emphasize features that make him unique; perform newborn physical examination with parents present
What was their "fantasized child"?	Emphasize the positive and unique features of their real child
Sibling Reactions	
What are the reactions of other siblings?	Maintain contact between mother and other siblings by phone or visit. Small gift from mother to other children. Emphasis on the uniqueness of each child: brother's ability to talk when baby can only cry; later other siblings will be able to teach new baby how to do the things they can do

tionship with the child may be long lasting. One example known to the authors is a woman who had desperately wanted a girl but had a boy, now 8 years old. She has consistently chosen feminine styles of boy's clothing (and sometimes girl's coats) for him to wear, and she has also painted his fingernails red when he was not in school.

Another important task parents face is determining their relationship to their infant. They must identify his obvious needs, assume responsibility for him, and in some way accommodate their life-style in order to care for him. This becomes readily apparent once the family goes home and assumes total responsibility for the baby. The mother, for instance, may realize she is in need of milk for the baby; she prepares to leave for the grocery store, only to realize that the baby cannot be left unattended. A couple may decide to go to the movies, and then realize they must find a babysitter, one who is able to take care of a newborn.

Parents are also faced with the tasks of reorganizing the family grouping to include the new member and establishing mutually satisfying roles for themselves. This must include regulating the demands of the infant and of the home environ-

Figure 12-2. Nurse performing routine newborn physical examination and explaining newborn variations to the parents. (Courtesy of Booth Maternity Center, Philadelphia, Pa.)

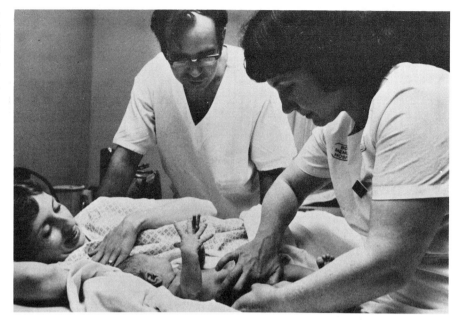

ment, and modifying those demands that parents impose upon themselves. What frustrations might now be generated in a compulsive house cleaner!

Siblings likewise may become frustrated. Young children often experience anger, guilt, and feelings of desertion when their mother disappears to bring back a new

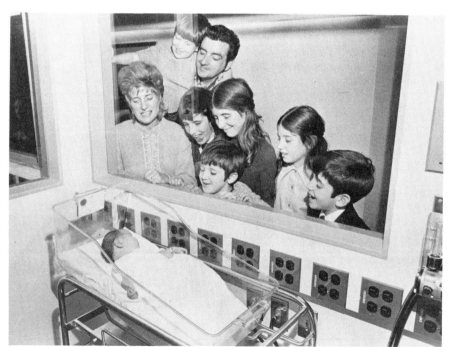

Figure 12-3. Children meeting their new brother. (Courtesy of Pennsylvania Hospital, Philadelphia, Pa.)

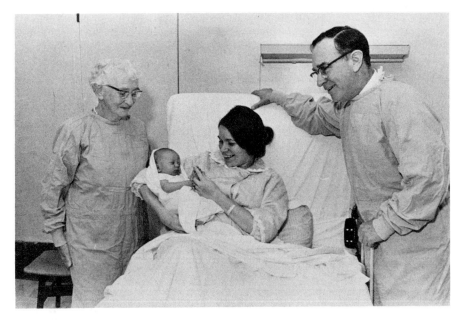

Figure 12-4. The infant develops warm supporting relationships with grandparents who are attuned to his needs. (Courtesy of Pennsylvania Hospital, Philadelphia, Pa.)

baby. After the new baby comes home, they may show jealousy and resentment and may act out these feelings in a variety of ways. Young children particularly may hesitate to approach their mother on her return, which can be very upsetting to her, especially if she is unaware that this is a common and very temporary reaction. Siblings are often more accepting of the new baby if they are able to visit the mother while she is in the hospital and to see the new baby (Figure 12-3). If this is not possible, if children are made to feel that they are still very special people, by being given extra love and attention and perhaps a small gift, they feel more secure and better able to relate to the new baby.

While all parents are faced with basically the same tasks, the quality of their performance differs. A child's normal development is fostered in the atmosphere that is created when parents have warm loving relationships with each other, with their children and with members of the extended family (Figure 12-4). It is further enhanced when the infant is able to develop long-lasting relationships with one or more people who are attuned to his needs. The strongest attachment, however, may not always be with the mother. The amount of warm adult-child interaction is an important stimulus in the development of intelligence and language [13], as well as in the development of his innate personality characteristics.

NEEDS OF THE INFANT

Parents are well aware that each infant communicates his individuality from the time of birth. Each infant's level of activity may differ, as well as the intensity of his responses to stimuli. Likewise the amount of stimuli needed to evoke a response in a particular infant may vary. It is possible to find in the same family one baby who is friendly and pleasant and who adapts easily to changes in his environment and another who responds in just the opposite manner. All of these factors do play an important part in the parents' reaction to their infant. If the parents' initial interactions with the baby are rewarded with his positive responses, the parents are more likely to continue with frequent and meaningful interactions.

While each infant exhibits different personality characteristics, infants do share patterns of behavior. Ribble [6] has investigated many of their early psychological needs. Babies receive most of their stimulation orally. For the first six months, sucking is their most satisfying and all-absorbing activity, and the baby requires frequent stimulation from it. Through it they satisfy their hunger and thirst, decrease tension, and receive comfort. Feeding serves as an important time for interaction between parents and their infant. The interaction is enhanced toward the end of the second month, when the baby is able to focus on them and on the sound of their voices, and by the end of the third month, when he turns his head and smiles at them. Babies who are not held and fondled show excessive sucking habits and frequently take in too much food, resulting in digestive upsets.

Spontaneous mouthing movements at birth are not always coordinated. Many infants breast-feeding for the first time fail to respond with effective coordinated sucking. This can be disconcerting to a mother, who may then think of herself as a failure, or may think that there is a defect in her child.

While the sense of touch is best developed in the mouth, the infant's face and head are also sensitive. Parents will find that gentle stroking of the head soothes a restless infant in a remarkable way. The sense of touch in the skin, while not so well developed at birth, is increased through the handling involved in baby care.

It is interesting to note that the tactile contact mothers first have with their infants proceeds in an orderly fashion [4]. The mother begins touching with her fingertips on the baby's extremities, and then proceeds to massage the baby's trunk with her palm. Still later the mother brings the baby closer to her own body and enfolds him. The activity changes from an exploratory kind of touching to a warm acceptance. Whether fathers follow this same progression of tactile contact has not been researched.

A sense of body position is well developed in many babies at birth. Gentle movement, firm holding, frequent changes of position, and rocking are important in the development of a sense of security in the infant. Some babies do not nurse well when they are not held securely.

Parents should be aware that the baby at birth is sensitive to light and readily adjusts himself to it. Staring is an important activity; in addition, eye-to-eye contact between parents and the infant appears to be important during the development of affectional ties. In one study, mothers stated that once the infants looked at them, they felt much closer to their babies [4] (Figure 12-5).

Sensitivity to sound is also well developed in the newborn. The human voice is important in bringing reassurance to the baby; nurses should encourage parents to talk frequently to their infants. While the infant gives a startled response to sudden loud noises, he may give an equally strong reaction to the stillness of a very quiet room.

The sensitivity of the infant to all of these stimuli is not usually appreciated by adults. The quality and quantity of his stimulation has to be as carefully considered as his food intake.

Figure 12-5. Eye-to-eye contact between parents and infants appears to be important during the development of affectional ties. (Courtesy of Pennsylvania Hospital, Philadelphia, Pa.)

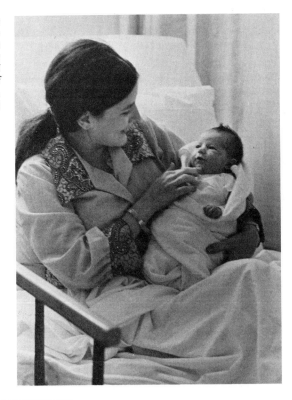

REFERENCES

1. Anderson, B., Camacho, M., and Stark, J. *Pregnancy and Family Health.* New York: McGraw-Hill, 1974.
2. Henning, E., Martoglio, G., Quita, M., Reinbrecht, J., and Strickland, M. A Dynamic Nursing Appraisal of the Puerperium. In N. Lytle (Ed.), *Maternal Health Nursing.* Dubuque, Iowa: W. C. Brown, 1967.
3. Hines, J. Father, the forgotten man. *Nursing Forum* 10:176, 1971.
4. Klaus, M., Kennell, J., Plumb, N., and Zuehlke, S. Human maternal behavior at the first contact with her young. *Pediatrics* 46:187, 1970.
5. Lesser, M., and Keane, V. *Nurse-Patient Relationships in a Hospital Maternity Service.* St. Louis: Mosby, 1956.
6. Ribble, M. *The Rights of Infants.* New York: Columbia University Press, 1965.
7. Rubin, R. Basic maternal behavior. *Nursing Outlook* 9:683, 1961.
8. Rubin, R. Puerperal change. *Nursing Outlook* 9:753, 1961.
9. Rubin, R. Maternal touch. *Nursing Outlook* 11:828, 1963.
10. Rubin, R. Attainment of the maternal role. 1. Processes. *Nursing Research* 16:237, 1967.
11. Rubin, R. Attainment of the maternal role. 2. Models and referrants. *Nursing Research* 16:342, 1967.
12. Rudolph, S. H. Notes from a maternity ward. *The Atlantic Monthly* 211:122, 1963.
13. Rutter, M. *Maternal Deprivation Reassessed.* Baltimore: Penguin, 1972.

FURTHER READING

Benedek, T. Psychobiological aspects of mothering. *American Journal of Orthopsychiatry* 26:272, 1956.

Bowlby, J. *Maternal Care and Mental Health.* New York: Schocken, 1966.

Brenton, B. *The Male in Crisis.* New York: Coward-McCann, 1966.

Clark, A. L.   The adaptation problems and patterns of an expanding family: the neonatal period. *Nursing Forum* 5:92, 1966.

Clark, A. L.   The beginning family. *American Journal of Nursing* 66:802, 1966.

Clausen, J., Flook, M., Ford, B., Green, M., and Popiel, E.   *Maternity Nursing Today.* New York: McGraw-Hill, 1973.

Eckes, S.   The significance of increased early contact between mother and newborn infant. *Journal of Obstetric, Gynecologic and Neonatal Nursing* 3:42, 1974.

Gordon, R., Kapostins, E., and Gordon, K.   Factors in postpartum emotional adjustment. *Obstetrics and Gynecology* 25:158, 1965.

Josselyn, I.   Cultural forces, motherliness and fatherliness. *American Journal of Orthopsychiatry* 26:264, 1956.

Kagan, J.   The child: His struggle for identity. *Saturday Review* 51:80, 1968.

Lidz, T.   *The Person.* New York: Basic Books, 1968.

Newton, N., and Newton, M.   Mothers' reactions to their newborn babies. *Journal of the American Medical Association* 181:206, 1962.

Rising, S.   The fourth stage of labor: Family Integration. *American Journal of Nursing* 74:870, 1974.

Thomas, A., Chess, S., and Birch, H.   The origin of personality. *Scientific American* 223:102, 1970.

Warrick, L.   Femininity, sexuality, and mothering. *Nursing Forum* 8:212, 1969.

Chapter 13 The Normal Newborn

PHYSICAL EXAMINATION OF THE NEWBORN

All newborns should be thoroughly examined immediately after birth, while the newborn is in the delivery room, and more thoroughly once he is taken to the nursery. On each of these occasions the results of the examination should be shared with the parents, if they cannot be present during it, so that they do not experience undue anxiety about the condition of their infant.

Nurses who are responsible for providing care to the newborn and the family should be able to do a competent physical examination of the newborn, whether it is in the hospital (when he is admitted to the nursery and prior to his discharge) or on follow-up visits in the home, clinic, or doctor's office. In addition to assessing the physical status of the baby, the data establish an initial baseline for the evaluation of future changes in the infant.

Prior to performing a physical examination, the nurse should review the estimated date of confinement, duration of labor, and type of delivery, as well as any problems such as maternal diabetes, rubella, hemolytic conditions, and addiction, that would place the infant at risk. The examination itself should be systematic and thorough, and the nurse should remember that just as newborns vary in temperament, so do they exhibit a variety of physical variations that are within normal ranges. When beginning the newborn examination, the nurse should first make those observations that can be done with minimal disturbance to the newborn.

Posture, Length, and Weight

Most normal newborns assume a characteristic symmetrical posture. When placed on his abdomen, the infant turns his face to one side, flexes his arms, and holds them close to his trunk. His hands are tightly fisted. His back is bent and his hips are flexed, with his knees drawn up on his abdomen and his pelvis raised off the examining table or mattress (Figure 13-1). Infants born in a breech position have a tendency to keep their knees and legs straightened rather than flexed, or they may maintain a frog-leg position, depending on the type of breech presentation. Infants born with a face presentation have a tendency to assume an arched posture (opisthotonus). Posture that is not symmetrical may be caused by fractures, commonly of the clavicle or humerus, or by nerve injuries, commonly to the brachial plexus.

The average length of the full-term infant is 51 centimeters (20 inches). Ninety-five percent of all full-term newborns measure in the range 46–56 centimeters (18–22 inches).

Figure 13-1. Normal posture of the full-term newborn.

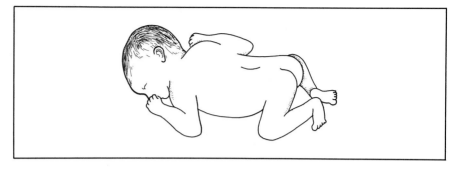

In most hospital nurseries, the baby's weight is checked at a fixed time each day. The average birth weight of white male infants in the United States is 3400 grams (7½ pounds); white female infants weigh approximately 3200 grams (7 pounds). The weight of 80 percent of full-term newborns falls within the range 2900–4100 grams (6 pounds, 5 ounces, to 9 pounds, 2 ounces). Negro and Asian infants are generally smaller at birth, while those of Northern European ancestry tend to be larger.

Newborns lose up to 10 percent of their birth weight in the first three to five days after birth but generally regain it in another week. The weight loss is attributed to a loss of fluid from body tissues and to a relatively low food and fluid intake.

Skin

The newborn's skin should be examined (under strong natural light) for color, edema, ecchymoses, pigmentary changes, scaliness and desquamation, and hemangiomas. During the first 24 hours after birth, the newborn's skin is generally smooth and reddish and may be covered with vernix caseosa, which disappears in about a day if it is not removed. The redness of the skin is due to a high concentration of red cells in the blood vessels, which are closer to the skin's surface because of the lack of subcutaneous fat [2]. The red skin blush changes to a pink hue in the following day or so, and the skin becomes more flaky. Marked scaliness and desquamation is a sign of postmaturity.

The infant's extremities may appear cyanotic after birth (acrocyanosis) due to immature peripheral circulation, with the feet usually showing more cyanosis than the hands. In addition to being cyanotic, the feet may be cold to touch. The infant who becomes cyanotic when crying may be showing signs of some forms of congenital heart disease; if he is cyanotic at rest with relief upon crying, he may be exhibiting signs of pulmonary dysfunction. An infant who has been previously well and suddenly becomes cyanotic and apneic may have thick mucus obstructing his upper respiratory tract. Any generalized pallor in the infant may be due to poor cardiac function, anemia from hemorrhagic disease, or acute blood loss. Pale conjunctiva and mucous membrane of the mouth may also indicate anemia.

Physiological jaundice is noticeable in less than one-half of all newborns. It generally appears on the second or third day, peaks at about a week, and has disappeared in two weeks. It first appears in the skin over the face or upper body and then progresses to encompass a larger area. The initial faint yellow may deepen into orange and become noticeable in the conjunctiva of the eyes. Jaundice may be difficult to observe in infants of low birth weight; because of their decreased subcutaneous fat, the capillaries are close to the surface of the skin, and the color of hemoglobin obscures the jaundice.

Jaundice in the newborn is caused by immaturity of the liver. As red blood cells are broken down, low levels of liver enzymes (mainly glucuronyl transferase) are not able to conjugate bilirubin, and its excretion is delayed. In the newborn, jaundice becomes noticeable when total serum bilirubin rises from a normal level of approximately 1 milligram per 100 milliliters to 5 milligrams per 100 milliliters. Unless there is a pathological hemolytic condition, the levels do not usually exceed 10–12 milligrams per 100 milliliters during the newborn period. The bilirubin levels in breast-fed infants are generally higher than in those who are bottle fed, presumably because the pregnanediol in breast milk inhibits the action of glucuronyl transferase. Some research indicates that if breast-feeding is discontinued for 24 hours, allowing glucuronyl transferase to become operative, resumption of breast-feeding no longer has the inhibitory effect [2, 16, 18].

The presence of edema in the newborn is another important observation for the nurse to make. The subcutaneous tissues around his eyes, legs, hands, and feet may occasionally be edematous for several days. The fine wrinkles over the dorsal aspect of the hands and feet of the normal newborn are not discernible in an edematous infant. Severe pitting edema may be due to heart failure, congenital heart disease, erythroblastosis, or electrolyte imbalance.

In the immediate period after birth, there may be marked edema and ecchymoses over the presenting part. In a vertex presentation there may be significant edema of the scalp (caput succedaneum), which regresses in about two days without treatment. This extravasation of serum into the soft tissues of the scalp occurs over the area that was encircled by the cervix; it is particularly evident when labor has been prolonged, causing membranes to rupture and the cervix to fail to dilate fully (Figure 13-2).

In breech presentations, there may be edema and ecchymoses of the buttocks or feet, while in shoulder presentations, the shoulder and arm may be affected. Ecchymoses may appear on other parts of the body following a difficult delivery, or they may indicate an infection or bleeding problem. The serum bilirubin may increase when ecchymoses are extensive [19].

Pinpoint hemorrhages (petechiae) may also be seen on the newborn's skin due to increased intravascular pressure, infection, or thrombocytopenia. These hemorrhages generally regress in 24–48 hours.

The nurse can test for petechiae, jaundice, and ecchymoses by applying direct pressure to the skin, either with the fingers or with a microscope slide. When both index fingers or both thumbs are placed on the baby's skin and then drawn apart while maintaining pressure, petechiae, jaundice, and ecchymoses will not disappear upon blanching, but red rashes caused by local vascular engorgement will disappear.

The most common red rash found on the newborn is called *newborn rash* or *erythema toxicum;* it usually appears on the trunk and diaper area. The rash con-

Figure 13-2. Caput succedaneum, a diffuse edematous swelling of the soft tissues of the scalp overlying the presenting part, which may cross the suture lines. It is caused by pressure of the cervix on the fetus' head during labor.

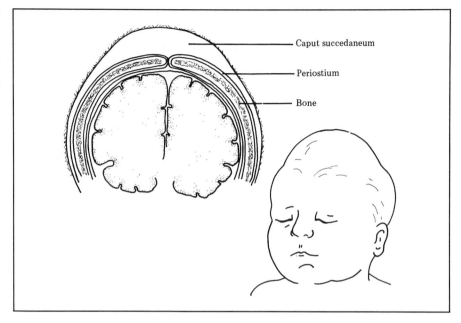

sists of pinkish-red papules, which frequently contain vesicles (Figure 13-3). Since the vesicles contain eosinophils, they give the appearance of being pathological and are often confused with staphylococcal infections. In order to differentiate between erythema toxicum and a staphylococcal infection, several of the lesions might be circled with a pen. Usually the lesions of erythema toxicum disappear in a few hours, whereas septic lesions will not. The entire rash usually regresses in 48 hours.

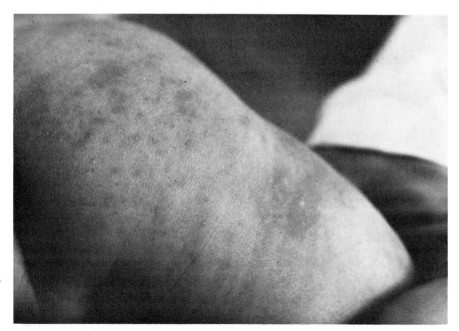

Figure 13-3. Newborn rash, or erythema toxicum. (Courtesy of Mead Johnson Laboratories, Evansville, Ind.)

Hemangiomas are vascular lesions that are usually present at birth in infants who have them. Port-wine stain (nevus flammeus) appears at birth as a flat, purple or dark-red lesion, appearing most commonly around the scalp and face. Those found over the bridge of the nose may fade, but the others usually do not and require cosmetics for concealment (Figure 13-4).

Strawberry hemangiomas may be present at birth, but most often they appear two or three weeks after birth. They are elevated bright-red lesions containing a collection of small immature blood vessels. They usually regress before the age of 4, but it may take as long as 10 years.

Stork bites (telangiectatic nevi) are flat red or purple lesions with irregular edges, found most often on the back of the neck, lower occiput, upper eyelid, and bridge of the nose. The lesions are areas of capillary dilatation that enlarge and fill when the infant cries. They are very common and disappear in approximately two years.

A rather rare nonpathological condition is *harlequin color change.* When the infant is placed on his side, the dependent half of his body turns red, while the upper half becomes pale. The color changes from the head to the pubic area and stops laterally, abruptly at the midline. Vasomotor instability and the effects of gravity are suggested as causes [23].

In Negro and Asian infants and those of southern European heritage, areas of blue pigmentation are commonly found over the lower back, sacrum, and buttocks. These *mongolian spots,* which parents often confuse with bruises, are nonpathological and usually regress by four years of age (Figure 13-5).

Another very common finding is *milia neonatorum* (Figure 13-6), which consists of enlarged sebaceous glands usually found about the nose but also on the chin, cheeks, and forehead. They usually regress in several days to a week or two. Because they resemble whiteheads, mothers are often tempted to squeeze them; they should be told of the risk of infection from squeezing and cautioned not to do so.

Head

The newborn's head and face should be examined for symmetry, paralysis, weakness, shape, swelling, and movement. The infant's head generally has a biparietal circumference of 33–35 centimeters (13–14 inches), approximately 2 centimeters (1 inch) larger than the chest. This measurement is made around the greatest circumference, over the occipital protuberance, and ending in the middle of the forehead (Figure 13-7).

During the first 24 hours after birth, the infant's head may be equal to or smaller than his chest because of the molding or overriding of the skull bones as the head attempted to accommodate itself to the birth canal (Figure 13-8). There is generally more molding when the infant's head is engaged for prolonged periods and in firstborn infants. There is relatively little or no molding with a breech presentation or in babies delivered by elective cesarean section. The molding generally regresses in 24–48 hours after birth.

If the newborn's head is over 4 centimeters (1.6 inches) larger than the chest, and this is true of successive measurements over several days, increased intracranial pressure is suspected. Malnourished infants have significantly larger heads in rela-

Figure 13-4. A. Port-wine stain (nevus flammeus). B. Strawberry hemangioma. C. Stork bites (telangiectatic nevi). (Courtesy of Mead Johnson Laboratories, Evansville, Ind.)

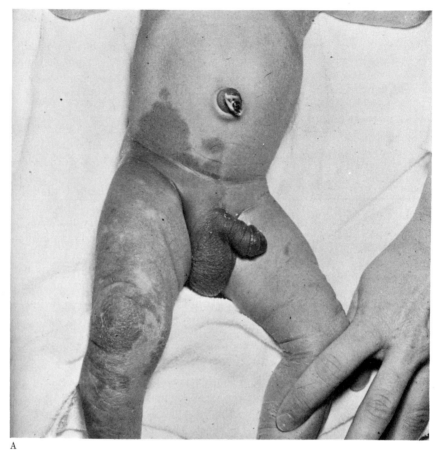

A

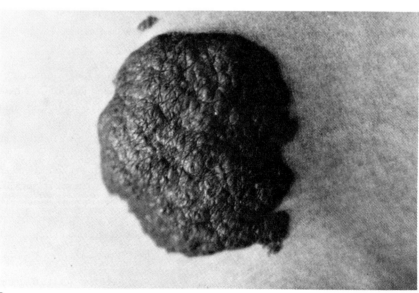

B

288

Figure 13-4 (Continued)

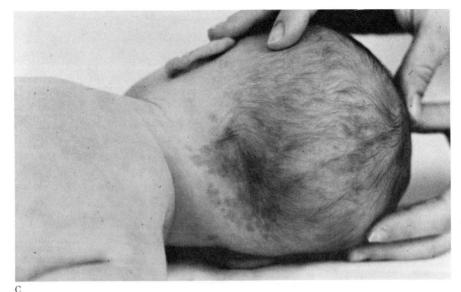

C

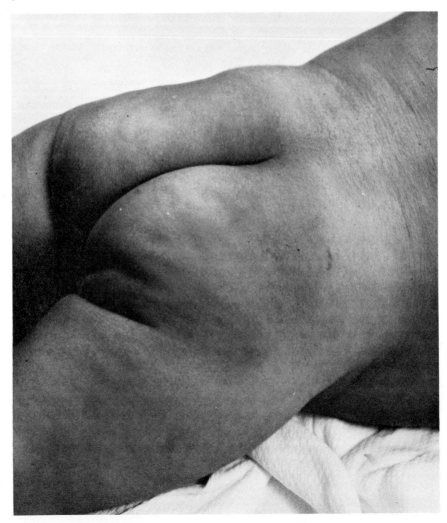

Figure 13-5. Mongolian spots. (Courtesy of Mead Johnson Laboratories, Evansville, Ind.)

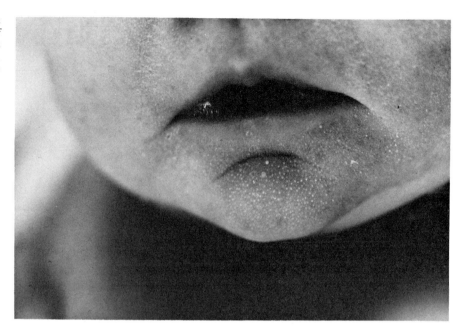

*Figure 13-6. Milia
neonatorum. (Courtesy of
Mead Johnson
Laboratories, Evansville,
Ind.)*

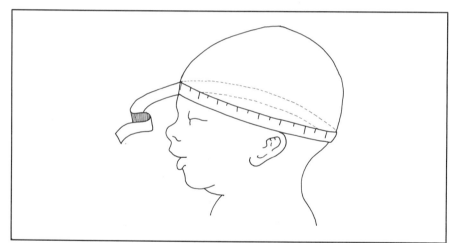

*Figure 13-7. Measuring
head circumference.*

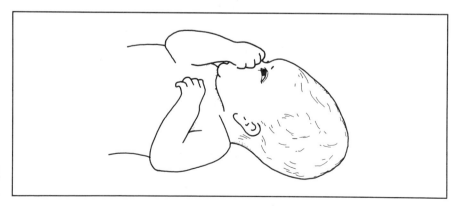

*Figure 13-8. Newborn
molding, or overriding of
the skull bones.*

290

tion to their chests than normal newborns; the smaller chest measurements may be due to depleted subcutaneous tissue [19].

In addition to measuring the newborn's head circumference, the nurse should palpate his fontanelles and suture lines. The anterior fontanelle should be open; the posterior may be closed. The size of the fontanelles may be decreased as a result of molding, but this disappears as molding regresses. The tension of the fontanelle should also be checked. Normally the anterior fontanelle is soft and concave or flat, but with increased intracranial pressure it becomes firm, convex, or bulging; with dehydration it may appear depressed. Parents are often concerned about touching the infant's "soft spot," and they should be informed that the fontanelle is covered with several layers of protective tissues, so that it can be touched and washed. The nurse should also explain to them that it will remain open for about the next year and a half to allow for brain growth.

The suture lines should be palpated to assess their degree of separation, which may be greater in malnourished infants, whose cranial bones may not have developed sufficiently. The separation may also be greater in infants with increased intracranial pressure due to hydrocephalus, subdural hematomas, cerebral edema, or meningitis.

The infant's head should be checked for *caput succedaneum* and should also be examined for *cephalohematomas,* which are collections of blood between the bones and the periosteum (Figure 13-9). These lesions are found most commonly in the parietal area and in infants who experienced prolonged head compression during labor or rapid traumatic passage through the birth canal. The incidence is also higher in first-born infants.

A cephalohematoma, which is rarely present at birth, may enlarge during the first three days. Unlike caput succedaneum, it does not extend across the suture lines, although more than one cranial bone may show a swelling. If the hematoma

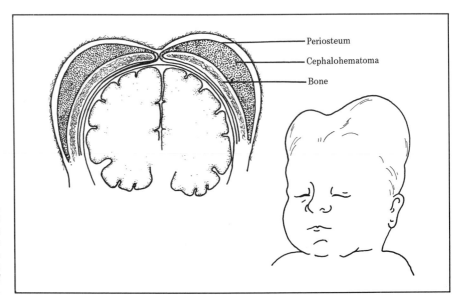

Figure 13-9. Cephalohematoma, a collection of blood between the bones and the periosteum. The swelling does not cross the suture lines and usually feels firm around the periphery and has a soft center.

crosses suture lines, it may indicate a skull fracture [3]. Upon palpation, a cephalohematoma usually is firm around the periphery, with a softer center.

These lesions are absorbed over variable periods of time, depending on their size. While smaller hematomas are rapidly absorbed, the larger ones calcify and are gradually incorporated into the enlarging skull.

The skull may also contain localized areas of softening (craniotabes), commonly along the suture lines in the flat cranial bones. Upon fingertip pressure these areas become indented but resume their shape when the pressure is removed. Craniotabes may be caused by an increase in intracranial pressure or by disturbances of the mother's calcium metabolism [10]. The areas of softening generally calcify rapidly after birth and seldom can be identified later.

The infant's facial movements should also be checked for symmetry. If there is injury to a facial nerve from trauma at delivery, the affected side of the mouth will fail to retract backward and upward when the infant cries (Figure 13-10). The majority of these paralyses resolve spontaneously within several days, although total recovery may require several weeks or months [8]; the paralysis may rarely be permanent.

Facial asymmetry may also be due to the position assumed in utero, for example, when the shoulder has been firmly pressed into the neck. This distortion generally regresses in a few weeks or months, depending on its severity.

Eyes

The newborn has a tendency to keep his eyes closed, making examination of them difficult. He also has a moderate photophobia and will promptly close his eyes on exposure to direct bright light. He will likewise close his eyes in response to loud noises or when his lashes are touched. However, a fully mature protective blink

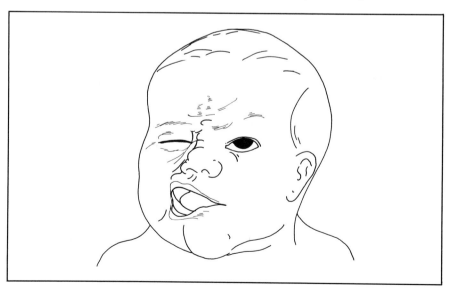

Figure 13-10. Facial paralysis.

reflex is absent in the newborn. When attempting to examine the infant's eyes, the nurse will find that trying to force his eyelids open meets with resistance. Shading his eyes by placing a hand on the side of his face may induce the infant to open them spontaneously. Slowly raising him from a supine to a sitting position may also be effective (baby-doll reflex). Once open, the infant's eyes should be checked for opacity of the pupil (congenital cataracts), color of the sclera, pupil size, and reaction to light. An unusually large cornea is likely to indicate congenital glaucoma.

Eye color is usually grayish-blue in white infants and brown in dark-skinned infants. Final deposition of pigment and final eye color do not appear for six to 12 months, although changes may be seen at three months. Likewise, the lacrimal apparatus is not mature at birth, and tears do not accompany crying for approximately one month.

Parents often inquire about the baby's ability to see in the immediate newborn period. They are often surprised to learn that their infant can perceive and differentiate between objects with different patterns, colors, and brightness. They are also often concerned with their newborn's transient "crossed-eyes" (strabismus) or jerky uneven eye movements (nystagmus). The parents need to be assured that these immature and uncoordinated eye movements are normal in the newborn and are the result of poor control of the eye muscles; the eye movements should become more coordinated by the third or fourth month. Infants exhibiting strabismus after the age of six months should generally be referred for treatment.

For approximately 48 hours after delivery the newborn's eyelids may be swollen, generally due to pressure on his head during delivery. The pressure may also cause rupture of capillaries in the sclera, resulting in subconjunctival hemorrhages, which appear as a red crescent band, either on the side of the iris or completely surrounding it. These hemorrhages are common; they appear in approximately 40 percent of all newborns and regress in about two weeks.

Another common finding is chemical conjunctivitis due to the instillation of silver nitrate drops at birth. The eyelids are edematous, the conjunctiva is red, and a purulent discharge may be present. The infant is usually treated with a warm saline eye irrigation several times a day, and the discharge usually disappears in a day or two. Similar discharges may be due to infections caused by staphylococcus, gonococcus, or a variety of gram-negative rods [19]. Generally these are not evident as soon after birth as chemical conjunctivitis, which may appear when the infant is admitted to the nursery from the delivery room.

Nose

Since the infant breathes through his nose and not through his mouth, obstructions such as mucus, choanal atresia, or stenosis will cause varying degrees of respiratory distress. It is important to examine the infant for adequate air flowing through his nose. This can be done by holding a wisp of cotton close to each nostril. As the baby exhales, the cotton will move away if there is adequate exchange.

Ears

In examining the infant's ears, the nurse should check their formation, position, and amount of cartilage present. Cartilage that gives the pinna a firm feeling is indicative of a full-term infant. The ears of a preterm baby are softer because they have less cartilage.

With the ear in a normal position, the helix is on the same plane as the angle of the eye (Figure 13-11). Ears that are twisted or rotated often appear to be low set but actually are not. Genuinely low-set ears may indicate Potter's syndrome (bilateral renal agenesis) or one of several other chromosomal abnormalities.

The formation as well as the position of the external ear should be examined closely. Significant flattening of the superior helix and large flabby ears that slant forward are often found in infants with unilateral absence of the kidney and congenital obstruction of the urinary tract [20]. Urogenital anomalies are often associated with malformations of the ear, since the embryonic development of both occurs during the same period.

Occasionally, accessory auricles are found around the ear in the form of small skin tags. They are usually treated by tying them off with a ligature.

Since the auditory nerve tracts are mature at birth, infants are able to hear well within a few days. By this time their eustachian tubes are clear of fluid and mucus.

Mouth

The infant's mouth should be checked for palate closure, size of tongue, presence of teeth, and signs of infection. When the newborn's mouth is examined, it is best to

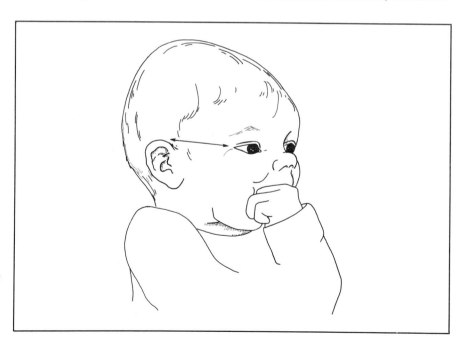

Figure 13-11. Normal position of the ears, with the helix on the same plane as the angle of the eye.

have the baby cry rather than to try to visualize his mouth and pharynx by depressing his tongue.

Occasionally the infant will be born with teeth (predeciduous), usually the lower central incisors. As a rule the roots are poorly formed or absent, and only the crowns are calcified. If the teeth become loose or interfere with feeding, they should be removed. Occasionally true deciduous teeth erupt shortly after birth; these can be differentiated from the predeciduous teeth by x-ray and should not be removed.

Epstein's pearls, which are small white nodules usually found on either side of the hard palate, are often mistaken for teeth by parents. They are of no significance and usually disappear a few weeks after birth.

Occasionally the frenulum of the tongue gives the appearance of what parents call "tongue tie" (frenulum linguae). This sharp thin ridge of tissue begins at the base of the tongue, runs along its undersurface, and extends far forward to the tip of the tongue. Previously it was clipped because it was thought to interfere with speech and eating; however, it is now known that this is not the case. In addition, because of the close proximity of a large vein, which may be severed when it is clipped, there is danger to the infant from bleeding and infection if the procedure is performed.

Sometimes sucking blisters, which appear as rounded thickened areas, may be found in the midline of the upper lip. Sucking calluses may also be seen, appearing as dried crusts or plaques, which run horizontally along the middle of the lips. During the first few weeks, the older ones are shed and new ones form.

The mouth should also be carefully inspected for signs of infection. A fungal infection (thrush), caused by *Candida albicans,* is occasionally found in the newborn; it is transmitted from the mother's vaginal secretions during birth. It appears as white or gray-white plaques on the tongue and mucous membrane and can easily be mistaken for curdled milk (Figure 13-12), but the plaques cannot be wiped off or brushed away as milk curds can. Thrush is treated with a solution of aqueous gentian violet or nystatin suspension (100,000 units per milliliter) swabbed over the mucous membranes three or four times a day.

The infant's tongue should be observed for size in relation to the size of his mouth. An excessively large tongue may be indicative of cretinism, mongolism, or other abnormalities.

Chest

When examining the newborn's chest, the nurse should check for breast enlargement and note the rate, quality, and type of his respirations. The average size of the newborn's chest is 30–33 centimeters (12–13 inches).

Frequently newborns experience breast enlargement at around the third day of life due to the withdrawal of maternal hormones, particularly estrogen, which have crossed the placental barrier during pregnancy. The engorged breasts may also secrete a thin white fluid known as *witch's milk,* probably related to the presence of prolactin in the newborn. Parents should be cautioned against massaging or squeezing their infant's engorged breasts, to prevent the occurrence of breast abscesses or mastitis. The enlargement generally regresses in about two weeks.

Both nipple and areola size should be noted, since they are far less pronounced in

Figure 13-12. Newborn thrush caused by Candida albicans. (*Courtesy of Mead Johnson Laboratories, Evansville, Ind.*)

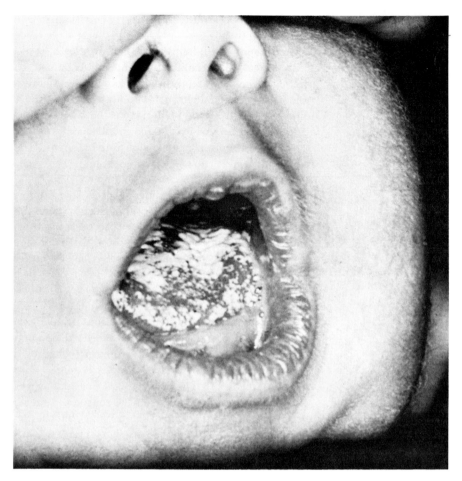

preterm babies and serve as an aid in estimating gestational age. There may also be supernumerary (accessory) nipples, which appear as pigmented spots of varying sizes and usually do not contain glandular tissue.

The infant's respiratory pattern should be observed before he is disturbed. Normal newborns breathe at a rate of between 40 and 60 breaths per minute. Rapid rates are usual for a few hours after birth; the respirations also tend to be shallow, with an irregular rhythm. The infant's respiratory movements are mainly diaphragmatic, since his thoracic muscles are weak. His chest remains relatively still as his abdomen expands with inspiration and falls with expiration. Frequently on inspiration the soft lower ribs tend to be drawn in as the abdomen protrudes, which is often apparent when the infant cries.

Abnormal respiratory signs include [19]:

1. Generalized cyanosis (most obvious and most serious).
2. Sustained respiratory rate in excess of 60 respirations per minute (tachypnea) when measured for 30 seconds or more on several occasions.

3. Irregular respirations associated with repeated apneic episodes often caused by central nervous system depression from hypoxia or intracranial hemorrhage.
4. Retractions, which indicate obstruction to the air flow through the respiratory tract. Upon inspiration the thoracic wall retracts between the ribs, above the clavicles, and below the inferior costal margins.
5. Respiratory grunt, in which the infant attempts to retain air and increase Po_2; an audible sigh during each expiration is equivalent.
6. Flaring of the nostrils (seen with air hunger).

Breath sounds may be difficult for the beginning practitioner to evaluate. The newborn's chest is small, and breath sounds are transmitted freely throughout. With practice, the exchange of air in the lungs can be detected, particularly if there is a difference in exchange between the two lungs. Decreased breath sounds are heard with shallow respirations, hyaline membrane disease, atelectasis, and emphysema.

The practitioner may also hear rales, which are caused as air rushes through fluid in the terminal bronchioles and alveoli. The sound is crackling in nature and may be heard in infants with hyaline membrane disease, pneumonia, and pulmonary edema, and occasionally is heard in normal babies. Rhonchi, which are coarse sounds that resemble snoring, are caused as air rushes through fluid contained in the large bronchi. They can be heard after aspiration of fluid or feedings [19].

The heart rate in the newborn ranges between 100 and 180 beats per minute. At birth the rate tends to be at the higher end of the scale, but it then falls; however during crying it may reach 200. On the average preterm babies have slower rates.

Normally the apical pulse can best be heard at the fifth intercostal space in line with the middle of the clavicle on the left chest. A shift in its location may indicate diaphragmatic hernia, pneumothorax, or dextrocardia. Occasionally the chest wall above the heart may be seen pulsating, especially in small babies with thin chest walls.

The newborn's heart sounds are usually clear, the second sound being higher in pitch and sharper than the first. Murmurs are also common, although the great majority of those detected in this period are transitory and not associated with anomalies. Most murmurs are systolic, occurring after the first heart sound and ending at or before the second sound [19]. In addition to checking the heart rate and sounds, the nurse should palpate the radial, brachial, and femoral pulses, which are indications of the adequacy of cardiac output. Absent femoral pulses may mean coarctation of the aorta, while significantly bounding ones may indicate congenital heart disease [14] (Table 13-1).

Abdomen and Back

The newborn's abdomen is cylindrical and appears to protrude slightly. If the abdomen is distended, the skin appears tightly drawn and the subcutaneous vessels can easily be seen. The liver can usually be palpated below the margin of the ribs on the right side. The kidneys may be palpated most easily within 6 hours after birth, before the intestines fill with air. The nurse may outline the kidney by placing a

Table 13-1. Newborn Blood Values

Blood Value	Preterm	Term
Hemoglobin (gm/100 ml)	15–17	17–19
Fetal hemoglobin (% of total)	80–90	70–80
Hematocrit (%)	45–55	57–58
White blood cells/ml	—	15,000
Reticulocytes (%)	≤ 10	3–7
Platelet count/ml	50,000–100,000	100,000–300,000
Blood gases (arterial, in first 24 hours)		
pH	7.30–7.39	7.30–7.39
Pco_2	33 mm Hg (range 31–35)	33 mm Hg (range 31–35)
Po_2	63–87 mm Hg	68–87 mm Hg

Source: S. Pierog and A. Ferrara. *Approach to the Medical Care of the Sick Newborn.* St. Louis: Mosby, 1971.

finger in the posterior flank for upward pressure, then using the fingers of the other hand to apply gentle downward pressure toward the posterior (Figure 13-13). Enlargement of the kidneys usually suggests hydronephrosis.

The ability of the kidney to concentrate urine and to excrete a solute load is considerably less in the newborn than in an older child or an adult. Uric acid crystals may sometimes be found in the urine, and appear on the diaper as reddish blotches that may be mistaken for blood. Uric acid crystals may yield false positives if the infant's urine is tested for albumin [27].

In addition to palpating the kidneys, the nurse should check for bladder distention, which appears as a firm globular mass that can be felt in the suprapubic region. Usually the infant voids within the first 24 hours; a record is kept of the number of voidings as well as any unusual characteristics. After the first few days, the infant voids from 10 to 15 times a day.

On the admission examination, the umbilical cord should be checked for the normal number of blood vessels. A single artery is often associated with congenital abnormalities, especially renal abnormalities. Occasionally a newborn may have an *umbilical hernia,* which is a defect in the anterior abdominal wall. All but the larger

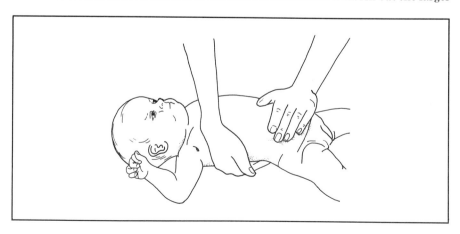

Figure 13-13. Palpating the kidney in the newborn.

Figure 13-14. Umbilical hernia and cutis navel.

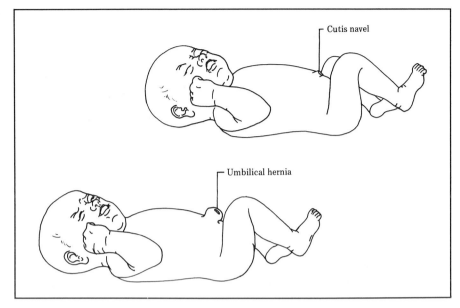

Cutis navel

Umbilical hernia

ones close spontaneously by approximately 2–3 years of age, as the child's abdominal muscles strengthen. The *cutis navel* (skin navel) is often confused with an umbilical hernia (Figure 13-14). In the cutis navel the cord stump protrudes from the abdominal wall and is covered by abdominal skin; it cannot be returned to the abdomen as an umbilical hernia can, and it becomes flatter with time.

The infant's anal sphincter should also be examined. Meconium is usually passed in the first 24 hours, but its appearance may be delayed. However, if there is no stool by the end of the first day, patency of the anus may be checked by passing a small tube into the anus no further than 1 centimeter (½ inch) [19]. The passage of meconium persists for about 48 hours, followed by transitional stools and milk stools. Transitional stools are a combination of the tarry black color of meconium and the yellow of milk stools. The stool gradually changes to a golden yellow of soft consistency if the infant is breast-fed or a light yellow of pasty consistency if the infant is bottle-fed. The number of stools decreases from six daily to two daily as the infant grows older.

While the infant is in a prone position, the nurse should check to see that the spinal column is of normal curvature. Sometimes a sacrococcygeal cleft or pilonidal dimple may be found; this is generally benign provided that it does not connect with an underlying sinus or deeper structure.

Genitalia

In examining a full-term male infant, the nurse should be able to palpate the testes in the scrotal sac, which is wrinkled and, provided that he is warm, hangs loosely from the infant's body. During the examination, it is important to close off the inguinal canal with the thumb and index finger to prevent the testes from slipping back into it (Figure 13-15). When the infant is chilled, the dartos muscle layer within

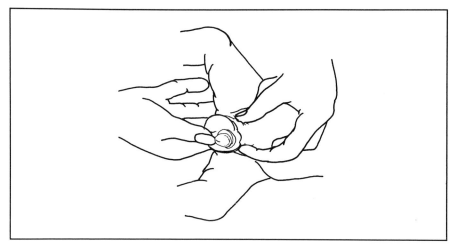

the scrotum contracts, making the sac appear rather small and very close to his body. Parents are often concerned when this happens and should be informed that the scrotum will appear larger and hang more loosely when their baby is warm. In preterm infants the testes may still be in the inguinal canal; the scrotal sac is smaller and less wrinkled and is held more closely to the body.

The glans penis of the newborn should be examined to locate the urethral opening. When the opening is ventral rather than central, it is known as *hypospadias;* when the urethra opens dorsally it is known as *epispadias.* If either of these congenital deformities are present, surgical repair is generally carried out by 2 years of age to prevent future embarrassment to the child. Since the foreskin is often used in making these repairs, these children are usually not circumcised. Hypospadias and epispadias are generally easily observed, so that there is no need to forcibly retract the tightly adherent prepuce covering the glans. The prepuce is usually retractable by 4–6 months of age [25]. If the urethral orifice is located far back on the penis and close to the perineum, adrenogenital syndrome should be considered. In this abnormality there is both failure to secrete cortisol and excessive androgen production by the adrenal glands. In female infants with the adrenogenital syndrome, the clitoris is enlarged.

Edema of the scrotal sac or a *hydrocele* may also be noted in a newborn male. Edema is more prevalent in babies born in breech presentations, and regresses within a few days. A hydrocele, a collection of fluid in the scrotal sac, usually regresses within one to three months.

In full-term female infants, the labia majora are generally larger than the labia minora, while the reverse is true for premature infants. Occasionally a piece of hymenal tissue may be seen protruding from the vagina; this hymenal tag regresses in several weeks. A white mucoid discharge and sometimes small amounts of blood (pseudomenstruation) may be seen on the infant's diaper or in her vagina. Both are due to a drop in maternal hormones, especially estrogen. While the bloody discharge appears for only a brief period, the white mucoid discharge may be present for a week or two.

Extremities

The infant's extremities should be examined for fractures; the most common sites are the clavicle, humerus, and femur. The entire length of the bone should be felt for knots or other irregularities. Movement and malposition should be noted, since newborns move fractured extremities less and often position them oddly.

The infant's hands and feet should be examined for *polydactyly* (extra digits), a

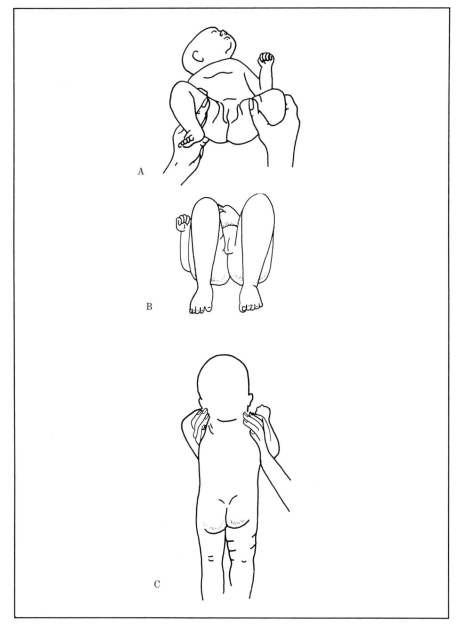

A

B

C

Figure 13-16. Examining for hip dislocation (see text for details).

disorder more commonly found in Negro newborns [10]. The most frequent form of polydactyly is an extra digit attached to the small finger of the hand. Usually the extra digit contains only soft tissue without bone and is treated by tying it off with a silk suture. In a few days it becomes gangrenous, dries, and falls off. If the extra digit contains bone, it must be surgically removed. *Syndactyly* (the fusing of two digits) is found infrequently and most commonly involves the toes; separation requires surgery.

All newborns should be carefully checked for hip dislocation, which is more common in girls, especially after breech deliveries; there is a high incidence in some families. Brown and Valman [12] report a racial predisposition, noting that the disorder is more common in Italians. The infant should be examined by placing him in a supine position and flexing his knees and abducting his hips out to the side and down toward the table's surface (Figure 13-16*A*). Hip dislocation is suspected if there is resistance to the abduction or if a click is heard, which signifies that the femur has slipped from the acetabulum. Another method is to flex the infant's knees, keeping his feet flat on the table (Figure 13-16*B*). The knee on the affected side will be lower (Allis' sign). A dislocated hip may also be indicated by unequal, higher, or extra gluteal or thigh folds on the affected side (Figure 13-16*C*).

Neurological Examination

Abnormal neurological signs in newborns may be transient phenomena, but must nevertheless be evaluated. As Korones [19] notes, predictions of later brain dysfunction cannot be made with consistent accuracy on the basis of neurological abnormalities during the newborn period.

In doing a neurological examination on a newborn, the nurse should first check those reflexes that cause the least disturbance to the baby. The observation should begin with his general level of activity, noting his spontaneous movements to see if he moves both sides equally well, and his lower extremities as well as his upper extremities.

The *tonic neck reflex* can easily be observed when the infant is at rest or asleep (Figure 13-17). When lying on his back, the newborn turns his head toward one side, with the arm and leg of that side extended while the opposite arm and leg are flexed. This has been described as the "fencing position." If the baby's head is gently turned toward the other side, often the position of the extremities can be reversed.

The *grasp reflex* is usually strong in full-term infants and weaker in premature or depressed newborns. The examiner tests this reflex by placing his finger across the infant's palm; the newborn grasps the finger so tightly that he can be pulled up almost to a sitting position (Figure 13-18).

The *rooting reflex* can be checked by lightly stroking the corner of the infant's mouth or cheek; his response is to turn his head toward the stimulated side in search of a nipple. Touching his upper lip causes him to open his mouth and turn his head slightly upward.

Sucking ability is tested by placing a nipple in the infant's mouth. The response of the normal newborn is an immediate forceful and coordinated suck, while preterm and depressed babies respond less, as do babies who have recently been fed.

Figure 13-17. Tonic neck reflex.

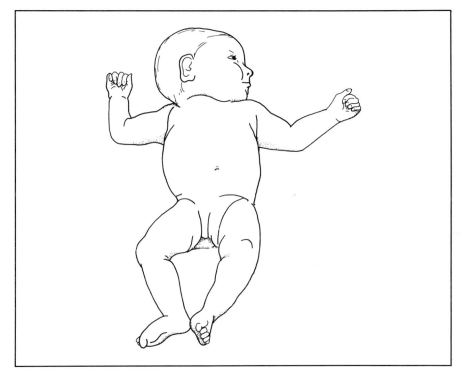

The Moro reflex and the stepping reflex may be tested after an evaluation of muscle tone, since eliciting the Moro reflex, in particular, does disturb the infant. In evaluating muscle tone the nurse should remember that normal newborns maintain some flexion in all extremities. When the examiner extends the infant's arm or leg, he normally responds by flexing it again when the extremity is released. Preterm infants and those who have suffered intrauterine hypoxia show less flexion at rest and little or no flexion in response to testing.

The examiner should always check head control. This can be done by lifting the infant and holding him by the wrists. If the baby has good head control, he contracts his shoulder and arm muscles and flexes his neck as he is pulled to a sitting position

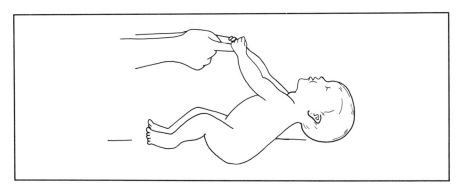

Figure 13-18. Grasp reflex.

*Figure 13-19. Evaluating
head control in the
newborn.*

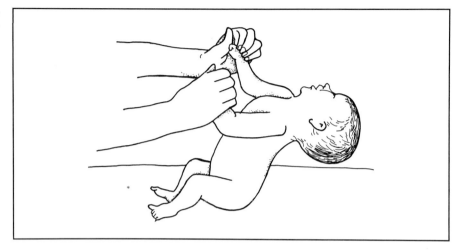

(Figure 13-19). When the infant reaches a sitting position, he should use his neck muscles to prevent his head from falling on his chest. Infants with Down's syndrome or intrauterine hypoxia show little head control or ability to contract their arm, shoulder, or neck muscles.

Muscle tone may also be checked by holding the infant horizontally in the prone position (ventral suspension), with the nurse's hand under the infant's chest (Figure 13-20). A full-term infant may momentarily hold his head in line with his trunk, but, for the most part, his head will remain at an angle of 45 degrees or less from the horizontal line. The maneuver allows the nurse to see the infant's control of his head, trunk, arms, and legs.

The *Moro reflex* (startle reflex) may be elicited by jarring the crib or by the preferred method of holding the newborn in a supine position with one hand under his head and one under his buttocks. When the hand under his head is moved to his back, allowing his head to drop slightly, the reflex is activated. The infant's arms,

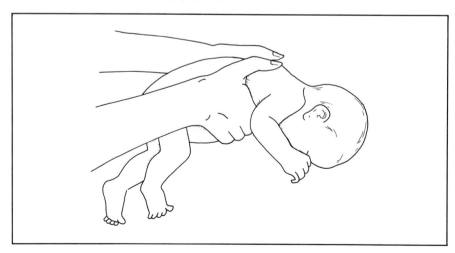

*Figure 13-20. Evaluating
muscle tone in the
newborn by holding him
in the prone position.*

Figure 13-21. Moro or startle reflex (see text for details).

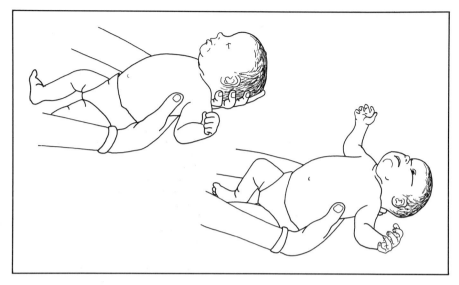

wrists, and fingers quickly extend and abduct, followed by flexion of his arms and legs in an embracing motion and usually a cry (Figure 13-21). It is important to check the response for symmetry. If one extremity does not respond it may indicate neurological damage or a fracture.

The *stepping reflex* may be checked by holding the infant in a standing position with his feet on the examining table. The normal baby's response will be to straighten his trunk and make alternate stepping movements with his legs.

Normal newborns also have a positive Babinski reflex. The presence of the previously discussed reflexes in the normal newborn indicates appropriate neurological response. Many reflexes, such as rooting, sucking, blinking, sneezing, coughing, gagging, and grasp, have an obvious functional value. Other reflexes, such as the Moro and the tonic neck reflexes, are thought to be vestigal reflexes handed down from the ancient past and still seen in lower animals. These primitive reflexes normally disappear in approximately three months (Table 13-2).

GENERAL HYGIENE

Nurses who work with newborns and their parents have numerous opportunities to incorporate many of the pertinent observations previously described into their care, teaching, and follow-up. They should remember that parents are extremely critical of minute anatomical and physiological variations in their babies. Anatomical asymmetries, such as one eye being open more than the other (especially on the side further from the source of light in the room), molding of the head, irregular breathing, engorged breasts (especially in the male), and variations in external genitalia, become magnified. One of the many times such variations can be discussed with the parents is in the hospital during the baby's bath.

Table 13-2. Examination of the Newborn	Body Part	Examination Procedures
	Head	Measure circumference
		Palpate suture lines and fontanelles
		Observe for indication of molding, caput succedanum, cephalohematoma
	Eyes	Observe for evidence of edema, discharge, conjunctivitis, subconjunctival hemorrhage, pupil capacity
	Ears	Observe position, size, and formation; note presence of cartilage
	Nose	Observe for patent nasal passages, nose breathing, nasal flaring, discharge
	Mouth	Check for palate closure, presence of teeth, Epstein's pearls, evidence of infection (thrush), size of tongue; note character of cry
	Chest	Measure circumference
		Examine heart and lung sounds; observe respirations
		Observe breasts for enlargement, discharge, development, supernumerary nipples
	Abdomen	Observe for symmetry
		Palpate liver and kidneys
		Observe condition of umbilical cord
	Genitalia	
	Female	Observe labia for development and protection provided by majora, clitoris for size; check for vaginal bleeding or discharge, presence of hymenal tag
	Male	Observe penis for evidence of epispadias or hypospadias; scrotum for rugae and presence of testes, evidence of swelling
	Back	Observe for straight spinal column, evidence of dimpling of skin over sacral vertebrae, patency of anus
	Extremities	Examine for fractures, polydactyly, syndactyly, club feet, posture and symmetrical use of extremities
		Observe creasing on hands and feet
		Examine for hip dislocation
	Skin	Observe color and thickness
		Check for indication of cyanosis, edema, ecchymoses, jaundice, lanugo, vernix caseosa, petechiae, desquamation, turgor
		Check for evidence of milia, mongolian spots, erythema toxicum, hemangiomas, infection
	Neurological	Check Moro's, grasp, suck, rooting, and tonic neck reflexes
		Observe muscle tone, head control, posture and movements

Bathing the Newborn

Babies can be cleansed in a variety of ways without violating basic underlying principles of safe care. Hospital policies concerning the bath have varied; at one time, daily soap and water and/or oil baths were the rule, but today complete baths are often not given. Instead in many nurseries blood, meconium, and excess vernix caseosa are wiped off with dry or water-moistened cotton balls and thereafter the diaper area is cleaned as necessary.

During the 1960s, in response to an increase in staphylococcal infections in newborn nurseries, the American Academy of Pediatrics recommended that infants be bathed in a liquid detergent containing 3% hexachlorophene after birth and then every other day. Subsequent research [5] has indicated that although the rate of staphylococcal colonization and staphylococcal skin diseases is indeed reduced, there is no documented proof that the use of 3% hexachlorophene ever arrested a serious nursery epidemic. In addition, its use has increased the colonization of gram-negative organisms and the incidence of gram-negative disease.

In recent years the actual safety of daily bathing of infants with a solution containing 3% hexachlorophene has been questioned, since it leaves protective residue that reaches a peak effectiveness after three baths and is absorbed through intact skin. When it was disclosed that blood levels found in newborns bathed daily in 3% hexachlorophene have been shown to approach levels known to be neurotoxic in experimental animals, the Food and Drug Administration ruled that hexachlorophene could be distributed only by prescription. Therefore, the routine prophylactic use of hexachlorophine for total body bathing of newborns in hospital nurseries or in the home is no longer recommended. The most actively promoted alternative, povidone-iodine (Betadine), can cause local and systemic reactions in hypersensitive infants, and there is no proof that it is safer [17].

Currently, the Committee on the Fetus and Newborn of the American Academy of Pediatrics [5] recommends dry skin care for newborns, which involves the use of plain nonmedicated soap and tap water, or tap water alone, on the baby's skin in the areas that need attention: face, neck, axillae, and groin, and the buttocks with each diaper change. If a nursery infection is present, once daily prophylactic bathing of the newborn with 3% hexachlorophene, followed by prompt and thorough rinsing, may be given on a short-term basis.

The Committee emphasizes that the two most important factors in the transmission of infection from infant to infant are hand contact and lapses in hygienic technique. Scrupulous handwashing with an iodine preparation, a 3% hexachlorophene emulsion, or any other cleansing agent before and between handling babies is essential.

It is important for the parents to have the opportunity to observe a bath being given to their baby and for one or both of them to give him a bath themselves before the family leaves the hospital. The nurse should take this opportunity to explore with the parents their plans for caring for the baby, the methods they have considered using, the facilities they have at home, so that, as a part of the dialogue, modifications can be suggested if necessary. All too often, demonstration baths become merely a lecture by the nurse concerning what *should* be done according to hospital policy, leaving little room for individual variation.

Parents who have other children are not necessarily uninterested in being taught to bathe their new infant in the hospital. Many times they are anxious to learn new techniques or to review their own, especially if some time has elapsed since their last child was born. In addition, the nurse should encourage them to share what they have learned from their past experiences, so that their "tips" might be passed on to new parents.

The baby's bath may be given at any time of the day but is usually given before a feeding. If the day is particularly warm, a sponge bath may be repeated two or three times during the day, taking care to rinse and dry all skin folds and creases thoroughly. Parents may not realize how active newborns really are; the nurse should stress the importance of never leaving the baby alone on an elevated surface where he could roll off; it is best for them to get into the habit of keeping one hand on him at all times.

Whether the nurse demonstrates the bath for the parents or they do it themselves, certain principles are basic. If all necessary supplies are organized before beginning the bath, the parent will be less likely to leave the baby alone or unduly exposed once the bath is begun. Safety pins should always be closed and put well out of the baby's reach. It is also preferable to have an area where dirty linen and soiled items can be placed. The room should be warm (75°–80° F) and free from drafts, and the bath water should feel warm to the elbow (98°–100° F).

The baby should be cleaned starting from the cleanest area and proceeding to the most soiled, in the following order: eyes, face, ears, scalp, neck, upper extremities, trunk, lower extremities, and finally genitalia and buttocks. The infant's eyes receive special care, and are gently cleaned with sterile water or tap water from the inner canthus to the outer canthus, to avoid contaminating the lacrimal ducts. A clean surface of the washcloth or a clean cotton ball is used for each stroke.

Throughout the procedure, various parts of the baby are washed, rinsed well, and dried thoroughly, with particular attention paid to the creases and body folds. Usually only one area of the infant is exposed at a time in order to avoid chilling, since the newborn's temperature-regulating mechanism is not fully developed at birth and his heat production is low. During the first few days his temperature is unstable, responding to slight stimuli with considerable fluctuation above or below the normal level. For this reason in many nurseries where a soap and water bath is routine, the baby's initial bath after birth is often delayed for several hours to allow his body temperature to stabilize.

Researchers [21] have demonstrated that the temperature of the newborn falls precipitously following delivery, to levels lower than are generally recognized. They suggest that temperature fluctuation and a decreased temperature may be desirable or even essential for a rapid and satisfactory adjustment to extrauterine life. Due to the extreme sensitivity of skin thermal receptors, a peripheral thermal stimulus, such as bathing, might be an important factor in heat production [26]. Some nursing research [28] has demonstrated that bathing the newborn did produce a greater initial drop (0.5° C, or 1° F) in body temperature than was seen in unbathed babies. However subsequent to this initial drop, the body temperature of the bathed newborn showed a significant increase (approximately 0.2° C, or 0.5° F), which was not seen in the control unbathed group of babies. This would seem to show that the bathing tended to produce a more rapid return toward the desired level of body temperature (36.1°–37.2° C, or 97°–99° F), although the researchers question whether or not the same effect might not have been achieved through stimulation by a light friction rub with a warm towel.

At the other end of the spectrum are those nurseries where no attempt is made to clean the baby, except for removing blood on his face and scalp. The vernix caseosa is not removed since most of it either rubs into his skin or rubs off onto his clothes within 12–24 hours. Sometimes it tends to remain longer in body creases and skin folds, such as the neck, axillae, and between the labia. This may encourage infection or irritation in these areas; therefore, the vernix caseosa is wiped away after 24–48 hours.

The baby is not given a tub bath until after the cord has dropped off, usually within two weeks. However, most parents are interested in learning how to support the baby's body during his tub bath. Usually this is done by placing the left arm under the baby's head and shoulders, grasping his left arm firmly. The right hand is used to grasp his ankles, and may be used to wash him after he is lowered into the tub. If a small towel is placed in the bottom of the tub, its surface will not be as slippery.

The so-called football carry is a useful hold for washing the baby's hair or to free one hand to arrange bath items. One arm is placed under the baby's body, with his head on that hand and his buttocks held securely between the adult's hip and elbow, leaving the other hand free.

Skin Care

The newborn's skin becomes irritated easily because the dermis and epidermis are very loosely connected. During the first two or three days after birth, the skin becomes increasingly dry; often cracks will appear, particularly around his wrists and ankles. Usually these are not significant and disappear spontaneously.

Because the newborn's skin is so easily irritated, the use of strong soap and excessive amounts of baby oil or baby powder should be avoided. Most of these products contain perfume, which, while it makes the baby smell nice, may actually have an irritating effect on his skin. Excessive use of powder, especially by shaking it on the baby, may leave large amounts of it to collect and become caked in his skin creases, and there is also the danger that he may inhale it. Parents should be advised to shake the powder on their own hands and smooth it on the baby. Many parents are interested to learn that cornstarch, a much less expensive substitute, provides the same effect as the commercially prepared baby powders. Baby oil is also perfumed and may be an irritant; it is also a good medium for bacterial growth if left on the skin in large amounts, and should therefore be used sparingly.

Cord Care

The baby's daily care involves not only bathing but also inspection and observation. One area which is routinely inspected is his umbilical cord, and parents are often concerned about its proper care.

Within 24 hours after birth, the evaporation of Wharton's jelly has caused the umbilical cord to lose its bluish-white moist appearance, and within a few days it becomes shriveled and almost black. Several days later the stump sloughs, leaving a small granulating wound, which after healing forms the umbilicus. Separation of the cord from the body most frequently occurs around the tenth day but occasionally takes several weeks; no attempt should be made to dislodge it before it separates naturally.

Formerly care of the cord was not given too much attention, and neglect of asepsis resulted in the transmission of infections through the umbilical vessels, with the eventual death of many infants. Sometimes even today serious umbilical infections are found, most frequently caused by *Staphylococcus aureus, Escherichia coli,* or *Pseudomonas aeruginosa.*

The blood vessels at the base of the cord are initially sealed off by formation of

Figure 13-22. A. Hollister
cord clamp. B. Clamp
closed on cord stump.

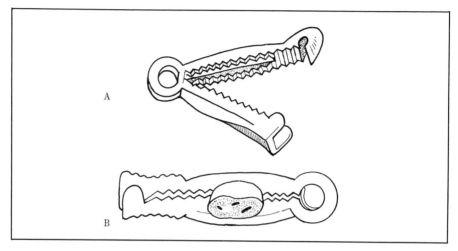

thrombi. Final obliteration does not occur until the end of the first month, when the vessels become fibrous cords. Until this anatomical closure occurs, the blood vessels may be portals of entry to pathogenic organisms. Signs of infection include any unusual or foul odors of the cord, red inflamed areas around the stump, and drainage from the cord, but the baby may have a serious umbilical cord infection without any local signs.

The newborn's cord is observed for bleeding as well as infection, particularly during the first 24 hours. Ziegel and Van Blarcom [29] note that bleeding seems to occur most often between the second and sixth hours of life, sometimes in association with crying or the passage of meconium. The danger appears to be greatest with a bleeding disorder or when the cord initially contains a large amount of Wharton's jelly; in the latter case, the cord shrinks, and the previously tight tie or clamp becomes loose. Usually a blood clot at the end of the cord stump prevents such bleeding, but if bleeding should occur, a hemostat should be placed on the cord as far away from the abdominal wall as possible, to allow for the application of another tie or clamp. As a rule, cord ties remain in place until the cord separates. Clamps are usually removed in 24 hours if the cord appears dry (Figure 13-22).

Since infants' cords dry more quickly and separate more readily when exposed to air, dressings are usually not applied. Diapers are usually placed below the cord for this reason and also to prevent urine from keeping the cord area moist. Cord care commonly involves wiping the cord stump with a cotton ball saturated with antiseptic solution or with a 70% solution of alcohol to further encourage drying until healing is complete. If the cord seems unusually moist, applying the alcohol several times a day enhances drying.

Genitalia

Parents should clean the genitalia of baby girls gently and carefully with moistened cotton balls or a soft cloth, wiping from front to back. A clean portion of the cloth or a new cotton ball is used for each stroke. Smegma, a thick cheesy secretion of the sebaceous glands, is removed from between the folds of the labia.

If a baby boy is not to be circumcised, parents are instructed to ease the foreskin back very gently during the daily bath in order to clean the smegma from around the glans. No force should be applied in attempting to retract the foreskin, since, as mentioned previously, it may be several months before it is easily retractable.

Circumcision, a sterile surgical procedure in which the foreskin (prepuce) of the penis is removed, traditionally has been done for religious or cultural reasons. In the United States it has been believed to be of medical value as well, and has been almost routinely performed on all male newborns. This is not the case in many other areas, including Europe, South America, and Japan. Physicians are now beginning to question the routine circumcision of newborns, and some of them are advising it only when a specific reason exists for the procedure.

In the past, circumcision has been routinely recommended to prevent the occurrence of disorders such as phimosis, cancer of the penis, and cancer of the cervix, and to save the "different" uncircumcised male "locker room embarrassment." It is also argued that the circumcised penis is cleaner and more aesthetic, and that it provides greater pleasure during sexual intercourse, although this latter fact is controversial.

Some physicians view circumcision as a basically unnecessary body mutilation, while others who argue against routine circumcision feel that circumcision, like any surgery, is associated with occasional hazards and complications. Primarily these complications involve infection, surgical trauma, and hemorrhage; the danger of hemorrhage seems particularly pertinent in light of the newborn's hypoprothrombinemia. It is generally felt, however, that the vitamin K injection given the newborn lessens the danger of hemorrhage.

Research [25] indicates that the increased incidence of genitourinary cancers in populations that do not practice circumcision appears to be related to poor genital hygiene, inadequate hygienic facilities, and venereal disease. The conclusion is that in groups where a high standard of cleanliness could presumably be expected, circumcision at birth would not seem to be justified.

At this time in the United States, circumcision of the newborn is still frequently performed, either in the delivery room shortly after birth, or on the second or third postnatal day, unless it is a religious ritual circumcision. The operation is usually performed without anesthesia, and the baby will cry probably as much from being restrained as from discomfort from the procedure. Sometimes he may be comforted by a sterile nipple pacifier or by a warm blanket.

The raw incision is usually covered with sterile petrolatum-saturated gauze. The main principle in circumcision care is to keep the wound clean and observe it for bleeding. In most instances, the circumcision dressing is carefully removed postoperatively when the infant voids for the first time and is then replaced. Dressings are usually not reapplied after 24 hours; the wound is cleaned with warm water following diaper changes, and the penis is sometimes coated with petrolatum until healing is complete, usually within a few days.

Because the newborn does have a transitory hypoprothrombinemia, the circumcision is particularly observed for bleeding every hour during the first 24 postoperative hours. Usually the baby's crib is tagged with a special sign, so that nursery personnel are alerted to the fact that he is newly circumcised. Only one layer of diaper should cover the penis, so that any bleeding will be evident; usually undue irritation is avoided by not placing the baby on his stomach. If bleeding does occur, it is usually stopped with very gentle pressure. Sometimes a 1 : 1000 solution of epinephrine is applied locally to the bleeding point. Of course, if the bleeding persists, the doctor is notified.

The parents are usually anxious when their baby has gone to be circumcised and want to see him on his return. This is a good time to show them the wound and begin the explanation of its care. After the circumcision, the baby finds comfort from being held, cuddled, and fed, since feedings are usually withheld prior to the procedure.

Diaper Rash

Another source of concern for parents is the diaper rash that babies often get, caused by a reaction of bacteria with the urea in the urine, resulting in an ammonia dermatitis. The best treatment consists of keeping the area clean and dry, with exposure to air and light several times a day. Additional warmth is provided by the use of a lamp (with a bulb no brighter than 40 watts) placed 30 centimeters (12 inches) or more from the buttocks for 30 minutes at a time. When the baby is being fed and has his diaper on, the area can be protected by ointments, such as petrolatum jelly, zinc oxide, or A and D ointment. This helps keep stool off the raw area and aids in the healing process. A frequent cause of diaper rashes at home is inadequate rinsing of the infant's diapers.

PARENTS' CONCERNS

Nurses can alleviate many of the concerns that parents have and will encounter in caring for their baby at home. This can only be done if they spend time with the parents, participating in the baby's care with them and giving them encouragement and positive reinforcement. This time is invaluable, for it is now that the nurse can review such topics as taking the baby's temperature, signs of hunger, normal occurrence of regurgitation, sneezing, hiccupping, and characteristics of normal stools. The nurse may also use this time to observe and evaluate the parents' comfort and ability in holding, dressing, feeding, bubbling, and positioning the baby.

In the hospital it is conceivable that if the baby is in a central nursery and is brought to the mother every four hours for feeding, the parents may take him home without ever having heard him cry. Sometimes they voice a concern about what his cry means or what to do if the baby does not stop crying when he is picked up. They should be told that the crying is his way of telling them that his diaper is dirty or that he is about to have a bowel movement, that he is hungry or has a gas bubble, or that he is being stuck by a pin. Sometimes a sudden noise will startle a baby; in this case cuddling usually quiets his crying. Often a warm bath will soothe and calm him. Parents need to be made aware of the fact that a certain amount of crying is normal and aerates the lungs.

Parents often ask when they can take the baby outside. Usually when the mother feels like going out for the first time, the baby may go along. This, of course, depends on the weather and often on the philosophy of their pediatrician. The baby should be well protected from temperature extremes and from direct exposure to sun or wind. The amount of clothing the baby needs is generally comparable to that which the parent is wearing.

If the parents will be travelling in a car, they should be reminded not to put the baby on the floor, where exhaust fumes tend to collect. Some physicians feel that flying should be postponed for the first several weeks, because the baby's middle ear is not developed enough to adapt to changes in pressure. It is important at take-off and landing that the baby be sucking on his bottle or nipple to assist in adjustment to changes in pressure.

NEONATAL IMMUNOLOGY

Before birth the infant is protected by the surrounding membranes, the uterus, and the biological defense mechanisms of the mother. At birth he leaves this sterile environment and enters one contaminated by infectious organisms. His own protective mechanisms, aided by antibodies passed across the placenta from the mother, should successfully defend him against the common infectious agents. However, since his general resistance remains low, he should be exposed to as few of these organisms as possible.

Several natural portals of entry exist in the newborn, for example, vessels of the umbilical cord, circumcision, and breaks in his skin. Opportunities for infection are inherent in certain anomalies, such as omphalocele and exstrophy of the bladder; in babies who receive repeated exchange transfusions or fluids or who have frequent blood sampling through the umbilical vein; in babies who require resuscitation; and in babies who are placed in isolettes that have not been thoroughly cleaned. Special precautions should be taken if the mother's membranes were ruptured more than 24 hours before delivery, or if she had a fever or infection during the last week of pregnancy, prolonged labor, foul smelling or purulent amniotic fluid, traumatic delivery, or an infectious disease, such as syphilis or tuberculosis.

The relative immune deficiency of the newborn makes him unusually able to develop serious infections, such as meningitis and septicemia, which are significant causes of severe disease or death in the neonate. He is also susceptible to the common viruses, such as cytomegalovirus and rubella.

The newborn's first line of defense is the surface protection provided by his intact skin and mucous membrane; there are also several basic host response mechanisms that operate in varying degrees [15, 19]. The initial inflammatory response of the newborn is delayed, and he cannot concentrate inflammatory cells at the site of infection as well as adults can, so it is less likely that his infection will remain localized.

The newborn's serum is deficient in its capacity to opsonize organisms (prepare organisms for phagocytosis by polymorphonuclear leukocytes). The part played by lymphocytes and macrophages in the newborn's defense is probably also decreased.

Serum immunoglobulins (IgG, IgM, and IgA) are important in the immunological defenses of the newborn because of their role in opsonizing bacteria for phagocytosis, in killing bacteria in specific systems, and in neutralizing viruses. IgG globulins contain antibodies to a majority of bacterial and viral organisms to which the mother has previously been exposed. These are the only globulins to cross the placental barrier, first appearing in the fetus around the third gestational month. They accumulate progressively, until they equal the mother's level at term. Therefore, the length of gestation as well as the mother's antibody complement are the determinants of the IgG level at birth; the average concentration in serum is 1000 milligrams per 100 milliliters at term, but lower levels are found in the premature infant. Most of these globulins are catabolized over the first three months of life; however, the infant's own synthesis of IgG increases gradually after the age of three months to cover the loss.

The fetus can produce IgM globulins at about the twentieth week of gestation. Since intrauterine infections may produce this immunological response in the fetus, the measurement of this globulin is used to establish the presence of such an infection. Some specific antibodies can be identified within the IgM fraction, including syphilis, toxoplasmosis, cytomegalovirus, rubella, and herpesvirus. Usually the IgM level at birth is below 20 milligrams per 100 milliliters of serum.

IgA globulins do not cross the placenta and are not detectable in most normal infants at birth. The fetus and neonate are slower to manufacture IgA than IgM globulins, so they are found less regularly in the serum of infected infants at birth.

Protection from Infection

Nothing administered to the newborn, including commercial gamma globulin, will improve the functioning of his immune defense system; consequently, it is important to protect him from undue exposure to organisms in the environment and to be alert for rapid diagnosis and treatment of infections when they develop. This is achieved by maintaining aseptic and clean technique in his care and by preventing his contact with persons who are themselves infected.

To further ensure protection from infection, the American Academy of Pediatrics sets certain standards and recommendations for hospital care of newborns [4]. Ideally the nursery itself should be enclosed and have some system of ventilation or air conditioning in which there is an adequate filtering device. The floor is always considered contaminated, and dropped objects must be discarded or sterilized before they are used again. All linen, clothing, formulas, and solutions used in infant care must be clean, or preferably sterilized, and each infant should have his own set of supplies. When the baby is moved to a common facility (scale or treatment table), a clean paper or sheet should be used for his protection. If he is in an incubator, he should be placed in a clean one every four days or every week.

Access to the nursery should be through a scrub room where personnel change clothes and thoroughly scrub their hands and arms, paying special attention to their nails. Handwashing is repeated when personnel move from one infant to another. These policies apply to each member of the nursing staff and to everyone else who enters the nursery, from cleaning personnel to aides, medical students, and physicians. Since exposure to agents most likely to make the newborn ill comes from persons in his environment, anyone who has infections of the skin or upper respiratory tract, diarrhea, or fever of unknown origin, is automatically excluded from the nursery. This ban includes parents and visitors as well as nursery staff. At home such hazards are fewer because of the relatively small number of individuals in contact with the baby.

In order to minimize the risk of infection when the baby is taken to his mother, some hospitals do not allow visitors on the unit during that time. The mother washes her hands before her baby is brought to her; if she has an infection, her baby can be taken to the door of her room so that she can see him, and she can be given reports of his progress.

Infection is not always indicated in the newborn by fever; hypothermia or marked temperature variations may be present, indicating the infant's inability to control his temperature. Infection may be suspected when the baby is inactive and/or does not eat well. Other indications of infection include jaundice beginning after the third day, a mottled appearance to his skin, abdominal distention, diarrhea, vomiting, changes in respiratory patterns, and skin lesions. A full fontanelle, a high-pitched cry, and irritability indicate an infection of the central nervous system.

NURSERY ARRANGEMENT

Nurseries may be constructed in various ways; there may be a centralized nursery where all babies of various ages stay, or the nursery may consist of a series of rooms through which babies progress as they grow older. The latter arrangement includes an admission area, a transitional care nursery adjacent to the delivery room (where an infant receives skilled intensive observation), and peripheral units to which the baby is moved for more routine observation and care. Such arrangements provide for rapid communication of information between personnel involved in delivery (nurses, obstetricians, and anesthesiologists) and those involved in newborn care (nurses and pediatricians). The elimination of long transportation routes between the delivery room and the nursery minimizes heat loss and respiratory emergencies enroute. The division of the nursery into more specialized areas ensures that skilled and motivated personnel see the infant first and provide high standards of *initial* care for all infants, including those with high Apgar scores. This is important since morbidity is not predictable in individual infants. This arrangement also concentrates equipment for resuscitation, ventilatory maintenance, and biochemical evaluation in the area immediately at hand.

DISCHARGE

Well before the family leaves the hospital, the nurse should explore with the parents their plans for follow-up health care for the infant and the mother. They should be made aware of community agencies nearby and the services they provide for continued health supervision and guidance. If the period of hospitalization is short, follow-up by a community health nurse may be welcome, especially in the absence of helpful relatives nearby. Parents should be helped to arrange for some form of continued health supervision, through a private physician, a hospital, or a community health center. Here the baby can be assessed for normal patterns of growth and development and given necessary regular immunizations when his immunological system is producing antibodies in good fashion, by the age of two or three months. In general, parents and their new infant make the first of many visits for continued health supervision within four to six weeks after leaving the hospital.

NEWBORN NUTRITION

Fluid

Normal nutrition for newborns includes providing water, electrolytes, and nutrients in adequate but not excessive amounts. Moore [22] outlines the main reasons why fluid balance is more precarious in the newborn than in older children and adults. Since metabolic rates of the newborn are higher, he utilizes a greater quantity of water. (The newborn produces 45–50 calories per kilogram of body weight per day, while adults produce 25–30 calories per kilogram per day.)

The newborn has a larger surface area in proportion to his body mass. Therefore he has a higher ratio of water loss through evaporation, about twice that of the adult. Because of this, his fluid balance is more susceptible to environmental temperature and humidity variations.

In the newborn the proportion of water in relation to total body mass is 70–75 percent, greater than at any other life period. Extracellular water comprises 30–35 percent of his total body weight, compared to 25 percent in an older infant, and 20 percent in an adult. In a 24-hour period he excretes 50 percent of his extracellular water, compared to the 14 percent an adult excretes; therefore, he has less reserve.

The kidneys of premature and full-term infants have about half the concentration power of the normal adult, and they function satisfactorily under usual conditions but not during times of stress. Since the newborn is not able to conserve water by concentrating urine, even in dehydration his output may not decrease. The normally higher levels of phosphate and potassium in his urine are also related to kidney immaturity.

The newborn's water requirement is 80–100 milliliters per kilogram of body weight per day during the first 10 days and 125–200 milliliters per kilogram per day thereafter. Babies must have at least 75–90 milliliters per kilogram of body weight per day to prevent dehydration. Otherwise they may exhibit the characteristic signs of dehydration: dry skin, loss of skin turgor, depressed fontanelle, weight loss, rapid and weak pulse, increased temperature, and soft eyeballs. When dehydration occurs, fluids are given intravenously and are carefully calculated to replace lost electrolytes. An infant's electrolyte balance is relatively unstable, especially sodium and potassium levels, because of the rapid exchange of water and the ease with which the balance is upset.

Nutrients

CALORIES

By the tenth day the infant needs 110–130 calories per kilogram of body weight per day (50–60 calories per pound) in order to provide energy for his relatively high basal metabolic rate, increasing activity, and rapid growth. However, needs will vary within the given range even for babies of the same age and size. The newborn should have 9 grams of protein daily (7–16 percent of calories) to provide for growth and to make up for losses from his skin and in his urine. (At one month he needs 14 grams of protein per day; at two months, 15 grams per day; and from three months to one year, 16 grams per day.)

About 40 percent of the newborn's calories should be in the form of carbohydrates. When carbohydrates comprise less than 20 percent of the calories, the baby will not be able to tolerate the high percentage of protein and fat in the formula. If over 50 percent of the calories are provided by carbohydrates, the baby will probably have loose stools due to his inability to hydrolize disaccharides, which will eventually result in impaired growth and development.

About 30–55 percent of the calories should be provided by fat, with the most acceptable proportion being around 40 percent. If fat content is too low, then either the protein intake will be so high that the renal solute load will be excessive, or the high level of carbohydrate will lead to diarrhea.

VITAMINS

Most babies in the United States receive supplementary vitamins, and as a result, vitamin deficiencies are relatively rare. In addition, in many hospitals babies are given vitamin K (0.5–1.0 milligrams) routinely at birth, since it is only after birth that normal intestinal flora are established and begin to synthesize vitamin K. Because formulas and breast milk contain B-group vitamins, it is felt that their deficiency would be unlikely in the newborn. Since the optimal amounts of B-group vitamins are not fully determined, however, many physicians believe that a supplement is desirable, if not essential. Folic acid deficiences may be overlooked because they can be masked by a common iron deficiency anemia.

On the other hand, with vitamin A the danger is overdosage. Healthy infants receiving human milk, cows' milk, and most commercial formulas do not need any extra vitamin A; 600 I.U. per day is adequate (most formulas have 1500–2700 I.U. per liter). If a milk-free or skim-milk formula is used, vitamin A must be supplemented since much of it is removed with the fat. However, a good concentration of vitamin A exists in the fish liver oils used to supply additional vitamin D.

With vitamin D there is a possibility of toxicity. In the United States, evaporated milk, most commercial formulas, and most fresh whole milk is fortified at least to the level of 400 I.U. per liter. Skim milk, some commercial milk, and human milk contain less than the 400 I.U. daily requirement; infants fed with these need supplemental vitamin D. The premature infant needs more vitamin D than does the full-term infant.

The minimum daily requirement of vitamin C is 25 milligrams; if the infant is breast-fed, his supply of this vitamin will be adequate if his mother has a sufficient quantity in her diet. Heated cows' milk has little or no vitamin C, but orange juice and other citrus juices supply it in good quantity. One ounce of fresh orange juice or two ounces of reconstituted frozen orange juice per day will satisfy the infant's requirement. However, the most common and easiest method of satisfying all his vitamin needs is through administration of a vitamin supplement in pill or liquid form. It should be emphasized that this is not really necessary for every infant, but depends on the quantity and quality of his intake.

MINERALS

The need for minerals is met with little difficulty, with the exception of iron. Over 75 percent of the total iron content in the newborn's body at birth is in erythrocytes, but a small amount is stored in other tissues. The iron from the erythrocytes is retained in the body when the red blood cells break down and is reclaimed later for hemoglobin synthesis. The amount of iron available depends on the initial hemoglobin mass and may be inadequate to meet the infant's needs in later months if the initial hemoglobin level was low or if the infant was of a low birth weight. After birth the hemoglobin drops steadily until it reaches a low of 11 grams per 100 milliliters with a hematocrit of 33 percent at about three months. A combination of factors accounts for this change, including lack of or slow hematopoiesis, breakdown of red blood cells, and growth and expansion of the circulatory system. In the full-term infant, the recovery of erythrocytes and hemoglobin levels begins at two months when the hematopoietic process resumes. In the premature baby, this physiological anemia persists for a longer period, up to four months, since he has a smaller hemoglobin mass initially and a rapid growth rate.

Iron deficiency (hemoglobin below 10 grams per 100 milliliters) may be found in 25–76 percent of infants over six months of age from economically deprived areas and in 1–2 percent of babies from more affluent families. Formulas fortified with iron are frequently used for babies who have a high risk of developing iron deficiency anemia. The use of iron-fortified cereals is also recommended.

Feeding

The newborn faces the task of adjusting to the change from fetal nutrition to that of taking in food, digesting it, and assimilating its nutrients on his own. His gastrointestinal tract previously has not been required to utilize much muscle, chemical, or absorptive activity in handling food. Now he must do this for himself with the help of his sucking, swallowing, and gagging reflexes.

As soon as the infant cries, he swallows a large amount of air into his stomach. Once he ingests liquid as well, his stomach may easily increase to a size four or five times that of its empty contracted state. Its capacity at birth is about 30–35 milliliters, about 75 milliliters by the second week, and 100 milliliters by the end of the first month (the average adult capacity is 1000 milliliters). The newborn has 2 million gastric glands (the adult has 25 million), which begin to secrete acid before birth. The proteolytic activity of these glands in the newborn is less than 20 percent of that in the two- or three-month-old baby. The stomach musculature, including the pyloric sphincter, is moderately developed at birth, but the elastic tissue is poorly developed. Peristaltic activity in the newborn does not occur in a progressive wave but rather in a simultaneous contraction of most of the stomach musculature.

The supporting musculature of the newborn's intestinal tract is poorly developed; since his abdominal wall is weak, his abdomen often appears distended. His intestinal tract does have well-developed secretory and absorbing surfaces, but peristalsis is weak and discontinuous.

The digestive system of the normal full-term infant has the functional capacity to propel, digest, and absorb every type of food in liquid form except complex carbohydrates. The major portion of the feeding leaves his stomach in 3–4 hours, most in $1\frac{1}{2}$–2 hours after the meal, but there are wide variations. Human milk leaves the stomach more rapidly than cows' milk, and formula made from unboiled cows' milk stays in the stomach longer than formula made from boiled cows' milk.

FEEDING SCHEDULE

It seems best to begin feeding each baby according to his individual need, which usually occurs within 4 to 12 hours after birth, instead of adhering to an established routine. Plain water is usually given first, followed by glucose water. First feedings test the infant's ability to suck and swallow adequately. If he aspirates the feeding, water will be less damaging to his lung tissue than milk. If the baby is in good condition and his mother is ready, he may nurse as soon as they leave the delivery room, or even while they are still there. How often and how much he is fed depends on the baby, and this is a somewhat unknown quantity in the beginning.

Many infants are placed on a demand schedule and are fed when they show signs of hunger: waking up, crying, refusing water with disgust, seizing the nipple, and nursing vigorously. The baby usually takes what he wishes and stops when he has had enough. Most babies eat six or eight times a day, with a time lapse of from 2–8 hours between feedings, which may vary from day to day. After three or four days, the infant may have several days on which he may want to eat very frequently. After a week or two, he establishes a fairly regular schedule.

It is not unusual for babies to dawdle over their feedings during the first few days. Parents must be patient then, and they will find that it is easier to feed their baby when he appears hungry. This is particularly true if the baby is breast-feeding since if he is not hungry, he is less likely to grasp the nipple well. This will be unpleasant for him and cause unnecessary concern for the mother. Nursing support helps the parents in the process of getting to know their newborn's eating patterns; this support can consist of help in holding the baby while he eats, adjusting his position, placing the nipple in the baby's mouth, or bubbling him.

CHOICE OF METHOD

Mothers usually request information on which to base their decision of whether to breast-feed or bottle-feed; this is a cultural decision rather than a medical one in most instances. Personal attitudes, social pressures, and psychological needs all play a part. The cultural values of some nurses are strongly in favor of one or the other method of feeding, and such an opinion can interfere with good nursing care if the mother is made to feel guilty or inadequate because of her choice. Prenatal counselors can do much to reassure the mother and to solve practical problems in advance; this may lead some hesitant mothers to give breast-feeding a trial. The danger of excessive persuasion does exist, however, and may result in the creation of a sense of guilt, defeat, or frustration in the mother who does her best to breast-feed but fails. If the mother has a chronic disease (heart, kidney, tuberculosis), breast-feeding can be an additional strain. Conditions of the infant that would be contra-indications include local deformities such as cleft lip and palate and sometimes jaundice. If the infant is premature and if active breast-feeding is delayed beyond three or four weeks, the likelihood of maintaining lactation is diminished.

Currently, the majority of infants in the United States are bottle-fed, with most of the mothers who breast-feed being in the upper and middle socioeconomic classes. This is the exact opposite of the situation 25 years ago, when the majority of infants were breast-fed, especially in the lower socioeconomic class. New social values make breast-feeding seem old fashioned or even vulgar to people in many geographical areas. Anthropologists in some countries even measure the level of acculturation by the incidence of artificial feeding—the less breast-feeding, the higher the sophistication level [9]. In developing countries where the water supply is often unsafe and sanitary facilities are not well established, breast-feeding is decreasing. This is especially unfortunate since gastrointestinal disease, a result of contaminated water and formula, is still a major cause of infant mortality. The *Lactobacillus* flora in the gastrointestinal tract of the breast-fed baby creates an environment unfavorable to *E. coli* growth and discourages this source of infant morbidity.

Formula Feeding

In general bottle-feeding is easier than breast-feeding since the position of the bottle can be more readily adjusted than that of the breast. The nipple of the bottle is usually of adequate length and size to fit the baby's mouth, and the flow is even and easily maintained. In addition, bottle-feeding allows someone other than the mother to participate in the infant's feeding, and thus permits the father an earlier and more active role in infant care.

Most hospitals purchase commercially prepared formula; served moderately cold or at room temperature, it is tolerated well by most babies. As mentioned previously, babies are best fed when they are hungry, dry, and comfortable. Whether it is the nurse or the parents who do the feeding, it is important that the baby be *held* throughout. This provides another opportunity to foster development of a feeling of closeness and security. Babies are usually held in a semireclining position, with the bottle tilted enough so that the nipple is constantly filled with milk (Figure 13-23). Since sucking is ineffective when the baby's tongue is raised, it is important to make sure that the nipple is placed over the tongue. If the baby is obtaining formula, there will be air bubbles in the bottle; sometimes a clogged nipple prevents this. Needless to say, the nipple is considered sterile and should not be handled when the baby is being fed. Normally the infant consumes his feeding in about 15–20 minutes.

The common practice of propping the bottle by the baby's side is potentially

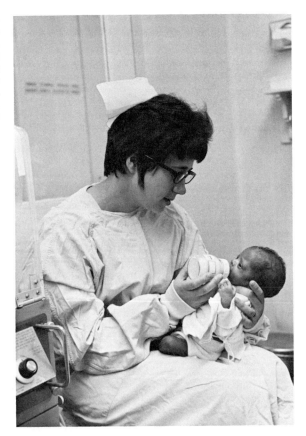

dangerous, since the baby may choke or suck in considerable air. Research [7] has also indicated that propping the bottle with the baby supine may predispose him to recurrent middle-ear infections. His eustachian tube is shorter and wider than in the adult, and it lies at such an angle that milk may be propelled to the middle ear through it following the tremendous amount of suction that the infant exerts when feeding.

When the baby goes home, his parents may choose to continue feeding him the particular formula he received in the hospital, or they may use one of a number of different preparations (Tables 13-3, 13-4, 13-5). A formula made with *evaporated milk* is still popular, low cost, generally available, sterile in the can, and convenient to store and handle; most brands of evaporated milk are equivalent in composition. For the newborn, evaporated milk is usually diluted with water in the ratio of 1:2 or 2:3, and the dilution for older infants is 1:1. The purpose of the dilution is to lessen the fat component of the milk; since the carbohydrate content is also diluted, additional sugar or corn syrup must be added. Nearly all brands are fortified with vitamin D (400 international units in a 13-ounce can). The amount of calories provided depends on dilution and on the amount of carbohydrate added. A dilution of 1:2 yields 14 calories per ounce; the 1:1 dilution yields 22 calories per ounce. Each 1 percent of carbohydrate added increases the energy value by 1.2 calories per ounce;

Table 13-3. Comparison of Components of Types of Milk

Type of Milk	Ratio	Calories/ Ounce	Grams per 100 Milliliters			
			Protein	Fat	Carbohydrate	Minerals
Human milk	Undiluted	20	1.1	4.5	6.8	0.2
Whole milk	Undiluted	20	3.3	3.5	4.8	0.72
Evaporated milk	1:1	22	3.6	4.2	5.3	0.75
Commercial preparations						
Enfamil	1:1	20	1.5	3.7	7.0	0.35
Similac	1:1	20	1.7	3.4	6.6	0.38

Table 13-4. Formula Preparation for Newborn

Basic Component	Daily Requirement
Calories	55 calories per pound of body weight (approximate)
Fluid	3 ounces per pound of body weight
Carbohydrates	40 percent of caloric daily requirement: cane sugar (48 calories per tablespoon) or corn syrup (60 calories per tablespoon)

Table 13-5. Formula for 6-Pound Baby, Using Undiluted Evaporated Milk, Corn Syrup, and Water

Basic Component	Daily Requirement
Calories	330 calories (approximate)
Fluid	18 ounces
Carbohydrates	132 calories[a]

6 ounces of evaporated milk[a] = 264 calories
1 tablespoon of corn syrup[a] = 60 calories
12 ounces of water ——
324 calories
18 ounces of fluid

[a] 1 ounce of evaporated milk contains approximately 3.1 grams of carbohydrate, so 6 ounces contains about 18 grams of carbohydrate. Each gram of carbohydrate represents 4 calories ($18 \times 4 = 72$ calories [in evaporated milk]). Corn syrup is all carbohydrate (1 tablespoon = 60 calories of carbohydrate). $60 + 72 = 132$ calories of carbohydrate.

the added carbohydrate allows normal metabolism of fats, permits protein to be used to build new tissues instead of to provide calories, and encourages normal water balance.

Fresh milk is usually boiled to modify the curd and to complete sterilization. Ordinarily water in amounts not exceeding half the volume of milk is used to dilute it for young infants. The added water is mixed with 5–8 percent carbohydrate (sugar or corn syrup). Fresh milk, likely to be fortified with vitamin D, is more expensive and cumbersome than evaporated milk, and it also requires refrigeration and a constant fresh supply. When fresh cows' milk is not modified, it yields 20 calories per ounce.

If *dried milk* is used, boiled water is used to reconstitute it to its original strength. Low-fat or nonfat dried milk will have a lower caloric value and will need a vitamin D supplement. The advantages of dried milk include low cost and the ability to be stored in bulk.

Hypoallergenic formulas are available when it becomes necessary to alter or avoid the protein fraction; these formulas use processes involving evaporating, drying, or boiling the milk, or consist of a nonmilk product, such as soybeans or almonds. These formulas have an unpalatable taste and are somewhat lower in nutritional value.

Low birth weight infants may fail to gain weight on an evaporated milk formula since they do not absorb butterfat well, and some formulas combine nonfat cows' milk and vegetable oil to solve this problem. Some of the commercial preparations (Similac and SMA) combine whey proteins, nonfat cows' milk, carbohydrate, vegetable oils, minerals, and vitamins, to achieve an end product resembling human milk in terms of the relation of whey proteins to casein and minerals.

PREPARATION OF FORMULA IN THE HOME

Artificial formula is usually made either by dilution of commercially prepared concentrated formula or by mixing an evaporated milk formula. If the baby is breast-fed, with only an occasional bottle, the commercial powdered formula is often used. It may be stored without refrigeration after opening.

The choice of preparation method depends on the kind of formula, the safety of the water and milk supply, the mother's ability to use the method, the presence of refrigeration in the home, and the number of bottles used each day. If safe milk and a pure municipal water supply are used, sterilization of the formula is usually unnecessary after the first few weeks.

With the *aseptic* method, the bottles, nipples, nipple-caps, and equipment used in making formula are sterilized (boiled for 10 minutes) before the formula is prepared. The formula is made according to directions, put into each bottle, nippled, capped, and refrigerated.

Terminal sterilization involves formula preparation under clean but not aseptic conditions. The equipment is washed thoroughly, the prepared formula is poured into the bottles, and the nipples and caps are applied loosely. They are placed in a sterilizer or large pot with a tight-fitting lid and boiled in water for 25 minutes. Prepared formula should not be left standing at room temperature but should be refrigerated as soon as it has cooled. Before refrigeration the screw caps are tightened.

When the baby does not take all of the formula from the bottle, what is left should either be discarded or used immediately in preparing cooked food, such as pudding. Generally this formula is considered unsafe for use for another feeding, even if it is refrigerated. Formula prepared for a single feeding should be used immediately.

Breast-Feeding

Many advantages are customarily attributed to breast milk: It is of correct chemical composition, it is constantly fresh and available at an even temperature, it is free from bacteria, it involves no preparation, and it causes a lower incidence of allergy. In addition, it is readily digested and assimilated, has a laxative effect on the baby, and results in less frequent and less severe feeding upsets. The flow of milk is well regulated, and the baby can suck until he is satisfied. Occasionally it is claimed that breast-feeding is cheaper, but in reality the recommended nutritional intake of the lactating mother makes breast-feeding a more expensive method of infant nutrition than some others. Poor maternal nutrition does not usually affect the quality of the milk, since the mother draws on the resources of her own tissues in its manufacture. Only the vitamin content is directly related to daily maternal intake. However, the quantity of milk can be affected; as a result, the malnourished mother probably will not have a sufficient amount of milk to adequately feed her infant.

Whether or not breast milk contains antibodies that are passed to the infant is a matter of controversy. Differences in the incidence of enteric infections in breast-fed and bottle-fed babies are documented, although some research [1] indicates that these differences fade in middle-class families with good hygiene. In populations where these differences do exist, it is hard to judge whether they are due to the beneficial effects of breast milk or to increased contamination during bottle-feeding.

There are certain components of breast milk that may provide protective properties [11]. It is suggested that IgA, the predominant immunoglobulin in milk, effects an antimicrobial protection of mucous membranes and probably acts locally on the gastrointestinal tract. Breast milk containing polio antibodies prevents successful oral immunization of the newborn with live polio virus vaccine by neutralizing the virus in the gut; therefore, the vaccine is given later. The content of IgA in early colostrum may be as high as 20–40 milligrams per milliliter; after the first two to four days, the IgA content of breast milk drops to 1 milligram per milliliter. It is postulated that an increase in milk production compensates for the drop. In addition to antibodies, breast milk is also thought to contain lymphoid cells, neutrophils, and macrophages with phagocytic activity. These may play a part in protecting the maternal lactiferous glands as well as the infant's gastrointestinal tract from infection. Breast milk contains a large amount of lactoferrin, which has a strong bacteriostatic effect on *E. coli.*

Colostrum, the first milk produced after the baby's birth, is a yellow substance with more protein (in the form of globulins) and salts than mature milk, and less fat and sugar. During this initial period of lactation the baby gets no more than $\frac{1}{2}$ ounce of colostrum at each nursing, so that it is of minimal nourishment. Its beneficial effects, other than the transfer of globulins, include the early establishment of the milk supply with a decreased possibility of subsequent breast engorgement. For these reasons many authorities advocate allowing the baby to start sucking as soon as possible after birth, with a delay of no more than 4 hours; however in many instances 12 hours elapse.

Mature milk, which appears about the third day, is a bluish-white liquid with an alkaline or possibly neutral reaction; colostrum cells are usually absent after the twelfth day. Fat globules are small, numerous, and of uniform size. For the first two weeks, mothers' milk is higher in protein and lower in fat, but in the following weeks, the protein decreases while the fat and carbohydrate content increases. The last milk the baby gets from the breast at each feeding is richest in fat.

Breast milk can be stored, usually by pasteurizing and freezing or canning it for future use. Throughout the country there are breast milk centers or banks for the collection of surplus breast milk, which is made available for premature infants or for those babies with special nutritional problems.

FEEDING TECHNIQUE

To successfully breast-feed, the infant must have both the areola and nipple in his mouth. To help the baby get a firm grasp on the nipple and areola, the mother may "point up" the nipple by gently pressing the areola between two fingers. As the baby begins to nurse, he should be prevented from pressing his nose against the breast and obstructing his nasal pathway. If this occurs, the mother should place her finger against her breast, pressing it back from the baby's nose. When the baby's jaws close, his gums compress the areola over the lacteal sinuses, squeezing the milk out. Air is sealed off by the baby's lips and flat cheek muscles. Breaking the infant's suction may be accomplished by placing a finger at the corner of the baby's mouth before pulling him away (Figure 13-24). This will prevent the nipple from becoming sore.

Periods of nursing interspersed with periods of rest are continued until the baby is satisfied. The baby nurses for 5 minutes on each breast initially, gradually increasing nursing time up to 15–20 minutes (total time). This varies considerably from baby to baby according to how hungry he is and how much he desires to suck. The baby may close his lips tightly around the nipple only and suck vigorously. With this method he obtains very little milk, and the nipple is likely to be injured by his vigorous sucking.

It is important that the mother be prepared for the initial grasp pain when the baby latches on to her breast. This will decrease as lactation becomes well established. She should also be aware of how to use the baby's rooting reflex to best advantage, since he will turn toward her breast and nipple when it touches his cheek. The nurse should refrain from trying to stimulate the rooting reflex manually, since the baby is likely to turn toward the nurse's hand rather than the mother's breast.

Successful breast-feeding also depends on frequent and complete emptying of the breasts, which stimulates the production of milk since the amount produced depends on the amount removed. Sucking itself is an important stimulus to milk production through its action on the pituitary, with subsequent release of prolactin. This stimulus is strong enough to allow a woman who has never been pregnant to

Figure 13-24. When the infant is finished eating, suction can be broken by placing a finger in one corner of the infant's mouth.

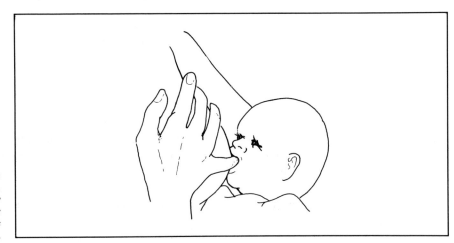

establish a milk supply for an adopted baby [13, 24]; however, this can only be achieved following persistent efforts on her part.

Sucking stimulation is greatest if the infant nurses on both breasts at each feeding, although some mothers prefer to use one breast per feeding. This choice also depends on the ease with which the baby takes the nipple, its condition, and the amount of milk produced. Usually the mother alternates which breast she offers the baby first at each feeding. Some nurseries offer a bottle to the baby after each feeding until the mother's milk supply is well established. This fluid supplement can be plain water, 5% glucose in water, low-calorie formula, or full-strength formula.

The initial filling of the mother's breasts may be accompanied by engorgement, but this varies considerably from mother to mother. The engorgement is partly due to increased vascularity and partly to the increased accumulation of milk. There may be secondary lymphatic and venous stasis if milk cannot be removed. Sometimes the ducts become occluded by congested tissues and/or blockage with earlier secretions that have become thickened. The mother needs reassurance that the discomfort of engorgement will subside in a day or two, since she may think that her breasts will remain uncomfortable for the entire time she will be nursing. If the areola is engorged and firm, the baby cannot compress the milk reservoirs underneath with his jaws. As a result, he may grasp the nipple alone, which will lead to tenderness, soreness, and cracking. Areolar massage will soften the area prior to nursing.

LET-DOWN REFLEX

When the nerve endings in the nipple are stimulated by the baby's sucking, prolactin, as mentioned previously, is released from the anterior pituitary. In addition, the posterior pituitary is stimulated to release oxytocin, which initiates the milk let-down (milk-ejection) reflex. Oxytocin stimulates the myoepithelial cells around each of the alveoli to contract, propelling the milk into the ducts so that it begins to flow from the nipple. Let-down is also often achieved through the psychological stimulus of hearing the baby cry or even thinking about him. It can become conditioned to the mother's emotion as she starts to nurse, and let-down can occur whenever she feels a sense of pleasurable anticipation, such as sitting down to a good dinner or stepping into a warm tub. Oxytocin is also involved in human sexual orgasm and its presence may account for the ready sexual arousal in some mothers during nursing. Conversely, sexual intercourse may result in an inadvertent production of a stream of milk with orgasm. Oxytocin, of course, also acts on the uterus and causes contractions for up to 20 minutes after feeding; consequently, breast-feeding aids involution.

The let-down reflex becomes stronger with increased sucking, and occurs regularly once it is firmly established, usually between the third and eighth weeks. When this happens there is less leaking of milk and occurrence of let-down at inopportune times. As a rule, good let-down is established earlier and more regularly in multiparas. The use of manual expression of colostrum two months before the baby is due may release more prolactin, which builds the colostrum supply and helps keep the ducts free from obstruction. As a result, the mother may build a more abundant milk supply more quickly and also establish a more efficient, stronger let-down within 24–48 hours after birth. Sometimes the stimulation of let-down is aided by manual expression of some milk before feeding.

HELPING THE MOTHER TO BREAST-FEED

Helping the mother to breast-feed is an important nursing function. For successful nursing, the mother needs sufficient rest and relaxation, adequate nutrition, enough fluid, and not too many social obligations or family problems. The nurse should be available at the mother's bedside the first time she nurses the baby and regularly thereafter, helping to make her comfortable, showing her how to handle the baby, helping the baby grasp the nipple, and praising and encouraging her. A breast-feeding mother often has difficulty finding a comfortable position for herself and the baby; sometimes the newborn may be successfully fed if he is lying in bed by his mother's side with the breast readily available. Another baby may do better cradled in his mother's arms as she sits in bed with her back supported, or as she sits in a rocking chair. Another baby may be more comfortable on his mother's lap, supported by a pillow (Figure 13-25).

Figure 13-25. A. Breast-feeding in sitting position. B. Lying on side while breast-feeding. (Courtesy of Booth Maternity Center, Philadelphia, Pa.)

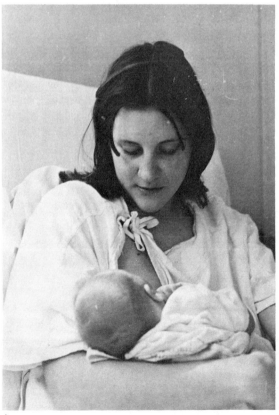

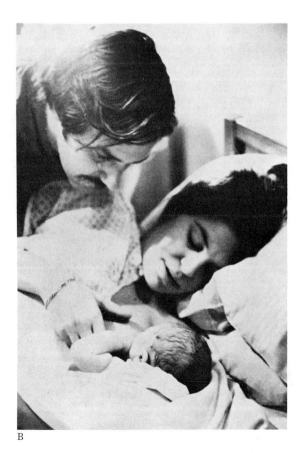

A

B

Many babies begin nursing easily and suck immediately, but occasionally a baby needs to experiment before he begins. Sometimes moistening the mother's nipple with a few drops of expressed colostrum or a few drops of formula or sugar water may prompt the baby to take the nipple more eagerly. If he does not nurse after approximately 10 minutes of trying, it is best to stop and try again at the next feeding or when he seems hungry.

It is difficult to determine the amount of milk a breast-feeding baby has taken. In some nurseries the baby is weighed before and after feeding to determine this, but most of the time other factors are used as indications that he is getting enough: his satisfaction, sleeping patterns, time between feedings, weight gain, and number of wet diapers.

Sometimes it is necessary for the mother to empty her breasts mechanically (other than by manual expression), in order to relieve engorgement, to maintain milk supply when the baby cannot empty her breasts in the early days of nursing, or to allow fissures to heal. In the hospital the mother may use an electric breast pump with intermittent suction. With this machine, pumping can be started with low suction, gradually increasing the pressure (not over 6–8 pounds) until the milk flows freely for about 10–15 minutes or until the breast is emptied.

A hand pump may also be used; with this, suction may be obtained by collapsing the rubber bulb at one end, placing the other, widened end over the nipple and areola, and releasing the bulb. The process is repeated until the desired amount of milk is emptied. This method is often used to soften the breast before the baby nurses.

It is not normal for there to be persistent pain upon nursing, other than the initial grasp pain; it is likely to be the result of an incorrect grasp by the baby. The discomfort could also be caused by cracks or blisters, which may provide a portal of entry for infection. Breast-feeding is usually decreased in time or discontinued for a day or two. Nipples will heal quickly if they are exposed to air, and sometimes A and D ointment promotes healing.

TRANSFER OF DRUGS AND OTHER SUBSTANCES IN BREAST MILK

Nearly all drugs that the mother takes may be found to some extent in her breast milk but not all of them appear in significant amounts. It is important, therefore, to consider not only what she is taking but how much. Unless the mother is taking large doses, alcohol, barbiturates, antibiotics, narcotics, salicylates, caffeine, and psychotherapeutic drugs appear in insignificant amounts in breast milk [6]. Mineral oil, milk of magnesia, and aspirin in the normal recommended doses may be safely taken. Atropine may decrease milk production and may cause intoxication in the baby. Ergot may cause vomiting, diarrhea, and weak pulse in the baby. If the mother is taking oral anticoagulants, her baby should be watched for bleeding tendencies. Steroids, bromides, cascara, and metronidazole (Flagyl) may cause symptoms in the baby. Radioactive iodine may be transmitted in the milk and may have a suppressive effect on the infant's developing thyroid; if the mother has had studies using it in the recent antepartal period, it is felt that it is wise to stop breast-feeding for a time. Smoking may decrease the mother's excretion of milk, but if she smokes only moderately, she should not be made to feel that she should give it up solely for the baby's sake. However, she should avoid smoking near the baby, since smoke inhaled by the baby increases the incidence and severity of respiratory diseases. As mentioned previously, oral contraceptives may inhibit lactation, particularly if they are begun before the fifth or sixth postpartum week. Long-range effects of marijuana on the infant have not been documented. The fact that breast milk contains more DDT than cows' milk is known; its medical importance depends on the amount received by the baby, who appears to be in no danger from present levels of DDT in breast milk.

Bubbling the Baby

When the baby's stomach is full, his sucking becomes slow and intermittent and he gradually falls asleep. Since he normally swallows air as he nurses, it is important to raise the air bubbles from his stomach. It is good practice to stop once or twice during each feeding to attempt to raise the bubble. If this is not done, the baby will burp when he is put back in bed and milk will be likely to come with it, increasing the danger of aspiration. Sometimes a baby stops sucking because a large air bubble has made his stomach feel full; after he is burped, he begins to suck with renewed interest.

Most babies are easily bubbled. If the infant is held in an upright position, the air will rise to the top of his stomach. If his body is supported against the nurse's or the mother's body or shoulder and he is gently patted or stroked on the back, the air comes up with a definite belch. Sometimes a change in position alone, from reclining to upright, is all that is needed. If the baby has not burped in 2 or 3 minutes, it probably would be wise to put him down and try again later. If this is still not successful in raising a bubble, he is put to bed and positioned either on his right side or on his abdomen. Hiccuping is common and is generally not significant.

Some babies, characterized as "spitters," regurgitate more than the usual amount; such a baby should be handled as gently as possible, fed in a calm relaxed atmosphere, and bubbled frequently. When he is placed in his crib, he should be put on his right side or abdomen in a reverse Trendelenburg position. It should be remembered that regurgitation relates to an overflow of milk, not to be confused with actual vomiting. The amount regurgitated is frequently less than it appears and the baby is usually retaining an adequate amount unless he fails to gain weight.

REFERENCES

1. Adebonojo, F. Artificial vs. breast feeding. *Clinical Pediatrics* (Philadelphia) 11:25, 1972.
2. Adlard, B. P. F., and Lathe, G. H. Breast milk jaundice: Effect of pregnanediol on bilirubin conjugation by human liver. *Archives of Diseases in Childhood* 45:186, 1970.
3. Alexander, M., and Brown, M. *Pediatric Physical Diagnosis for Nurses*. New York: McGraw-Hill, 1974.
4. American Academy of Pediatrics. *Standards and Recommendations for Hospital Care of Newborn Infants*. Evanston, Ill., 1967.
5. American Academy of Pediatrics, Committee on Fetus and Newborn. Hexachlorophene and skin care of newborn infants. *Pediatrics* 49:625, 1972.

6. Arena, J.   Contamination of the ideal food. *Nutrition Today* 5:2, 1970.
7. Beauregard, W.   Positional otitis media. *Journal of Pediatrics.* 79:294, 1971.
8. Behrman, R., and Mangurten, H.   Birth Injuries. In R. Behrman (Ed.), *Neonatology.* St. Louis: Mosby, 1973.
9. Berg, A.   The economics of breast-feeding. *Saturday Review of the Sciences* 1:29, May 1973.
10. Blake, F., Wright, F. H., and Waechter, E.   *Nursing Care of Children.* Philadelphia: Lippincott, 1970.
11. Breast milk and defence against infection in the newborn. *Archives of Diseases in Childhood* 47:845, 1972.
12. Brown, R. J. K., and Valman, H. B.   *Practical Neonatal Pediatrics.* Oxford: Blackwell Scientific, 1973.
13. Buckner, J.   Breastfeeding adopted child: She knew it was possible. *Philadelphia Inquirer,* September 1, 1972.
14. Driscoll, J. M.   Physical Examination. In R. Behrman (Ed.), *Neonatology.* St. Louis: Mosby, 1973.
15. Gordon, R.   Neonatal immunology: A review of host response to infection. *Michigan Medicine* 72:219, 1973.
16. Hargreaves, T., and Piper, R. F.   Breast-milk jaundice. *Archives of Diseases in Childhood* 46:195, 1971.
17. Hexachlorophene in the nursery. *Medical Letter on Drugs and Therapeutics* 15:1, 1973.
18. Jaundice. *LaLeche League News* 13(4), July–August, 1971.
19. Korones, S.   *High-Risk Newborn Infants.* St. Louis: Mosby, 1972.
20. Longenecker, C. G., Ryan, R. F., and Vincent, R. W.   Malformation of ear as clue to urogenital anomalies. *Plastic and Reconstructive Surgery* 35:303, 1965.
21. McClure, J. H., and Caton, W. L.   Newborn temperature: Temperature of term normal infants. *Journal of Pediatrics* 47:583, 1955.
22. Moore, M. L.   *The Newborn and the Nurse.* Philadelphia: Saunders, 1972.
23. Neonatologists and the critical first hours. *Journal of the American Medical Association* 202:41, 1967.
24. Newton, M.   Breast feeding by adoptive mother. *Journal of the American Medical Association* 212:1967, 1970.
25. Preston, E. N.   Whither the foreskin. *Journal of the American Medical Association* 213:1853, 1970.
26. Ross Conference on Pediatric Research.   *Thermoregulation of the Newly Born.* Columbus, Ohio: Ross Laboratories, 1964.
27. Vulliamy, D.   *The Newborn Child.* Baltimore: Williams & Wilkins, 1972.
28. Whitner, W., and Thompson, M.   The influence of bathing on the newborn infant's body temperature. *Nursing Research* 19:30, 1970.
29. Ziegel, E., and Van Blarcom, C.   *Obstetric Nursing.* New York: Macmillan, 1972.

FURTHER READING

Applebaum, R. M.   The modern management of successful breast feeding. *Pediatric Clinics of North America* 17:203, 1970.
Bornstein, M., Kessen, W., and Weiskopf, S.   The categories of hue in infancy. *Science* 191:201, 1976.
Crelin, E.   *Functional Anatomy of the Newborn.* New Haven: Yale University Press, 1973.
Eiger, M., and Olds, S.   *The Complete Book of Breastfeeding.* New York: Workman, 1973.
Fomon, S.   Nutrition in Infancy. In D. Lauler (Ed.), *Infant Nutrition.* New York: Medcom, 1972.
LaLeche League International.   *The Womanly Art of Breastfeeding.* Franklin Park, Ill., 1963.
Meyer, H.   What parents worry about in their newborn infants. *Medical Times* 100:51, 1972.
Pryor, K.   *Nursing Your Baby.* New York: Harper & Row, 1973.
Schaffer, A., and Avery, M. E.   *Diseases of the Newborn.* Philadelphia: Saunders, 1971.
Stevenson, R.   *The Fetus and Newly Born Infant.* St. Louis: Mosby, 1973.

Chapter 14 Complications of Pregnancy

FETAL DIAGNOSIS

In the past, there were relatively few ways of determining fetal maturity or well-being apart from determining estimated date of confinement, carefully observing uterine growth, and listening to fetal heart sounds. Currently a number of diagnostic methods are available to determine fetal maturity, the presence of sex-linked disorders, chromosomal abnormalities, hemolytic disease, and various enzyme deficiencies. The list of disorders that can be diagnosed in utero is growing rapidly as methods of detection become more sophisticated (Table 14-1). This knowledge provides the parents of severely affected fetuses with the option of abortion if they so choose, and for the parents of infants who must be delivered prematurely, provides a much greater chance of having their infant delivered when he is viable. Much of this testing, as well as counseling on genetic matters, is done in centers located throughout the country and financed in part by the National Foundation of the March of Dimes. Nurses working with childbearing families should be aware of the nearest center that provides these services in case referral is necessary.

Fetal Maturity

Tests to determine fetal maturity generally involve amniocentesis. In this commonly used procedure, the obstetrician anesthetizes the woman's skin over her lower abdominal wall and inserts a needle through it and through the wall of her uterus into the amniotic cavity. A syringe is attached to the needle, and amniotic fluid is withdrawn. This procedure can be done successfully as early as the second trimester when amniotic fluid is plentiful enough so that it can be obtained with minimal danger to the pregnant woman and/or fetus. The fluid may be tested for lecithin-sphingomyelin (L/S) ratio, creatinine and uric acid levels, bilirubin levels, and the presence of fat cells. Other tests to determine fetal maturity include ultrasonic scan and x-ray.

Lecithin-sphingomyelin. As the fetus matures, phospholipid protein matter necessary for lung expansion and gas exchange at birth is deposited in the alveoli of the lung; this material can be detected in amniotic fluid in the later months of gestation. Prior to lung maturity, the two important lipoproteins, lecithin and sphingomyelin, are in equal concentrations. Lecithin is produced in two major pathways, the choline and methylation pathways; until the thirty-fifth week of gestation, methylation is the primary pathway, while after 36 weeks of gestation lecithin is produced through the choline pathway. The choline pathway produces a more stable and

*Table 14-1. Prenatal
Diagnosis by
Amniocentesis*[a]

Chromosomal disorders
  Down's syndrome
Metabolic disorders
  Maple syrup urine disease
  Galactosemia
  Glycogen storage disease
  Glucose-6-phosphate dehydrogenase deficiency
  Tay-Sach's disease
  Niemann-Pick disease
  Mucopolysaccharidoses
    Hunter's syndrome
    Hurler's syndrome
Miscellaneous
  Adrenogenital syndrome
  Lesch-Nyhan syndrome
  Cystic fibrosis
  Anencephaly

[a]Partial list.
Source: Data from J. Thompson and M. Thompson. *Genetics in Medicine.* Philadelphia: Saunders, 1973; J. P. Greenhill and E. A. Friedman. *Biological Principles and Modern Practice of Obstetrics.* Philadelphia: Saunders, 1974.

effective form of lecithin, while lecithin produced by the methylation reaction is easily inhibited by hypothermia, hypoxia, and acidosis, and possibly by cesarean section. After 35 weeks of gestation the concentration of lecithin usually increases, while that of sphingomyelin decreases. When the ratio of lecithin to sphingomyelin in amniotic fluid is 2:1, the choline pathway of lecithin synthesis is activated, the fetal lung is considered mature, and the chances that the infant will develop respiratory distress syndrome are low [5].

A rapid foam test is in use that indicates the presence of lecithin in amniotic fluid. When the fluid is mixed with ethanol and is shaken vigorously, a stable foam forms in the presence of adequate amounts of lecithin, while lesser amounts form varying degrees of bubbling [11].

Creatinine and Uric Acid. Creatinine levels found in amniotic fluid are considered by many physicians to be reliable measures of gestational age. After 34 weeks' gestation, the concentration in amniotic fluid rises progressively and rapidly. Most amniotic fluid specimens with levels in excess of 1.8 milligrams per 100 milliliters of fluid correlate with gestational ages over 36 weeks [10, 11]. The concentration, however, depends on fetal muscle mass, kidney excretion, amniotic fluid volume, and maternal serum levels [25].

Uric acid levels are often ascertained with creatinine levels to determine fetal age. Uric acid, like creatinine, increases significantly as gestation increases, reflecting an increased urinary output and muscle mass of the maturing fetus [35].

Bilirubin. By using spectrophotometric analysis of amniotic fluid, it is possible to measure minute quantities of bilirubin and other breakdown products of hemoglobin. Bilirubin normally appears in the amniotic fluid as early as the twelfth week, and the level decreases as gestation advances (particularly after the thirty-fifth week), presumably as the liver matures and is able to conjugate bilirubin. Bilirubin levels remain high or increase in the presence of hemolytic disease. It is difficult to obtain good test results if there is meconium or blood in the amniotic fluid specimen or if hydramnios is present [10, 25].

Fat Cells. Amniotic fluid may also be tested for the presence of fat cells in determining fetal maturity. There is a sharp rise in the number of these cells after 36 weeks, possibly due to the functional maturity of fetal sebaceous glands. The fetus is considered mature when a 20-percent fat cell count is found in amniotic fluid. These same fat cells, which stain orange with a 1% Nile blue sulfate stain, can be identified in vaginal smears when the woman's membranes have ruptured [11, 15].

ULTRASOUND TESTING

Ultrasound testing involves using reflected sound waves as they travel in tissue; it can be used to produce an echocardiogram. When the ultrasonic pulse beam is directed appropriately through the fetal head, the biparietal diameter may be measured accurately. A cross section can be obtained using an oscilloscopic beam and the ultrasonic beam so that the echo dots yield a cross-sectional anatomical picture (Figure 14-1).

Ultrasound can detect pregnancy (as early as the eighth week), multiple pregnancy, fetal abnormalities (such as anencephaly and hydrocephalus), hydatidiform mole, fetal death, fetal soft tissue abnormalities, and hydramnios. It can also be used to determine placental position, as well as to estimate fetal weight. Thompson [34] found that 91 percent of fetuses with biparietal diameters of 8.5 centimeters (3.3 inches) or greater weighed over 2500 grams (5.5 pounds), and Stocker, et al. [32] found that 90 percent of fetuses weighed over 3000 grams (6.6 pounds) when the diameter was 9.1 centimeters (3.6 inches). Weight determinations have been inaccurate with fetuses who were small or large for their gestational age, unless serial determinations were performed. Problems measuring the biparietal diameter are also encountered when the fetal head is deep in the pelvis, in breech presentations, or when the mother is obese or has hydramnios.

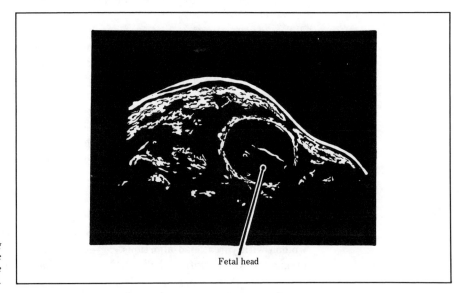

Fetal head

Figure 14-1. Drawing simulating ultrasonic transverse scan of the fetal head.

X-RAY

X-rays have been used to determine fetal maturity based on specific epiphyseal centers of ossification, the size of the fetal skull, and fetal length. This method has the inherent problem of exposure to radiation for the fetus and mother, as well as intrinsic inaccuracies resulting from variations in growth rate and skeletal maturation.

In general, the distal femoral epiphysis is apparent at 36 weeks and the proximal tibial epiphysis at 38 weeks; however, female fetuses are more advanced in bony development than males. The skeletal maturation of black fetuses develops more rapidly than that of white fetuses [7, 15]. The use of x-ray to determine fetal maturity is being replaced today by use of ultrasound measurements.

Fetal Well-Being

Tests to determine fetal well-being may require a blood specimen from the mother, a 24-hour urine collection, and an endoscopic examination, or amniocentesis may be done.

ESTRIOL

One test of fetal well-being depends on the determination of estriol levels from samples of maternal urine collected over a 24-hour period. Serial estriol determinations provide information about the fetoplacental unit, since the biosynthesis of estriol within the placenta cannot occur without precursor substances produced in the fetal adrenal gland. As pregnancy advances, the low urinary values found in the first and second trimesters increase, particularly during the last three to four weeks. Levels above 12 milligrams per day after 34 weeks are considered adequate [11]. Levels that drop 50 percent or more in a week signify danger to the fetus, and levels of 4 milligrams per day or less indicate that fetal death is possible within 48 hours [11].

The level of estriol excretion shown by the test is influenced by the length of gestation, fetal and placental size, existence of multiple pregnancy, maternal renal function, and adequacy of the urine collection. There is reported to be poor correlation between fetal well-being and estriol levels when erythroblastosis is present, and estriol levels are low with fetal malformation. Because of these problems, estriol levels in amniotic fluid specimens have been studied, but reports indicate that correlations using this method are not any better than those using specimens from urinary collections [15]. Plasma estriol levels are being studied, but to date the technique remains complex and is not in widespread use.

PLACENTAL POLYPEPTIDES

Placental function can be monitored by determining levels of human chorionic gonadotropin (HCG) and human placental lactogen (HPL). In early pregnancy, women with threatened abortions excrete decreasing amounts of HCG. In later pregnancy, women with diabetes, Rh immunization, and preeclampsia excrete high levels of HCG, suggesting that near term, high levels may signify impending fetal death.

It has been reported that as pregnancy advances there is a linear increase in the production of HPL (chorionic somatomammotropin). Levels falling below 4 micrograms per milliliter after 30 weeks of gestation indicate fetal danger. Rather than a single test, serial determinations (as in estriol studies) should be performed to follow the progress of the pregnancy in diabetes, hypertensive disorders, isoimmunization, intrauterine growth retardation, and threatened abortion. Since this test merely indicates placental function, it is used in conjunction with other tests that indicate fetal status or maturity [30].

HORMONAL CYTOLOGY

Hormonal cytology has also been used to determine the status of the pregnancy, as reflected in the morphological appearance of desquamated vaginal cells. When abortion threatens, there is an increase in the number of karyopyknotic cells. Fetal death is associated with a decrease in small cells and the appearance of parabasal cells. Persistent ferning of cervical mucus beyond the first two to three months of pregnancy confirms a poor prognosis for that pregnancy [15].

ENZYME STUDIES

Maternal plasma levels of diamine oxidose (histaminase) may be used to evaluate fetal well-being in the first two trimesters. The amount increases normally during the first 20 weeks of pregnancy, while falling levels during this time indicate threatened or missed abortion. Enzyme titers greater than 500 units per milliliter indicate that pregnancy will be maintained into the third trimester [15].

Enzyme studies may also be carried out on cultures of fetal cells obtained from amniocentesis. Results of these studies can establish the presence of enzyme deficiencies in the fetus, such as the deficiencies found in galactosemia and the Lesch-Nyhan syndrome. Other enzyme deficiencies, such as the low levels of hexosaminidase A found in Tay-Sachs disease, may be detected in amniotic fluid cells as well as the liquor itself.

The karyotyping of cultured cells can demonstrate the presence of various chromosomal abnormalities, including mongolism. Some hospitals routinely do karyotype screening on pregnant women who are 40 years of age or older, because of the increased incidence of trisomy in this age group. Karyotyping also establishes the fetal sex, which may be helpful for couples who have a history of sex-linked disorders such as hemophilia.

ALPHA-FETOPROTEIN

Alpha-fetoprotein, which is currently receiving much attention in the determination of fetal well-being, is a major plasma protein of early fetuses, synthesized by the fetal liver and yolk sac but not the placenta. Its function is not known but it may bind estrogens. Alpha-fetoprotein levels are highest in fetal serum during the first 12–14 weeks of gestation; after this period the concentration of alpha-fetoprotein decreases and that of albumin increases. Increased levels in maternal serum are associated with maternal immunization against Rh and ABO blood factors, severe fetoplacental dysfunction, and intrauterine death. Levels in amniotic fluid normally decrease as pregnancy progresses, while greatly increased levels have been found in fetuses with spina bifida, anencephaly, and other neural tube defects [23, 29].

CORTISOL

In addition to alpha-fetoprotein, cortisol has been the subject of much research to determine its role in fetal development and the use of cortisol as a measure of fetal well-being. Experimental and clinical observations suggest that glucocorticoids have an important role in the normal process of fetal lung maturation. Receptors for glucocorticosteroids have been demonstrated in fetal lung tissue. There is indirect evidence that glucocorticoids stimulate acceleration of pulmonary surfactant and enhance fetal lung maturation. Premature birth, prior to the 24 to 48 hours of increased cortisol levels in utero that is found in full-term births, is associated with respiratory distress syndrome. Although the treatment remains controversial, premature infants have a lower incidence of respiratory distress syndrome (even though as fetuses in utero they were shown to have low L/S ratios) if the mother receives glucocorticoids 24 hours prior to the birth [2]. One study [12] reported amniotic fluid cortisol levels 2.4 times higher at 35 to 40 weeks of gestation than those found at 20 to 34 weeks. Respiratory distress syndrome did not occur when total amniotic fluid cortisol was greater than 60 milligrams per milliliter. Pregnancies over 40 weeks were reported to have further increases in total cortisol, and values over 120 milligrams per milliliter were found in this group.

AMNIOSCOPY

Amnioscopy has limited value in determining fetal well-being. An amnioscope may be passed by aseptic technique into the cervical canal to visualize the amniotic fluid for the presence of blood or meconium. However, the procedure may cause cervical trauma and vaginal bleeding and possibly premature rupture of membranes or premature induction of labor [1].

OXYTOCIN CHALLENGE TEST

In order to assess the fetus' ability to withstand the stress of labor, the woman may undergo a short period of simulated labor contractions. This test may be carried out anytime after the thirty-fourth week of gestation; contractions are started and maintained by giving the woman an intravenous infusion of oxytocin for 15 minutes or until she has had about eight contractions. The fetal monitor records the fetal response to each uterine contraction, showing type II dips when placental insufficiency is present (see Chapter 15). If the fetal heart rate shows intolerance to the test, the intravenous infusion is discontinued; the baby is delivered by cesarean section, since he might not survive the stress of labor.

FIRST-TRIMESTER COMPLICATIONS

Spontaneous Abortion

Spontaneous abortion, the loss of a fetus up to 20 weeks of gestation or weighing less than 500 grams (1.1 pounds), accounts for the loss of 1 in every 5–7 pregnancies [15]. It is not known what causes most spontaneous abortions; however, it is known that in the early months of pregnancy, spontaneous expulsion of the conceptus is preceded by fetal death.

Spontaneous abortions have been attributed to abnormal uterine environment, defects in germ plasm, and defects in early development, possibly due to teratogens such as chemicals, viruses, radiation, or poisoning from heavy metals, anesthetic or illuminating gases. They have also been attributed to systemic disease in either parent, maternal thyroid dysfunction, and severe maternal anemia. In one study, 76 percent of the spontaneously aborted fetuses were abnormal [18]. Depending on the population studied, chromosomal abnormalities were found in 22–50 percent of the aborted fetuses; the earlier the abortion occurred, the more severe the associated anomaly was [31]. It has also been documented that women over the age of 35 have a higher incidence of spontaneous abortion and of infants born with congenital malformations [15].

One maternal factor believed to favor abortion is decreased amounts of progesterone produced by the corpus luteum early in pregnancy or by the placenta later in pregnancy. Early in pregnancy the deficient progesterone is unfavorable to implantation and development, while deficiency later may increase uterine sensitivity and allow coordinated uterine contractions to expel the pregnancy.

Maternal infection has also been cited as a cause of spontaneous abortion, which may result from a transfer of bacterial toxins and microorganisms that affect the fetus. It is also possible that the infectious process in the mother may increase her temperature and metabolic needs while compromising those of the fetus and placenta. Chronic infections with *Listeria monocytogenes* and *Toxoplasma* have been cited as causes of abortion.

Perhaps surprisingly, a woman may undergo anesthesia and surgery without spontaneous abortion, provided that hypoxia is avoided. Likewise, while abortion may result from trauma, it is an extremely rare occurrence.

Abortions early in pregnancy result in the loss of the entire products of conception, while abortions later in pregnancy usually result in the loss of the fetus but retention of the placenta or portions of the membranes. Pregnancy tests may continue to yield positive results as long as portions of the placenta continue to produce HCG.

When *threatened abortion* occurs, most physicians prescribe bed rest and abstinence from intercourse, although many would agree this treatment has no basis in fact. Diethylstilbestrol had been used as a treatment for threatened abortion in the past, but vaginal clear-cell carcinoma has been reported among the female children of these pregnancies [8]. Some physicians will give progesterone if a pregnanediol test shows decreased progesterone excretion, and some of them have reported improved fetal survival rates. Progesterone, however, can cause masculinization of the female fetus if given before the twelfth week, or phallic enlargement when given over longer periods.

If rest does not relieve her symptoms, the woman may be asked to resume some of her activities, in the belief that the pregnancy will be lost and the activity may shorten the time. Many clinicians, citing the high percentage of abnormal fetuses expelled in spontaneous abortion, question whether any attempt should be made to try to retain a pregnancy once an abortion threatens. It should also be noted that approximately one out of every five women has some spotting of blood during the early months of pregnancy, and only one-half of these pregnancies are lost [17].

When abortion becomes *inevitable* as the external cervical os dilates and the membranes rupture, pieces of the conceptus may be expelled. When a portion of the conceptus remains in the uterus (*incomplete abortion*) bleeding continues; if it is not removed, infection can ensue. The uterus is evacuated with a curette or a vacuum extractor. If the pregnancy has advanced past the first trimester and the cervix is not open, saline instillation may be used.

Habitual abortions (which are said to have occurred when women have lost three or more pregnancies), have been attributed to thyroid dysfunction, uterine abnormalities, pathological ova, hormonal imbalance, tumors, and an incompetent cervical os. With treatment, 70–80 percent of all women who experienced habitual abortion successfully carry a pregnancy [17].

In habitual abortion caused by an *incompetent cervical os,* the woman loses the pregnancy during the second trimester as the cervix silently dilates, the membranes rupture, and the fetus is expelled. The cervix rarely dilates prior to the sixteenth week, since the products of conception are believed to be too small to cause cervical dilatation prior to that time. Therefore, the treatment consists of surgical reinforcement of the weak cervix with a purse-string suture prior to this time or before the cervix has dilated 4 centimeters (Figure 14-2). There are two similar surgical procedures that are used, the McDonald and the Shirodkar procedures. When the McDonald procedure is used, the cervical suture is removed at 38–39 weeks, allowing the woman to progress through labor and vaginal delivery. With the Shirodkar procedure, either the suture is snipped prior to or at the beginning of labor, or it may be left in place for the next pregnancy, in which case a cesarean section is performed. The nurse working with a laboring woman who has had either of these procedures performed may find that progress is slow due to fibrotic changes in the cervix, but this slow progress may be followed by very sudden cervical dilatation and delivery. Cervical lacerations may also occur.

A woman who experiences a *missed abortion* retains her dead fetus in utero without undergoing uterine contractions that would expel it; the reasons for this are unknown. The fetus becomes macerated, developing flabby skin, soft tissues, and loose bones, or more rarely becomes mummified as it dries and becomes leathery. With fetal death, pregnancy tests may remain positive if villi are still active. The woman experiences a regression in breast and uterine size; after three weeks, blood fibrinogen decreases as a result of intravascular coagulation. The latter problem may be averted by intermittent administration of heparin subcutaneously [13]. If spontaneous abortion does not occur soon after diagnosis, intra-amniotic injection of saline is used in an effort to expel the uterine contents.

*Figure 14-2. Shirodkar
procedure for reinforcing
a weak cervix.*

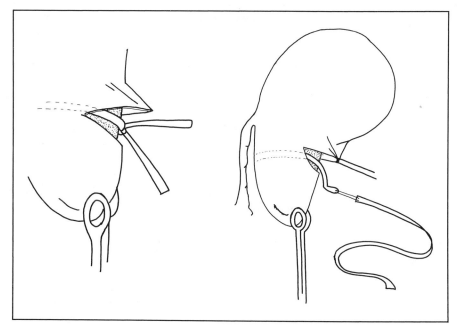

Figure 14-2. Shirodkar procedure for reinforcing a weak cervix.

Ectopic Pregnancy

Ectopic pregnancy, or pregnancy outside of the normal uterine environment, is a complication which ranks seventh among the causes of maternal mortality. Because its symptoms are sometimes vague, it may be confused with other abdominal conditions, resulting in a delay in diagnosis and treatment. In about three or four out of 1000 cases of ectopic pregnancy, the woman disregards vaginal staining for several days or weeks and then she collapses and dies as a result of hemorrhagic shock before she can be treated surgically.

An ectopic pregnancy occurs once in every 87–300 deliveries, and 98 percent of the time implantation takes place in one of the fallopian tubes [28]. Causes of ectopic pregnancy vary, but many such pregnancies result from a congenital anatomical irregularity in the tube or the presence of diverticula, either of which may impede or prevent the progress of the dividing trophoblast through the tube. Other factors that may contribute to the incidence of ectopic pregnancy are endometriosis of the oviduct, previous tuboplasty, previous tubal pregnancy, or the use of an intrauterine contraceptive device. The current increase in cases of venereal disease may actually result in an increased incidence of ectopic pregnancies, since the accompanying pelvic inflammatory complications and formation of scar tissue result in narrowed tubal lumens. The use of the antibiotics in treatment has also probably contributed to the incidence of ectopic pregnancy by preventing tubal occlusion (sterility) but not preventing injured mucosa and scar formation. There is some evidence that postabortion infections may produce a similar result [27].

The trophoblast may implant in the interstitial, isthmic, or ampullary portion of the oviduct. An interstitial or cornual implantation occurs least often and is the most dangerous, since diagnosis is often not made before rupture occurs. Hypertrophy of the cornua allows the conceptus to reach sizable proportions before the trophoblast penetrates the uterine and tubal walls and causes rupture. Sometimes signs and symptoms do not appear before the beginning of the second trimester. The rupture is similar to rupture of the uterus, and the intra-abdominal hemorrhage is sudden, massive, and an immediate threat to life.

Implantation in the tubal isthmus is more common. Hypertrophy of the tubal musculature at the isthmus is insufficient to accommodate the growing ovum, and the wall at the placental site is weakened. Any trauma—straining at stool, coitus, or bimanual examination—may cause slight hemorrhage in this area. Within two or three weeks after the first missed period, the tube bursts from overdistention of the thinned necrotic wall, and there is bleeding into the peritoneal cavity. Although the rupture is usually on the abdominal surface, occasionally it is into the broad ligament. Sometimes a hematoma will form there, resulting in mild discomfort. Further growth of the pregnancy and hematoma will result in rupture of the broad ligament and its contents into the abdominal cavity.

Ampullary implantations are the most frequent form of tubal pregnancy. When the implantation occurs near the distensible fimbria, the conceptus may grow for six to 12 weeks before it is lost. It may be extruded into the abdominal cavity without injury to the tube, and transient pelvic pain for only a few hours may be the only symptom. If bleeding is extensive, signs of intra-abdominal hemorrhage will be present. Sometimes the conceptus may reimplant in the abdominal cavity or in a mass of adhesions and continue to grow as a secondary abdominal or tuboabdominal pregnancy. If the implant is medial to the fimbria, the woman's clinical course is comparable to an isthmic pregnancy.

Ovarian pregnancies, which are very rare, result from the implantation of the egg within the follicle; usually surgery becomes necessary by the end of the first trimester. Very rarely the implantation site is the cervix, and the initial diagnosis is likely to be placenta previa. Cervical implantation usually results in hemorrhage severe enough to necessitate a hysterectomy.

An abdominal ectopic pregnancy, an exceedingly rare event, occurs when the egg implants on the surface of the ovary, on another reproductive structure, or on the pelvic peritoneum. It may be a primary implant or secondary to a tubal abortion. This pregnancy may go to term, but the fetal prognosis is very poor due to hemorrhage or separation of the placenta. The universal symptom is pain, and a soft tissue x-ray is usually diagnostic. The placenta is absorbed if left in place, but it may separate before the vessels completely thrombose. Sometimes the condition may go completely undetected, in which case the fetus becomes a small lithopedion (calcified fetus), only to be identified years later during abdominal surgery or autopsy.

Unfortunately there are as yet no reliable diagnostic laboratory procedures that definitely establish or exclude ectopic pregnancy, and the diagnosis is rarely made before tubal rupture or hemorrhage takes place. The woman with an ectopic pregnancy may have a history of longstanding infertility or pelvic inflammatory disease. She will give a history of irregular vaginal staining, possibly dysuria or dyspareunia, one or more missed or scanty periods, and the sudden onset of abdominal pain and syncope while doing something strenuous. Her other symptoms of lower abdominal and pelvic discomfort may be vague but may also be localized to the side of gestation.

If rupture has occurred, her signs and symptoms will be governed by the amount of hemorrhage. She may have abdominal tenderness, rigidity, and generalized, sharp, knifelike abdominal pain. Her uterus is likely to be enlarged because of the trophoblastic estrogen and progesterone, and movement of her cervix will elicit a sharp localized pelvic pain because blood has irritated the pelvic peritoneum. This cervical movement may also give her the urge to void, defecate, or vomit. If the blood has irritated the diaphragm, her pain may be referred to her shoulder or chest. Pain in the flank, rectum, or suprapubic region is not uncommon. Blue skin about the umbilicus (Cullen's sign) appears late and is present only if the hemorrhage is extensive. If the rupture occurs gradually, her symptoms will be less characteristic and may vary from hours to weeks in their appearance. Culdoscopy, culdocentesis, and laparoscopy are useful diagnostic procedures for the visualization of the pelvic structures or for detection of blood in the peritoneal cavity.

In most cases the treatment is immediate surgery to establish hemostasis and combat shock. Blood replacement is begun and blood volume is monitored by central venous pressure. The affected tube is usually removed, although if one tube has already been lost, there is usually an attempt to save the remaining one by resection. The ultimate prognosis is good for the woman in whom rupture occurs early. Surgical removal of an unruptured ectopic pregnancy carries no more risk than the hazards of anesthesia and laparotomy. It should be remembered that Rh isoimmunization may follow an ectopic pregnancy.

Care of the woman with an ectopic pregnancy revolves specifically around the prevention of a life-threatening hemorrhage. Therefore she is very carefully monitored, with bed rest, pad counts, and frequent vital signs. Since this is a completely unexpected event most of the time, many couples are completely overwhelmed once they understand the seriousness of what is happening. They often need a chance to discuss their fears and concerns, particularly regarding their chances for a subsequent successful pregnancy.

SECOND-TRIMESTER COMPLICATIONS

Gestational Trophoblastic Disease

A hydatidiform mole is a hydropic swelling or "degeneration" of the connective tissue of immature chorionic villi resulting in segmental grapelike accumulations of fluid within the villous branches (Figure 14-3). These grapelike clusters are grossly visible and tend to develop when the villous circulation fails to develop normally. Vesicles become attached by fibrous strands to one another, distending the entire uterus. There may also be the remains of a degenerating fetus if embryogenesis has proceeded normally for some time. One theory regarding the development of a mole is that an initially normal placenta undergoes villous degeneration when a fetal death occurs and circulation ceases, but no abortion occurs promptly [28].

A hydatidiform mole occurs once in 1500–2000 pregnancies in the United States.

Figure 14-3. Hydatidiform mole.

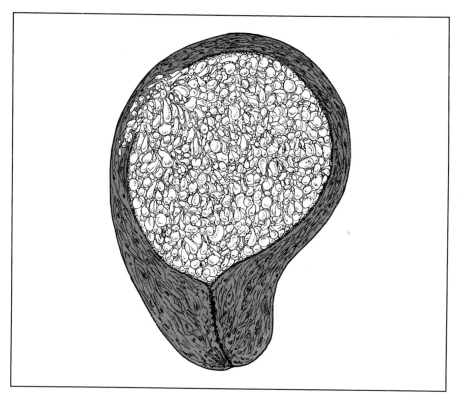

The incidence is much greater in the Far East, especially China, the Philippines, and Malaya, where it occurs once in every 145–500 pregnancies [15]. The diagnosis of a benign hydatid mole may be confused with multiple pregnancy or with a threatened abortion accompanied by concealed hemorrhage, both of which cause one of the signs of a molar pregnancy: a uterus which is unusually large for the time of gestation. In addition, there is vaginal bleeding, which may be slight or profuse, as part of the mole becomes separated from its attachment. Bleeding may be brown (like prune juice) or bright red and will probably result in anemia, so the woman may appear pale and weak. Usually the HCG titer is markedly increased beyond the ninetieth day of gestation, when it would normally be expected to drop. About 30 percent of women with molar pregnancies have hyperemesis. About 10 percent have hyperthyroidism as the trophoblastic cells produce a molar thyrotropin, similar to the hormone isolated from the pituitary gland and placenta [24]. About 20 percent of the time, symptoms of preeclampsia present before the twentieth week of gestation.

Vaginal bleeding, usually the first symptom of a molar pregnancy, commonly occurs at the beginning of the second trimester, but it may not occur until the sixth month. Occasionally the bleeding may be accompanied by the passage of some of the hydropic villi. When the woman is examined, no fetal heart tones can be detected by auscultation and electrocardiography, and no fetal skeleton is shown on ultrasound and x-ray.

Once the diagnosis is made and the woman's blood loss is replaced, the mole is removed by dilatation and curettage, suction curettage, or if it is more advanced than 14 weeks, by hysterotomy. Hysterectomy is considered if the woman is 40 years or older, since the potential for development of subsequent malignancy is high in this group. Development of subsequent malignancy is one of the complications of molar pregnancy, along with the possibility of preeclampsia, recurrent hemorrhage, and perforation of the uterus.

The cure rate, once the mole is removed, is 85–90 percent. The antimetabolite drugs, methotrexate or actinomycin-D, may be given both before and after removal of the mole, to prevent the development of trophoblastic disease. This type of prophylaxis is used especially when the incidence of malignant disease is high and the chances of follow-up poor. Because of the toxic side effects of these drugs, they are not administered unless the woman is kept under close observation, with appropriate blood and kidney studies.

A woman who has had a molar pregnancy is observed routinely for one year for gonadotropin activity; HCG levels should be negative within six weeks after evacuation. Chest x-rays are done at intervals to determine if any metastasis of molar tissue has occurred. To avoid masking the HCG levels with those of a subsequent pregnancy, the woman should wait for at least six months to one year before attempting another pregnancy. The incidence of a repeat mole is minimal. As a rule there is no specific follow-up treatment for women whose titers fall quickly and do not rise again.

Chorioadenoma Destruens (Invasive Mole)

If the mole retains the invasive qualities of the trophoblast, it may invade deeply into the myometrium and perforate blood vessels and may also invade the vagina or parametrium. This invasive phenomenon occurs in 1 out of every 6 to 10 patients who have a mole, and is diagnosed by biopsy. Chemotherapy yields good results, although in some cases hysterectomy may be advocated. Chorioadenoma destruens is more malignant than the benign mole but less malignant than choriocarcinoma.

Choriocarcinoma

Choriocarcinoma is one of the most malignant neoplasms affecting women, but fortunately it is very rare. About one-third of the cases of choriocarcinoma develop from a normal pregnancy after the twentieth week of gestation, and about one-third develop from a molar pregnancy [28]. The woman's symptoms are similar to those of a woman who has a mole, but the disease is accompanied by early metastasis to the lung and the vagina. It is diagnosed by an increased HCG titer and by x-ray demonstration of metastatic lung lesions. Treatment includes chemotherapy and hysterectomy, but even with chemotherapy, about half of these women cannot be cured.

Feelings of fear and anxiety run high in the woman with trophoblastic disease while tests are made that will determine her freedom from malignant disease. If the affected pregnancy has been a first one, it might be more difficult for her to resolve her feelings about producing an abnormal growth rather than a baby. She may well question her feminine identity or her future childbearing ability, and she may feel guilty about having done something wrong to cause the abnormal pregnancy. If she has to have a hysterectomy, there may be additional feelings resulting from alteration of body image and loss of sexual identity. Severe depressive reactions may result from the combination of side effects of the chemotherapy and separation from family members and perhaps from the psychological impact of the baby's arrival. Effective emotional support from the nursing staff is a necessity.

Hyperemesis Gravidarum

A dangerous and abnormal situation exists when a woman's vomiting continues after the first trimester and interferes with fluid balance and other phases of nutrition. Fortunately, hyperemesis gravidarum is rare today.

The specific etiology of hyperemesis is unknown. It may be related to an increased amount of HCG, although the increase is probably a result of the state of dehydration rather than being caused by increased secretion. However, in molar pregnancies, the increased HCG levels are associated with a greater incidence of hyperemesis. No foreign or specific protein substance has been identified as a possible cause of hyperemesis; one suggestion is that it may be a reflex from uterine displacement [28]. It is generally accepted that there is a psychosomatic component in hyperemesis, resulting from insecurity, anxiety, or a negative attitude toward the pregnancy [15]. However, in some cases the vomiting may have actual physical causes not necessarily related to the pregnancy.

The woman with hyperemesis experiences vomiting, especially when the stomach is empty; her other symptoms may include nausea at the mention or sight of food, weight loss, increased pulse, dehydration, signs of vitamin deficiency, thirst, hiccups, heartburn, ptyalism, constipation, and scanty, concentrated urine. With treatment nearly all women respond well. Therapeutic abortion is rarely necessary.

Most of the time women with hyperemesis are hospitalized for treatment, and nurses play a vital role in their eventual recovery. Their initial assessment of the woman's physical condition and feelings about herself and her pregnancy forms the basis for further care. The nurses' attitudes of confidence in the effectiveness of the treatment and their reassurance, concern, warmth, firmness, and understanding are important elements in the woman's positive response.

Women with hyperemesis are usually restricted from oral intake and given intravenous fluids for 48 hours. Then, if symptoms have subsided, they are permitted frequent small meals, which they choose themselves but which are predominantly carbohydrate. Small doses of sedatives and tranquilizers, and the frequent use of mouthwash will contribute to recovery, which may be slow.

Hospitalization removes the woman from pressing duties and responsibilities, which is often essential to improvement in her condition. Usually no visitors are permitted in this protected environment, occasionally not even the husband. Family members should be encouraged to call the nurse for progress reports during this period of separation.

THIRD-TRIMESTER COMPLICATIONS

Placenta Previa

About 5–6 percent of pregnant women have vaginal bleeding or staining in the latter half of pregnancy. Sometimes the open blood vessels thrombose and the bleeding ceases, but occasionally the hemorrhage is of such magnitude that the death of the mother and fetus results.

One of the major causes of hemorrhage in the latter half of pregnancy is placenta previa, which occurs when the ovum implants on or near the isthmic portion of the uterus. During the following growth and development, the placenta covers a portion of the lower uterine segment, including the cervix. Placenta previa occurs in about 1 percent of patients who are beyond the twentieth week of gestation; about 75 percent of these will be multiparas. As parity increases, placenta previa becomes more frequent, presumably due to atrophic changes of the endometrium.

Although the etiology of placenta previa is uncertain, it may develop when the ovum encounters an area of healthy endometrium in the lower portion of the uterus. It could develop following implantation in the upper segment owing to faulty or poorly vascularized endometrium. In the presence of this relative ischemia, the placenta will spread over a large area and will extend into the lower uterine segment. The placenta is likely to be thin with a large surface area and additional cotyledons in the form of succenturiate lobe formation. Marginal insertion of the cord commonly occurs. Since the lower uterine segment is covered with significantly less endometrium than the uterine body, the development of placenta accreta (a placenta that is abnormally adherent to the uterine wall) occurs with some frequency. It may be that placenta previa develops from a portion of the decidua capsularis located near or in contact with the lower uterine segment, in which case the villi of the chorion laeve beneath the particular area of the capsularis persist [28].

DIAGNOSIS AND INITIAL CARE

The woman's care depends on the type of placenta previa, the length of her gestation, and the amount her cervix is dilated (Figure 14-4). In total placenta previa, the internal cervical os is completely covered; in partial placenta previa, it is partially covered; and in a low placental implantation (marginal placenta previa), a margin of the internal os is covered by the placenta.

Placenta previa is characterized by painless vaginal bleeding in the latter half of pregnancy, especially in the last trimester. It occurs without warning and in the absence of trauma; very often the woman will awake in a pool of blood of varying amounts, usually about a cupful. In cases of total placenta previa the bleeding is usually greater and appears earlier than in partial placenta previa. Most often the mother contacts the clinic nurse, midwife, or obstetrician by telephone, and she is advised to come to the hospital immediately by ambulance, even though the initial episode of bleeding is rarely fatal.

Since she is likely to be taken to the labor floor, the nurse there is the one who usually will give her initial care [22]. The amount of her bleeding is checked (50

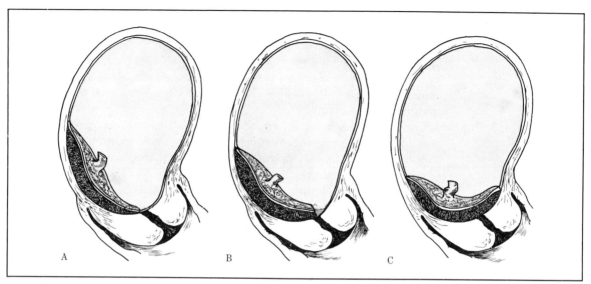

Figure 14-4. Types of placenta previa. A. Marginal placenta. B. Partial placenta previa. C. Total placenta previa.

milliliters, small amount; 100 milliliters, moderate amount; 500 milliliters, profuse amount), and a decision is made regarding which labor bed will be best for close observation of her condition. En route to her room she is asked about the bleeding: When did it start? More or less than a menstrual period? Any previous episodes? Pain, cramping, contractions? Was the doctor notified? Did she have any accidents? When is the baby due? After she is transferred to her bed, her vital signs are checked (blood pressure, temperature, pulse, respiration, and fetal heart tone), and her abdomen is palpated for tenderness, rigidity, and fetal position. Often the placental souffle can be heard above the symphysis pubis. The mother's emotional status is also noted.

This initial nursing assessment is communicated to the doctor, and the nurse can inform both of the expectant parents of the care and treatment to come. This usually includes blood work, an intravenous infusion, close monitoring, oxygen if necessary, a possible speculum examination, and diagnostic tests for placental localization. If the same nurse remains with the couple throughout these procedures, even accompanying them to the x-ray department, they may identify with a familiar individual and not have the extra emotional burden of relating to more than one member of the nursing team.

Abnormal fetal presentations are common with placenta previa and can be identified early. They often provide the first clue, before the initial bleeding episode, that tests to localize the placenta should be done. This is especially useful prior to the thirty-fifth or thirty-sixth weeks of pregnancy. After this point, the diagnosis is established by a vaginal examination in the operating room or delivery room, with everything in preparation for an immediate cesarean section (double set-up). If a vaginal examination is done before this time, it may precipitate serious bleeding and necessitate immediate termination of the pregnancy.

Placental localization can be achieved in a number of ways. X-ray methods include cystography, with a contrast medium in the bladder, and femoral angiography, a test that outlines the intervillous spaces and is 97 percent accurate. Soft tissue x-ray is 90–95 percent accurate, and a radioactive isotope scan, which is also highly accurate. Ultrasound can be used to outline the boundaries of the placenta. Thermography, probably just as accurate as ultrasound, depends on the presence of warmth over the highly vascularized placenta. Angiography and ultrasound are accurate by the early and middle portions of the third trimester. Isotope scans and soft tissue x-ray are less accurate before the thirty-fourth week [15].

In the complete form of placenta previa, extensive placental detachment occurs. With lesser forms, more of the placenta will remain attached. Placenta previa has a 1.5 percent maternal death rate, from hemorrhage, infection, traumatic rupture of the uterus, and air embolism. Overall perinatal mortality is below 15 percent, primarily resulting from prematurity and intrauterine asphyxia due to the placental position and the chance of cord prolapse. When the delivery occurs after the thirty-fifth week of gestation, perinatal mortality does not exceed 5 percent. The relatively low mortality is attributable to overall improvements in anesthesia, adequate blood replacement prior to the termination of the pregnancy, and expert care of the premature infant.

It is estimated that about half of the placenta can become detached but the infant will still have a chance of being delivered alive [28]. Through the eighth month of pregnancy, delivery is delayed whenever possible to increase fetal maturity and enhance both fetal and maternal prognosis. This may mean a prolonged hospitalization for the woman, or she may be sent home with instructions for decreased activity.

The nurse's role in the continuing care of this woman includes making appropriate referrals to other agencies for homemaking services or financial assistance. In addition, telephone contact or home visits will provide an on-going assessment of her condition [22]. This may include planning activities at home, helping to prepare the children for the mother's next hospitalization, preparing the family for a possible premature baby and evaluating the home for his care, beginning preoperative teaching (since the woman may eventually need a cesarean section), and possibly drawing blood for hemoglobin and hematocrit.

At the second episode of bleeding or when delivery is anticipated, the expectant parents are probably frightened but they should be prepared for what is to come. If the woman is within four weeks of term, active treatment is instituted even though the bleeding may be slight. If there is a complete or partial placenta previa, a cesarean section is done. The classic approach (through the upper uterine segment) is often used to avoid incising the placental site to decrease blood loss (since with placenta previa the lower uterine segment is rather vascular and easily traumatized) and to provide greater access to the fetus who is high in the uterus.

If the placenta is marginal or attached low in the uterus, the usual plan includes artificial rupture of membranes and vaginal delivery. This presupposes that the release of amniotic fluid will allow the presenting part to enter the pelvis and tamponade the portion of the placenta comprising the previa, thus producing hemostasis. Oxytocin may be given very carefully. The hazard that accompanies vaginal delivery in a woman with placenta previa is the interference with fetal circulation by pressure of the presenting part against the placenta or umbilical cord. Constant monitoring of fetal heart tones is imperative, and preparations should be made for an immediate cesarean section in case it becomes necessary. Fetal distress or recurrent bleeding during the course of labor necessitates cesarean section in about half of the cases of placenta previa in which vaginal delivery is attempted. Postpartum hemorrhage may occur, since the placental site is in the lower uterine segment, where there are not as many muscle fibers to contract and occlude blood vessels. There is an increased risk of uterine infection from prolonged rupture of membranes, retained placental fragments, and anemia. Rupture of the uterus may occur if the muscle has been weakened by the ingrowth of the placenta and the presence of blood sinuses. Since there may also be a significant loss of blood from the fetal circulation via placental hemorrhage, it is wise to make routine checks of the infant's hematocrit.

Abruptio Placentae

Abruptio placentae refers to the premature detachment of a normally implanted placenta during the latter half of pregnancy, particularly during the last trimester. It is one of the most serious complications of pregnancy, occurring in about one of 150–200 pregnancies. In about 10 percent of cases, the separation is severe enough to contribute to maternal mortality from hemorrhagic shock. In the other 90 percent of cases, only a small area of the placenta is detached and the result is not as serious. Abruptio placentae appears to be more common in women with toxemia and vascular and renal disease. Its incidence increases in women over 30; in women over 40, the frequency is double that in women under 30. The frequency of abruptio placentae is also increased in women with a parity of five or more [14].

Although the etiology is largely unknown, a popular theory attributes it to interference with the afferent flow of blood to the intervillous space. Some degeneration and necrosis of the decidua near its junction with the trophoblast occurs normally in the last trimester. If it becomes pronounced, the vascular channels lose support and collapse, causing bleeding from the placental site. It is also postulated that a folic acid deficiency or tension on a short umbilical cord may be contributory. Although it is possible that the vena cava syndrome (obstruction of vena cava) may increase venous pressure in the intervillous space sufficiently to detach the placenta, through the formation of a retroplacental hematoma, most of the time a human adaptive mechanism stabilizes the uterine circulation. Excessive intrauterine pressure, as in marked hydramnios or multiple pregnancy, can produce pressure necrosis of the decidua. A sudden and marked decrease in intrauterine pressure, as in spontaneous rupture of membranes in hydramnios, might also be contributory. In about 33–50 percent of women with abruptio placentae, there is some degree of hypertension and proteinuria. Associated constricted arterioles may lead to decidual degeneration.

Placental separation may occur at the periphery, in which case bleeding may be visible as the blood flows from the edge of the placenta under the membranes, through the cervix into the vagina. Sometimes the amniotic fluid is a burgundy red color. Separation may also be initiated centrally by the formation of a blood clot behind the placenta; the clot may sometimes measure as much as 1000 cubic centimeters. In severe cases the myometrium may be infiltrated with blood (Couvelaire uterus). If the hemorrhage is concealed, the amount of bleeding cannot be estimated and the situation is potentially very serious. If the amount of bleeding is great, it may distend the uterine wall toward the abdominal cavity.

DIAGNOSIS AND INITIAL CARE

The diagnosis of abruptio placentae is usually not difficult for the physican to make, but the extent of the separation is hard to estimate. Usually the woman reports some vaginal bleeding, the sudden onset of severe continuous abdominal pain and/ or low back pain, and a rigid, tender, irritable uterus. As in placenta previa, she is hospitalized immediately (Table 14-2).

Nursing assessment begins with the admission of the mother to the hospital; since the placenta may separate during labor, nurses should be alert for a significant change in her condition. The first indication of danger may be her complaint of a charleyhorse type of pain in her abdomen [22], and her uterus may become irritable, rigid, and boardlike. Fetal heart rate may become irregular or absent, and there may be a definite increase in fetal activity. Sometimes the fundal height increases, and active bleeding may or may not be observable. Shock may appear disproportionate to the evident blood loss. Since maternal apprehension increases greatly, it is important for the nurse to explain everything that is happening to both of the expectant parents. They should be mentally prepared for a possible cesarean section. While not giving false reassurances, the nurse can reinforce the positive aspects of the woman's care by having them listen to the fetal heart tones and telling them when vital signs are stable and when there is no evidence of further bleeding. The seriousness of the situation demands constant nursing supervision.

If the abruption is mild and if the mother is near term, labor may be induced and the mother delivered vaginally as quickly and as atraumatically as possible. If labor does not begin in 8 hours or less, a cesarean section is usually done. The longer the

	Characteristic	Abruptio Placentae	Placenta Previa
Table 14-2. *Characteristics of* *Abruptio Placentae and* *Placenta Previa*	Onset	Third trimester	Third trimester (commonly in eighth month)
	Bleeding	May be concealed, external dark hemorrhage, or bloody amniotic fluid	Mostly external, small to profuse in amount, bright red
	Pain and uterine tenderness	Usually present; irritable uterus, progresses to board-like consistency	Usually absent; uterus soft
	Fetal heart tone	May be irregular or absent	Usually normal
	Presenting part	May or may not be engaged	Usually not engaged
	Shock	Moderate to severe depending on extent of concealed and external hemorrhage	Usually not present unless bleeding is excessive
	Delivery	Immediate delivery, usually by cesarean section	Delivery may be delayed, depending on size of fetus and amount of bleeding

delay, the greater is the likelihood of increased placental separation, increased bleeding, and increased risk of hypofibrinogenemia.

Hypofibrinogenemia is the result of consumption of fibrinogen by disseminated intravascular coagulation (DIC), caused by absorption of thromboplastin-like material from the placental site. Fibrinogen levels, ordinarily elevated in pregnancy, may drop to incoagulable amounts (below 100 milligrams per 100 milliliters) within a matter of minutes in rapidly developing premature separation of the placenta. Prompt delivery usually limits the progression of this disorder and eliminates the need for further therapy if uterine tone is maintained. Supportive treatment includes type and crossmatch, blood transfusions, clotting mechanism evaluation, and intravenous fluids.

If the placental separation is moderately severe or severe, a cesarean section is done in order to save the fetus and the mother after hypofibrinogenemia, if present, is corrected. If a Couvelaire uterus has developed, it will not contract sufficiently during labor, making vaginal delivery impossible. If maternal hemorrhage is uncontrollable, a cesarean section should be performed to allow an immediate hysterectomy.

Perinatal mortality accompanying abruptio placentae is around 15 percent; fetal complications arise from premature birth, anemia, and hypoxia, but early cesarean section increases the chances of fetal survival. The maternal mortality for this disorder is 6 percent. Late postpartum hemorrhage may be a subsequent problem.

Coagulation Defects

The terms used for coagulation defects include the defibrination syndrome, consumptive coagulopathy, and DIC, the last of which is the most common. Coagulation defects are associated with longstanding intrauterine fetal death and severe abruptio placentae. DIC may be a secondary effect of amniotic fluid embolism and is seen in association with some cases of sepsis or endotoxin shock; it involves a decrease in plasma fibrinogen concentration and other clotting factors, with a sharp fall in platelets.

DIC is more common in women with Rh-negative sensitization, hypertension, or preeclampsia; in these patients, fetal death in utero and abruptio placentae are fairly common. The incidence is estimated at 3 to 5 in 1000 pregnancies.

The etiology is controversial but definitely involves a reduction in circulating fibrinogen to levels of 100 milligrams per 100 milliliters or less [28]. It is due either to the direct effect of primary fibrinolysis or to intravascular clotting with resultant activation of the fibrinolytic system. In either case, hemorrhage is the end result. The most consistent findings are decreased fibrinogen, decreased plasminogen, and varying degrees of thrombocytopenia. Most cases involve disseminated intravascular clotting, with fibrinolytic activity appearing in response to fibrin deposition (Figure 14-5).

It is possible that in normal pregnancy some intravascular clotting may occur in undetectable amounts due to the increase in Factors VII, VIII, and X, and fibrinogen [19, 28]. The process of fibrin deposition may normally be required to maintain

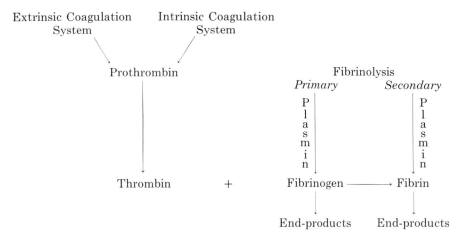

Figure 14-5. Disseminated intravascular coagulation. (Modified from C. McLennan and E. Sandberg. Synopsis of Obstetrics. St. Louis: Mosby, 1974.)

the integrity of the intervillous space, which is constantly being challenged by myometrial contractions. Fibrin deposition may also keep the placental surface intact [28], but occasionally it reaches pathological proportions and decreases placental transport.

DIC is rarely encountered before the twentieth week of pregnancy. Many intra-uterine fetal deaths occur between five and eight months of pregnancy, when the spontaneous onset of labor is less likely. DIC more often occurs when a dead fetus is retained for five or more weeks. Fortunately most women deliver within this time, but about 40 percent of women in whom the dead fetus is retained longer will develop DIC. It is often heralded by the appearance of ecchymoses and bleeding from mucous membranes, which may first present during delivery.

A clot observation test is a rapid and practical method of identifying a clotting defect. Normal blood clots in 8–12 minutes, and the clot remains intact for 24 hours. If a clotting defect is present, the blood may not clot, or if it does, the clot may undergo partial or complete dissolution within 30–60 minutes [28]. This indicates a low fibrinogen level and/or fibrinolytic activity; a fibrinogen level determination confirms the diagnosis.

With the diagnosis of DIC, the mother is given fibrinogen (Factor I), together with whole fresh blood. Minimal treatment of women with severe cases consists of the administration of 2–4 units of blood with 4–8 grams of fibrinogen. Heparin is often used to offset the lethal effect of the thromboplastic substances entering the circulation from the degenerating fetus or placenta, the amniotic fluid, or the blood clot behind an abruptio placentae [13]. Heparin produces this effect by inhibiting the function of the intrinsic coagulation system and by accelerating the neutralization of thrombin. Overheparinization can be controlled by protamine.

Evacuation of the uterine contents helps to control the loss of blood and removes the stimulus to clotting. However, effective hemostasis at the time of delivery does require a stable clot. Bleeding in severe cases in the past may have been attributed to atony, when it has actually been the result of a defect in the clotting mechanism. The process may become irreversible, in which case maternal death ensues.

Hypertensive Disorders in Pregnancy

Hypertensive disorders in pregnancy rank among the three leading causes of maternal mortality and make a significant contribution to perinatal mortality. Preeclampsia and eclampsia (formerly termed toxemia) are two major hypertensive disorders, which are characterized by the development of hypertension, edema, and proteinuria and are usually relieved by termination of the pregnancy.

PREECLAMPSIA AND ECLAMPSIA

Preeclampsia, unique to human gestation, appears almost exclusively in the third trimester, most often in the last 10 weeks of pregnancy, during labor, or within the first 12–48 hours post partum. It appears most frequently in young primigravidas and in women with molar pregnancies, diabetes, multiple pregnancies, or hydramnios.

Preeclampsia may be mild or severe. Women with mild preeclampsia may be comparatively symptom-free and may have little or no peripheral edema remaining after bed rest. Their blood pressure is usually near or above 140/90, or about 30 millimeters of mercury above normal systolic and 15 millimeters of mercury above normal diastolic pressures. Young women who normally have blood pressures of 90/60 may have significant problems when their blood pressures approach 120/80 [15]. It is essential that a baseline blood pressure reading be recorded early in pregnancy. In the woman with mild preeclampsia, a 24-hour urine collection contains about 1 gram of albumin. A random, clean, midstream specimen shows +1 or +2 albumin (Table 14-3).

Mild preeclampsia may rapidly progress to severe preeclampsia and possibly eclampsia. Generalized edema is apparent, and there may be pitting edema over the lower extremities, abdominal wall, face, hands, and sacral area. Severe preeclampsia is characterized by a sudden and marked weight gain of more than 0.9 kilogram (2 pounds) over a period of a few days or a week. Blood pressure is 160/100 or higher and the daily 24-hour urine albumin is 5 grams or more, or +3 or +4. The woman may also experience frontal headache, nausea, vomiting, cerebral or visual disturbances, listlessness, hyperreflexia, oliguria (less than 400 milliliters per 24 hours, or less than 30 milliliters per hour), increased hematocrit, and finally epigastric pain. Eclampsia is said to have developed when convulsions are superimposed on severe preeclampsia.

Preeclampsia appears in about 7 percent of all pregnancies. Because of improved antepartal care, better general health and nutrition, and early detection and treatment of the disorder, the incidence of preeclampsia has decreased by 25–50 percent, and the incidence of eclampsia has decreased by 60–95 percent. Unfortunately the cause of these conditions is essentially unknown, but functioning trophoblastic tissue is apparently necessary to their development. Environmental factors, such as climate and socioeconomic status, and personal factors, such as diet, activity, and health habits, may be contributory, since the incidence appears to be increased in the southern states [15]. The exact relationship of good nutrition to the development of preeclampsia is obscure, but the frequency of the disorder appears to be higher in populations in which diets are deficient (see page 354). It may also be that

Symptom	Definition
Mild preeclampsia	
Hypertension	Increase of 30 mm Hg or more systolic, or systolic level of 140 mm Hg or more; increase of 15 mm Hg or more diastolic, or diastolic level of 90 mm Hg or more
Proteinuria	+1 or +2 or 1 gm/liter in midstream or catheterized urine specimen (found in two specimens at least six hours apart)
Edema	Generalized, facial, hand and fingers; reflected in a rapid weight gain of over 0.7 kg (1.5 pounds) per week
Severe Preeclampsia	
Hypertension	160/110 or above
Proteinuria	5 gm or more in 24-hour urine collection or +3 or +4 reading on turbidometric analysis
Edema	In addition to generalized edema, possibly pitting edema; weight gain may be 0.9 kg (2 pounds) or more over a period of a week or less
Headache	
Blurred vision	
Oliguria (less than 400 ml in 24-hour urine collection)	
Epigastric pain	

Table 14-3. Symptoms of Preeclampsia

preeclampsia is an autoimmune disease, since the placenta may be considered antigenic [28]. DIC may also be a mechanism involved.

A currently favored theory is that preeclampsia is caused by uterine ischemia, although it is possible that the ischemia is a result, rather than a cause, of the disease. Mechanical factors in or around the uterus fail to allow the blood flow to adapt to the requirements of the uterus and fetus [15]. Decreased uterine blood flow leads to the production by the ischemic placenta (or by ischemia-induced decidual degeneration) of pressor polypeptides, thromboplastin, or thromboplastin-like substances. Ischemia is augmented by mechanical factors, such as increased myometrial tension (resulting from multiple pregnancy or during labor), or excessive amounts of trophoblast (hydatid mole). Primigravidas have decreased vascular hypertrophy. Women with chronic hypertensive vascular disease already have arteriolar sclerosis and increased vascular resistance.

Some studies show an imbalance in the renin–angiotensin–aldosterone system to be a cause of preeclampsia [33, 37]. It may be that the increase in renin and angiotensin levels in normal pregnancy are not always controlled. The source of the increase (placenta and/or erythrocyte) fails to maintain plasma angiotensinase at levels necessary to balance the angiotensin production and destruction, with a resulting pressor effect [28].

The kidney consistently shows the effects of preeclampsia or eclampsia with decreased renal blood flow and decreased glomerular filtration rate. Tubular capacity for reabsorption of sodium appears to be increased, and cardiac output is increased. In severe cases, the cardiac load is significantly increased because of increased peripheral vascular resistance and elevated viscosity of the blood, as a result of hemo-concentration. Uterine blood flow decreases with hypertension, and the decreased uteroplacental blood flow is a principal cause of fetal death and of the tendency for infants to be small for gestational age. The placenta shows an increased number of infarcts. Pulmonary edema, conjestive heart failure, cerebral hemorrhage, and complications of operative obstetrics are major causes of death in women with preeclampsia and eclampsia. Retinal edema and spasm of retinal arteries may result in actual detachment of the retina. Increased cerebrovascular resistance may lead to dulling of the sensorium.

All care of the woman with severe preeclampsia is directed toward the prevention of convulsions by decreasing blood pressure, establishing diuresis, and continuing the pregnancy to viability. The woman is hospitalized and placed on bed rest, and sedatives or hypotensive agents may be necessary. When she lies on her side, renal and uterine blood flow increases, which may result in diuresis and the return of blood pressure to normal levels. Vital signs are monitored every 4 hours; her weight and her intake and output are recorded daily, but fluids are not necessarily restricted. Under this regimen her symptoms usually diminish.

NUTRITIONAL ASPECTS

There is some evidence that the development of preeclampsia or eclampsia may be related to nutrition, specifically protein deficiency [39]. It is no longer regarded as valid to restrict calorie intake to avoid large weight gain (accumulation of fat) in the hope of avoiding preeclampsia. Another common practice, based on rather dubious evidence, has been the routine restriction of salt in the hope of preventing edema. Actually, the restriction of sodium intensifies the normal renin-angiotensin-aldosterone mechanism, which results in a positive sodium balance [26]. Therefore, sodium restriction should probably not be a major part of the routine treatment of preeclampsia, and there is some question, as well, about the routine use of diuretics. However, some preeclamptic women may not handle sodium well, and on *this* basis, the restriction is indicated when hypertension develops [15].

TREATMENT

The woman's pregnancy is maintained until at least the thirty-sixth week, if possible. Urinary estriol determinations and ultrasound measurements of fetal growth are used to monitor the condition of the fetus. In the management of severe preeclampsia, blood pressure is usually lowered by a pharmacological agent. Magnesium sulfate, commonly administered intramuscularly in a 50% solution with 1% procaine, is a popular choice. It has a depressant action on the myoneural junction, decreasing hyperreflexia and resulting in some vasodilatation. It also depresses the central nervous system and may cause osmotic diuresis, secondarily decreasing intracranial pressure.

Magnesium sulfate (usually 5–10 grams in 10–20 milliliters) is injected deep into the gluteal muscle (Figure 14-6). Because the solution is very irritating to tissues, the needle used to draw it up should be discarded. As the injection is made, the needle is rotated like a wheel, because of the large amount of solution. Usually the

*Figure 14-6. Technique for
injecting magnesium
sulfate (see text for
details).*

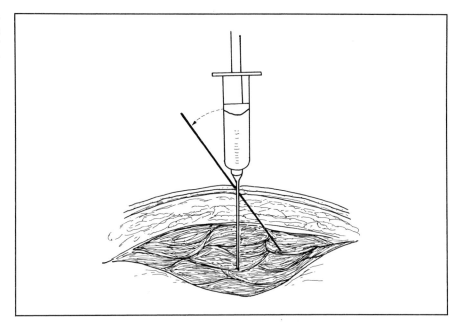

Figure 14-6. Technique for injecting magnesium sulfate (see text for details).

dose is divided equally between the two buttocks, and the tissue is massaged well following the injection. Since magnesium sulfate is eliminated chiefly by the kidneys, a high serum concentration may be reached if urine output is low. As a result, respiration or cardiac action may be depressed, although respiratory depression does not occur until after the patellar reflex disappears. If this reflex is absent, or if respirations are below 16 per minute or urine output is under 30 milliliters per hour, repeat doses of magnesium sulfate are not given. Calcium gluconate is an effective metabolic antagonist and should be kept available. Other medications used to decrease hypertension are hydralazine (which decreases arteriolar resistance) and morphine or other sedatives.

If eclampsia develops (i.e., if convulsions occur), the woman is monitored very carefully. She is put on bed rest with padded side rails, intravenous fluids, a central venous pressure line, and a Foley catheter. She is restricted from oral intake, her output is recorded hourly, and vital signs are recorded frequently. The foot of the bed may be elevated to facilitate tracheobronchial drainage. Suction to prevent aspiration, oxygen, and padded tongue blades should be readily available. Every effort is made to decrease the woman's sensory stimulation, promote a quiet environment, and give her only the care that is absolutely necessary. When her convulsions cease, irritability decreases, blood pressure decreases from 140/100 to 105/100, and her pulse is below 100, then some thought is given to the termination of her pregnancy. If her cervix is favorable for labor, her membranes are ruptured and oxytocin is given. A cesarean section is usually performed if the induction fails, her labor slows, her condition worsens, or fetal distress develops.

The pathophysiological changes associated with preeclampsia and eclampsia tend to regress rapidly. Diuresis in the first 12 hours following delivery is often a first and valuable sign of recovery. Mothers are supervised carefully for about 10 days post partum. Usually edema and proteinuria decrease progressively and are gone by the fifth postpartum day.

Maternal mortality increases with the severity of the disorder; the mortality in preeclampsia is nearly three times that for mothers in general, and the mortality in eclampsia is 7 percent. For the fetus, the average perinatal mortality is 10 percent, primarily due to prematurity, and this rate also increases with the severity of the maternal condition.

It is uncertain whether preeclampsia and eclampsia can be prevented. Antepartal care is given the most credit for alerting health personnel to signs and symptoms that can be treated. Dietary salt restriction and the use of thiazide diuretics have no documented value in prevention. Weight control is not thought to be of any value in this regard either. In some research, early manifestations of preeclampsia have actually been relieved by an increased salt intake [15]. Needless to say, pregnant women should be aware of the symptoms that should be reported to the nurse, midwife, or obstetrician so that they can be more carefully monitored.

Chronic Hypertensive Vascular Disease

About half of the women who have hypertensive disorders have chronic hypertensive vascular disease (CHVD). The hypertension precedes the pregnancy and exists during the first half as well as the last half of pregnancy. Sometimes it is hard to differentiate CHVD from chronic renal disease.

Women with CHVD are placed on bed rest, sodium restriction, diuretics, sedatives, and hypotensive drugs, and they return for weekly visits. The pregnancy is terminated as soon as possible, but every effort is made to prolong it to 34 weeks or more.

A high fetal loss is associated, especially if preeclampsia is superimposed; many infants are small for their gestational age. CHVD is also associated with abruptio placentae, stillbirth, and late abortion. Most women survive, but there is a tendency for their condition to be more severe with succeeding pregnancies. Therefore a discussion of contraception is an important element of the nurse's teaching plan for them.

MULTIPLE PREGNANCY

On the average, multiple pregnancy resulting in twins occurs in 1 of 80 pregnancies; triplets occur in 1 of 6400 pregnancies; and quadruplets occur in 1 of 512,000 pregnancies. Monozygotic twinning occurs apparently at random in 1 of about 200 pregnancies. Dizygotic twinning is controlled by various factors, especially ethnic and familial, and is subject to pituitary secretion of follicle-stimulating hormone (FSH), with the ova coming from the same graafian follicle or from separate ones, in the same or opposite ovary. The number of mature ova released from the ovary depends on the balance between the action of the pituitary gonadotropins and the inhibiting action of ripening follicles on the maturation of other follicles. If such inhibition does not occur (due to endocrine imbalance, such as excessive pituitary stimulation), two or more ova can be released [16].

Twinning is most common among blacks, less common among whites, and least common among Orientals. Dizygotic twinning is familial, and families that have a history of dizygotic twins have a higher incidence of multiple births. The twin-bearing mother probably has a higher FSH secretion rate, leading to polyovulation. The trait may be inherited through the father; however, accurate studies to support the above assumption have not been made [28].

Multiple births may also be the result of treatment for infertility with human FSH. Twinning appears to be increased with advancing maternal age up to 39 years, probably due to higher levels of gonadotropin. The incidence is decreased after the age of 39, probably due to a decline in ovarian function. Higher frequency of twinning with increasing parity may be due to permanent changes in the activity of the pituitary gland or ovary during pregnancy [16].

Figure 14-7.
A. Monozygotic twins—one chorion, two amnions, and one placenta.
B. Dizygotic twins—two chorions, two amnions, and two placentas.
C. Dizygotic twins—two chorions, two amnions, and a single fused placenta.

Dizygotic (fraternal) twins always have two chorions and two amnions. Genetically as dissimilar as any other siblings, fraternal twins are definitely diagnosed as such if one twin is male and one female (Figure 14-7).

Monozygotic (identical) twins have one chorion and two amnions about 70 percent of the time, and two chorions and two amnions about 30 percent of the time. This is dependent on the time of the twinning impetus (splitting of the ovum). If it is on day 3 or after, when the chorion is established, they will be monochorionic. If it is on day 8 or after, they will be monoamnionic, since by then the amnion

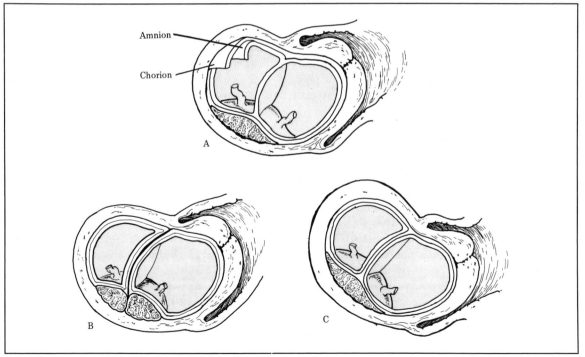

is established. Once the embryonic axis is formed, after day 14, true twinning is presumably impossible; if it does occur, the twins are likely to be conjoined [28].

The diagnosis of monozygotic twinning can be made with certainty at birth when the placenta is available, or later, using blood groups and skin grafting. A single placenta is usually associated with identical twins, although dizygotic placentas may fuse and appear as one. Triplets may be monozygotic, dizygotic, or trizygotic.

Both perinatal mortality and maternal mortality are greater in multiple births than in single ones; in pregnancies lasting over 20 weeks, 14 percent of twins die in the perinatal period, compared to 3 percent of singletons. Since 50–80 percent of all twin pregnancies are delivered before term, prematurity is the major cause of the increased mortality. Monoamnionic twins have the highest mortality, often due to entangled umbilical cords and blocked circulation. There may be a significantly greater hazard for the second twin as a result of prolonged exposure to anesthesia, uterine contraction with detached placenta, or the greater likelihood of breech presentation. Abnormal placental insertions of the cord occur in about 7 percent of twin pregnancies, compared to 1 percent in singletons. Congenital anomalies tend to appear more frequently as well.

Maternal complications of hypertensive disorders and hydramnios are more common, and overdistention of the uterus may contribute to a greater incidence of postpartum hemorrhage. Labor may be abnormal, since overstretching of the myometrium may cause uterine contractions to be ineffective in dilating the cervix during the active phase. This, plus the resulting increase in operative deliveries, tends to increase the incidence of infection.

Care of the Mother

The primary goal in caring for the woman with a multiple pregnancy is to bring the pregnancy beyond the point at which each twin weighs 2000 grams (4.4 pounds). If she gets adequate rest, nutrition, and antepartal care, it is likely that she will not develop preeclampsia or have premature dilatation of her cervix. The presence of a skilled pediatrician in the delivery room will benefit the infants.

Multiple pregnancy is diagnosed when the woman's abdomen is larger than expected for the length of gestation. It is often associated with rapid uterine growth, pronounced edema, proteinuria, and fetal motion over her entire abdomen. Two fetal heart tones can be counted simultaneously, but since fetal size is small, the heart tones are less likely to be audible at a time when the size of the uterus would indicate they should be heard. Abdominal palpation yields many small parts by six or seven months. Ultrasonography or x-ray is used for a positive diagnosis. Twinning may not be suspected or diagnosed until after the birth of the first infant, when the mother's uterus remains almost as large as before.

Women who are carrying twins are on a rigid prenatal regimen and are seen more frequently for check-ups. Good general hygiene and preadmission to the hospital for bed rest between the twenty-eighth and thirty-sixth weeks of gestation may prolong pregnancy and prevent premature labor. Since hypertensive disorders may accompany multiple pregnancy, such women should be made aware of the pertinent signs and symptoms that they should report to the nurse, midwife, or obstetrician.

The excessive abdominal distention leads to digestion difficulties, constipation, and dyspnea, especially if hydramnios is present. Varicose veins and urinary stasis (resulting in chronic urinary tract infection) may also develop. Pressure symptoms are relieved if the woman lies on her side whenever she is taking one of her frequent rest periods. Small frequent meals will make digestion easier.

Delivery

Since the mother's delivery is likely to be early and complex, the nurse should prepare her for the possible procedures she will go through and for the appearance of her babies, should they be premature. Since the mother is unlikely to be able to take care of two or more babies at home without some amount of help, the nurse should investigate the resources which the mother has at her disposal, making appropriate referrals or doing follow-up visits. Sometimes parents need to be reminded of the uniqueness of each of their infants.

The interval between the actual delivery of each twin is usually three to 15 minutes. Since the uterus contracts to accommodate to the decreased intrauterine volume, there is the danger of placental separation while the second twin is still inside the uterus. In many cases the second twin is in a transverse lie, or his presenting part is above the inlet. In both instances prolapse of the cord or dystocia is more likely to occur. Therefore, an internal podalic version is done and the second twin is delivered breech.

Both twins are vertex about 45 percent of the time; one vertex and one breech, 38 percent; both breech, 9 percent; one transverse, 7 percent [15]. If they happen to be interlocked, the delivery is by cesarean section, or a very difficult vaginal delivery results, many times with the loss of one twin. If labor must be stimulated in multiple pregnancy, oxytocin is used very cautiously.

Transfusion Syndrome and Blood Chimerism

Sometimes in monochorionic (monozygotic) twins there is an interfetal anastomotic vascular connection (transfusion syndrome). During the development of a single placenta, some blood vessels almost regularly join, whether artery to artery, vein to vein, or artery to vein. The most significant degree of transfusion syndrome results when a single arteriovenous communication exists. An artery from one fetus supplies a cotyledon, which is drained by a vein from the other fetus. As a result, one fetus (A) continuously loses blood to the other (B). Therefore, B gets hypervolemia and presumably hypertension, cardiac hypertrophy, and occasionally edema, and he generally grows larger. B may urinate excessively, resulting in hydramnios. Nourishment for the two twins is, of course, unequally divided. When the process occurs very early in gestation, one twin (B) will tend to overpower the other, with the weaker heart dilating into a tortuous vessel. This fetus remains undeveloped. At times one of the twins dies before birth. Gradually the fluid constituents are resorbed, and the twin becomes a shriveled, compressed appendage (fetus papyraceus) of the placenta. If the A twin survives, he is likely to be small and to suffer from microcardia, anemia, dehydration, and perhaps oligohydramnios. Such a different prenatal environment may cause such "identical" twins to remain different for quite some time.

Postnatally, if the donor twin (A) has a hemoglobin of below 13.3 grams per 100 milliliters in the first 24 hours, a transfusion is usually given [38]; this infant may have an early iron deficiency anemia. The recipient twin (B) has polycythemia, and jaundice and hyperbilirubinemia are postnatal threats. He is prone to dehydration because of frequent urination. Treatment aims to decrease polycythemia and blood viscosity. A hematocrit over 75 percent warrants phlebotomy or partial exchange of plasma for blood, which will also help to correct the hyperbilirubinemia.

Sometimes dizygotic twins who have an anastomoses of their fetal circulations will show a blood group chimerism, which means that they contain a mixture of two distinct types of blood. Blood chimerism has been detected in only a few sets of monozygotic twins.

HYDRAMNIOS AND OLIGOHYDRAMNIOS

An excessive amount of amniotic fluid (hydramnios) or a very small amount (oligohydramnios) may be associated with maternal disease, such as diabetes mellitus, heart disease, kidney disease; with multiple gestation; or, in 25–33 percent of the cases, with fetal abnormalities. In about half of the cases of hydramnios and oligohydramnios there is no demonstrable cause.

Amniotic fluid is constantly changing, and the fetus contributes to this by swallowing about 450 milliliters in 24 hours and by urinating into it. The cells of the amnion appear to be secretory, and it has been suggested that their secretory function may be altered in some way when the amount of fluid is abnormal [28].

Cases of hydramnios (Figure 14-8), in which the amount of amniotic fluid is 2–4 liters or more, are often associated with particular fetal anomalies. In esophageal and duodenal atresia an insignificant amount of fluid may be swallowed, and in anencephaly or hydrocephaly the swallowing reflex may be disturbed through an alteration in brain structure. In spina bifida, it is thought that cerebrospinal fluid may be added to the amniotic cavity through the exposed meninges.

Chronic hydramnios is usually noticed around 28–38 weeks of gestation. Acute hydramnios, the result of a very rapid process, is usually noticed around 20–24 weeks of gestation. Spontaneous labor often results before the end of the second trimester as a result of rapid uterine expansion. Premature delivery is common not only for that reason, but also because the cervix is often effaced and considerably dilated due to the pressure exerted on it. However, 2 or 3 liters of fluid may be removed by amniocentesis, which may maintain the pregnancy to viability. In extreme cases, repeat amniocentesis may have to be done. In addition, some authorities recommend the use of diuretics, although diuretics are regarded as ineffectual by others [15]. It is rarely necessary to terminate the pregnancy.

The woman experiences pain in her abdomen, back, and thighs, caused by increased pressure. She may complain of dyspnea, nausea, and vomiting, and she may have edema of her abdominal wall, vulva, and lower extremities. Usually it is difficult to hear the fetal heart tones, and the fetus cannot be palpated easily.

Figure 14-8. Woman with extreme case of hydramnios (5500 mililiters of amniotic fluid was measured at delivery). (From L. M. Hellman and J. A. Pritchard. Williams Obstetrics *[14th ed.], 1971. Courtesy of Appleton-Century-Crofts, Publishing Division of Prentice-Hall, Inc.)*

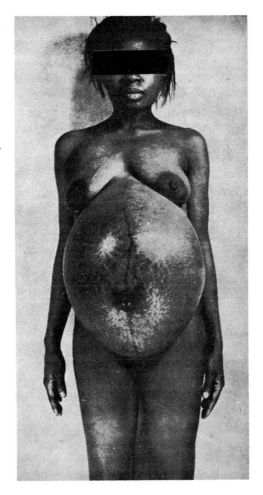

The maternal prognosis is usually good, although abruptio placentae and hemorrhage may result if the uterine volume decreases suddenly. Shock may result from a sudden decrease in intra-abdominal pressure. Fetal prognosis is poor, since in many cases the baby will be born prematurely and have anomalies and prolapsed cord, or he may be the victim of abruptio placentae.

Oligohydramnios, a rare condition in which the amount of amniotic fluid may be only 100–200 milliliters, is sometimes associated with fetal renal agensis or postmaturity. If it occurs early in pregnancy, the amnion may adhere to the fetus, or amniotic bands may form around one of his arms or legs, with resulting deformities in either case. If oligohydramnios occurs late in pregnancy, the fetal skin may be leathery and dry. The infant may be born with a club foot or hand or with amputated digits, and shortness of muscles may lead to torticollis (wry neck).

In some cases labor may also be premature. As a rule uterine contractions are ineffectual, and the labor may be prolonged. Fetal hypoxia may occur because the decreased surrounding fluid results in cord compression.

ABNORMALITIES OF THE PLACENTA AND CORD

Placental Abnormalities

It is believed that flat subchorial infarcts form the basis for two placental abnormalities: placenta marginata and placenta circumvallata [15]. If these infarcts occur at the edge of the placenta, they may form a more or less complete white infarcted ring (placenta marginata). In this case the membranes may adhere to the decidua and the placenta may be delivered without them, with postpartum hemorrhage resulting from the retention of the membranes.

If the infarcted ring is raised from the surface, the attached membranes may double back over its edge, resulting in a dense ring of tissue (placenta circumvallata) (Figure 14-9). Often this condition is asymptomatic, but it may be associated with premature bleeding during the second and third trimesters of pregnancy and premature delivery.

Placenta succenturiata occurs when one or more accessory lobes are attached to the main placenta. Usually it is not symptomatic until the third stage of labor, when

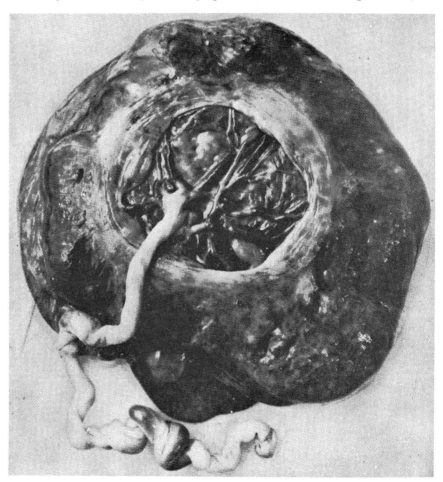

Figure 14-9. Placenta circumvallata. (From L. M. Hellman and J. A. Pritchard. Williams Obstetrics [14th ed.], 1971. Courtesy of Appleton-Century-Crofts, Publishing Division of Prentice-Hall, Inc.)

the lobes may be inadvertently left in the uterus, predisposing the mother to hemorrhage.

If infarcts occur within the placenta itself, they may compromise fetal oxygenation or nutrition; if they involve a substantial portion of tissue, they may even cause fetal death. Calcium deposits on the basalis surface of the placenta are a sign of its normal aging process and are frequently found in term pregnancies, particularly if the gestation has been prolonged. Usually they are of no clinical importance, but extensive calcification is associated with a poor fetal prognosis.

Abnormalities of the Cord

Ordinarily the cord inserts at or near the center of the placenta, although an insertion at a different position is not uncommon. If the cord is inserted at the placental periphery (battledore placenta), there may be slight bleeding, which could be confused with placenta previa.

A velamentous insertion occurs when the cord inserts into the membranes in such a way that the umbilical vessels travel between the amnion and the chorion to the placenta (Figure 14-10). This is often accompanied by other placental anomalies, such as infarcts, placenta succenturiata, or placenta previa. Its occurrence is nine times more frequent with twins than with single births, and it occurs very frequently with triplets. This type of cord insertion is particularly dangerous to the fetus when the vessels travel along the lower uterine segment and cross over the internal cervical os (vasa praevia). The vessels are usually torn when the membranes are ruptured.

Since the umbilical vein is longer than the arteries and since the vessels are longer than the cord itself, the vessels become twisted and coiled in an effort to accommodate to the available space. Usually at these points the Wharton's jelly is a little thicker, and false knots or nodes tend to appear in the cord. True knots are very rare, and occur when the fetus passes through loops in the cord.

About 20 percent of the time, the fetus is so active in utero that the cord becomes coiled around its neck (nuchal cord). This is a potentially serious complication, since it may make the cord functionally short and may interfere with the mechanism of descent. Cord compression during labor and delivery may cause fetal asphyxia. For these reasons the midwife or obstetrician will feel for the cord immediately after delivering the baby's head; if loops are present, they should be uncoiled before attempting to deliver the baby's shoulders.

DIABETES

Pregnancy represents an additional physiological stress to the woman with a chronic illness. Helping this woman and her family through a pregnancy that results in delivery of a healthy infant requires much teaching and support, a knowledge of appropriate community agencies, and a thorough knowledge of the interaction of pregnancy and chronic illness.

The number of women with diabetes who are choosing to have children is increas-

Figure 14-10. Velamentous insertion of umbilical cord. (From K. L. Moore, The Developing Human: Clinically Oriented Embryology. Philadelphia: Saunders, 1973.)

margin of placenta

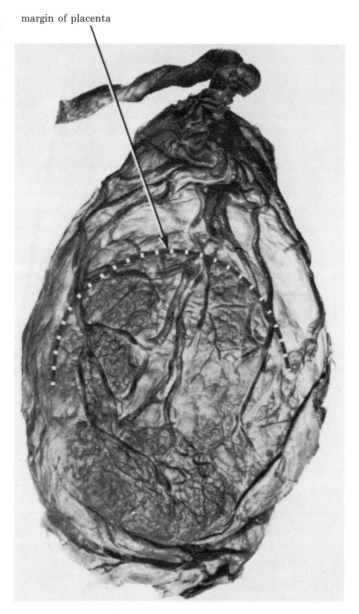

ing each year. Prior to the advent of insulin, pregnancy for these women was rare. Many diabetics never lived to reproductive age and the women who did were very frequently infertile. Diabetic women who did become pregnant faced a 25 percent chance of dying during childbearing and only a 50 percent chance of having a living child [17]. Today diabetic women are becoming pregnant and, with good health care, are delivering live, healthy infants. This requires coordinated and comprehensive care.

A diabetic woman who wishes to become pregnant should be counseled about getting ready for pregnancy. Her diabetes should be in good control, and she should be in good nutritional status and know how to avoid infections.

If the diabetes does not remain in control, the woman may abort, usually because of ketoacidosis and placental insufficiency. Controlling the diabetes is not always easy, since pregnancy causes an increased peripheral resistance to insulin, and a placental insulinase increases the rate of destruction of insulin. In addition, chorionic somatomammotropin mobilizes lipids while sparing carbohydrates for fetal use, thereby antagonizing the action of insulin [3]. The problems with insulin regulation may be compounded by nausea and vomiting in early pregnancy, and further compounded if the woman develops an infection of any kind.

Care of the Pregnant Diabetic

During the course of the pregnancy, the woman, as well as the family, needs much support in coping with the changes in her diabetic state, as well as with the usual changes of pregnancy. The woman may have been doing well at regulating her blood sugar for a number of years and may now find it far harder to control. The effects of progesterone on gastrointestinal motility and the increased pressure of the growing uterus increase absorption time of food. This effect and the effects on insulin noted above may leave the woman feeling as though she has lost control of the diabetes. The nurse can reassure her by explaining the changes in food absorption and insulin that occur during pregnancy and can tell her that after delivery her diabetes will respond as it did prior to her pregnancy.

The woman's insulin requirements will also change during pregnancy. Many women find that their insulin requirements will remain the same or even decrease during the first half or two-thirds of pregnancy, only to increase tremendously during the last trimester. This presumably occurs as the effects of chorionic somatomammotropin increase. Some women find their insulin requirements gradually increasing throughout the pregnancy, and other women who had been controlled by diet alone may require insulin for the course of the pregnancy. Oral hypoglycemics are not as effective during pregnancy, are teratogenic in some species, and may cause hypoglycemia in the newborn [15]. Some women who show no signs or symptoms of diabetes in the nonpregnant state will become symptomatic when pregnant, a condition known as gestational diabetes. When not treated, this condition may lead to fetuses who are large for their gestational age and who often die in utero [21]. The diabetes disappears in these women following the pregnancy, but many become overt diabetics later in life [3] (Table 14-4).

Women who have been diabetic for some time are aware of periods throughout the day when their blood sugar is low. During pregnancy they will find that this pattern has changed and that hypoglycemia may occur at very unexpected times. Likewise, it may take much more fast-acting available carbohydrates, such as fruit sugar or glucose, to raise the blood sugar. Because of this, care of this pregnant woman must include an assessment of her knowledge of the symptoms of insulin shock and diabetic ketoacidosis, and her awareness of what she should do at the onset of such

4-4. *Classification*
of Diabetes

Class	Definition
A	Abnormal glucose tolerance test only; also called latent, chemical, gestational diabetes
B	Diabetes of adult onset (after age 20), with less than 10 years' duration and no vascular involvement
C	Diabetes for 10–19 years, or beginning in adolescence between ages 10–19, without vascular involvement
D	Diabetes of long duration (duration of 20 years or more, or onset before 10 years of age), with evidence of vascular involvement
E	Evidence of calcification of iliac or uterine arteries
F	Evidence of diabetic neuropathy

Source: Modified from P. White. Pregnancy and Diabetes. *Medical Clinics of North America* 49:1015, 1965.

symptoms. The immediate family members also should be aware of these signs and symptoms, and someone should be able to administer an injection to the woman if needed.

Insulin Shock

Not infrequently, pregnant diabetics will experience insulin shock, which may result from changes in intestinal absorption and insulin action. Another contributing factor may exist when the woman regulates her insulin dose according to the amount of glucosuria. During pregnancy there is a tremendous increase in glomerular filtration without a concomitant increase in tubular reabsorption of solutes. As a result, some glucose may be lost in the urine. Lactose may also appear in the urine and will yield a positive reaction when glucose testing is done. The diabetic woman who wants to be well-controlled during her pregnancy may well adjust her insulin dose on her own, or she may not eat as much at her next meal when she tests her urine and finds a positive reaction to glucose. Her blood sugar may already be low, and she may soon be in shock. Many of these episodes can be avoided if the woman is aware of the changes that occur in pregnancy. She should be told that it may be safer for her to have small amounts of sugar in her urine and that she need not be concerned unless she has a large amount (+3 or +4) of sugar or any trace of acetone. If she feels shocky, 2 tablespoons of honey or corn syrup mixed in a glass of fruit juice should help. If she is not at home, cola is usually available and should be effective. The woman who has been having repeated episodes of shock may need to carry a dose of glucagon in her handbag, or keep one at home where a member of the family can administer it. She should also carry a card in her wallet that identifies her as a diabetic and preferably wear a Medic Alert bracelet during pregnancy. If she has been having repeated episodes of shock, her husband, a family member, or a neighbor should phone or visit periodically during the day.

   The woman and members of her family are always concerned about the fetal effects of an episode of insulin shock or acidosis. They should be told that the fetus seems not to be affected by hypoglycemic episodes, but episodes of ketoacidosis are tolerated poorly by the fetus [15].

Concerns of the Family

One of the most essential components of care for the family is listening to their concerns. In addition to worrying about the status of the baby, the woman may be very concerned about loss of control over her diabetes. Her husband may also be very concerned about this, wondering if this lability will continue after the baby is born and if they will be able to care for the infant in that case. He may also wonder if he can cope with the lability on a continuing basis. The family may also have financial concerns, especially if the woman is hospitalized during the course of pregnancy in order to get her diabetes better controlled. If there are other children in the family, arrangements must be made to care for them in mother's absence. Costly tests to determine serial urinary estriol levels will be made in the later months of pregnancy. The woman will usually be hospitalized a week prior to delivery to assess her status, as well as that of the fetus, and to prepare her for delivery.

Delivery

Delivery of the infant of a diabetic woman is also costly. In the past, all diabetic women were delivered by cesarean section prior to their expected date of confinement, since many fetuses died in utero. The fetal deaths may result from premature placental aging and consequent insufficiency, which is common among diabetic women. Currently many physicians allow a woman to go to term and deliver vaginally, provided that the fetal status is not compromised. Labor may begin spontaneously, or it may be induced. Estriol levels provide a measure of the functioning of the placenta and fetus, and fetal monitoring during labor allows an assessment of fetal response during this period. If these testing methods are not available, or if there is a sudden change in insulin requirements during this period, women with overt diabetes are usually delivered between 36 and 38 weeks of gestation, either by induction or by cesarean section. On the day of delivery, long-acting insulin is usually not given. The woman is generally kept hydrated with intravenous fluids of 5% dextrose in water, and regular insulin is used to control blood sugar and ketone levels. The physical exertion of labor decreases her insulin requirements.

During the first few days post partum, the mother's insulin requirements may fluctuate markedly, often dropping abruptly following delivery. This fluctuation stabilizes within a few days.

The diabetic woman is also more likely than the nondiabetic woman to encounter complications during pregnancy and delivery. Pregnant diabetics encounter an increased incidence of hypertensive disorders, infection, hydraminos, and postpartum hemorrhage. The infant born to the diabetic mother may be larger, encounter respiratory difficulties after birth, and have an increased tendency to inherit diabetes. It has been reported that children of diabetic mothers who had acetonuria (reflecting ketoacidosis) during pregnancy have lower IQs than the general population and than children of diabetic mothers who did not have this complication [6]. It also has been reported that infants of diabetic mothers tend to be more immature than would be expected for their gestational age, possibly due to an immature enzyme system [9]. They have delayed development of ossification centers, a high incidence of hyperbilirubinemia and respiratory distress syndrome, and a higher concentration of fetal hemoglobin than other infants of similar gestational age. The perinatal death rate ranges between 10 and 15 percent. All of these factors can severely tax the coping ability of the family, which should make clear the need this family has for support and comprehensive care during the pregnancy and in the postpartum period.

CARDIAC COMPLICATIONS

The woman with cardiac disease should be counseled prior to becoming pregnant. She should be aware of the reason for the restrictions that will be placed on her activities and her diet, and she should be aware of the statistical chances of delivering a live infant. However, she should also be told that there is no evidence to date that normal childbearing causes any permanent deterioration of cardiac status or that giving birth shortens her life expectancy [15]. She and her partner may then thoughtfully consider pregnancy as well as other options in starting their family. If they do decide on pregnancy, they will then begin with a knowledge of what the woman's care will involve.

Pregnancy imposes a significant circulatory burden on the woman, due to increases in her cardiac output, oxygen consumption, and blood volume. The burden begins in the first trimester, increases throughout the second, and persists to term. Cardiac output peaks at 25–28 weeks and blood volume peaks at 32–34 weeks. During labor, cardiac output increases 20–30 percent during each uterine contraction. The pulse rate, blood pressure, and left ventricular work also increase. In women receiving saddle block or caudal anesthesia, however, these changes were not seen according to one study, prompting Greenhill and Friedman [15] to comment that this finding suggests that response to pain, anxiety, and muscular activity play a more important role in raising cardiac output than any autotransfusion from the uterine sinuses into the systemic circulation. This should emphasize the importance of supportive nursing measures to relieve the anxiety and pain of all women in labor.

Following delivery the woman usually has bradycardia as she becomes more relaxed and is relieved of pain and as the venous return is augmented. The first uterine contraction following birth of the infant puts a significant amount of blood into the general circulation and gives a brief rise in plasma volume. Blood loss over the next few hours reduces the plasma volume. However, this reduction is brief, since the fluid that has accumulated in interstitial spaces during pregnancy begins to enter the general circulation, raising the plasma volume to abnormally high levels [15]. This explains the normal diuresis in the first few days post partum. The woman with cardiac disease must be watched very carefully during this period of increased cardiac burden. The elevated plasma volume continues for approximately two weeks.

Maternal mortality associated with heart disease ranges between 1 and 5 percent, the major cause of death being cardiac decompensation and heart failure. The majority of problems occur in the periods during pregnancy, labor, and puerperium

when the cardiac burden is greatest. If the woman is cyanotic during pregna
is likely to deliver an infant who is small for his gestational age or to go in⌄o labor
prematurely; if the woman is very severely cyanotic, the fetus may die in utero. The
woman who is acyanotic and does not experience cardiac failure generally delivers a
healthy infant.

In the past, most heart disease found in pregnant women was the result of rheumatic fever. Today the incidence of congenital heart disease is increasing, as children with congenital heart defects have corrective surgery and reach their reproductive years, and women with such defects run the risk of delivering infants who are also congenitally deformed.

The functional classification of the American Heart Association serves as an important guide in caring for the pregnant woman with cardiac disease (Table 14-5). Most women in classes I and II are able to handle the physiological demands of pregnancy. As is the case for women in any of the classifications, they will have their cardiac status evaluated very early in pregnancy, if not before. This usually includes chest x-rays, an electrocardiogram, and tests for vital capacity. They will continue under close medical supervision throughout pregnancy and for some time following delivery. They must get adequate rest, at least 10 hours of sleep at night as well as rest periods throughout the day, since physical exertion is an important cause of heart failure. Only light housework is recommended, and climbing stairs is restricted. One study [36] suggests that even women with classes I and II heart disease have limited blood flow and oxygen supply to the fetus and should substantially restrict physical activity. It is also suggested that women avoid abdominal compression and the supine position and wear support hose to prevent venous pooling in the legs. All stresses, emotional as well as physical, must be avoided. Infection is one of the more serious stresses; pregnant women with cardiac disease should be treated immediately if they experience infection of any kind. Upper respiratory infections, especially bronchitis and pneumonia, are leading causes of severe heart failure in pregnancy. Dental caries may also become foci of infection. The woman should have a well-balanced diet to prevent anemia, which also would severely tax her heart.

Women in classes I and II often are hospitalized a week before labor is expected, so their cardiac status may be evaluated again. Particularly during the later months of

Table 14-5. Classification of Patients with Cardiac Disease

Class	Definition
I	No limitation of physical activity; no symptoms of cardiac insufficiency or anginal pain
II	Slight limitation of physical activity; comfortable at rest; excessive fatigue, palpitations, dyspnea, or anginal pain with ordinary physical activity
III	Marked limitation of physical activity; comfortable at rest; excessive fatigue, palpitations, dyspnea, or anginal pain with less than ordinary physical activity
IV	Inability to perform any physical activity without discomfort; symptoms of cardiac insufficiency or anginal syndrome possible at rest; discomfort increased with physical activity

Source: Based on Functional Classifications of the New York Heart Association.

pregnancy, the women should be assessed for signs of impending cardiac decompensation. How is her color? Does she have signs of edema in her ankles or hands? Is her respiration labored, her pulse fast? How is she handling restrictions placed on her activities? All of these assessments should be made each time she visits.

Labor and Delivery

Women with cardiac complications must be followed very carefully during labor. The importance of relieving anxiety and pain already has been mentioned; the nurse should also carefully monitor and record the woman's vital signs every 15 minutes, or more often as labor progresses, noting any signs of beginning cardiac failure. If a pulse rate taken between contractions and in the absence of fever reaches 110 per minute or greater, this suggests approaching cardiac failure. The nurse also should be alert for dyspnea, rales, and tachypnea. Fetal monitoring also is used.

When analgesics are needed, the mother should receive them promptly; combinations of a narcotic analgesic and a synergistic tranquilizer are used. Regional anesthesia may be used for pain relief during labor and delivery except in those mothers where hypotension may be life-threatening.

They should labor upright in bed or on their side in a semirecumbent position. Many of them also will need oxygen during the course of labor. Since bearing down increases the cardiac burden, these women are delivered as soon as possible after they are fully dilated. They are allowed to deliver spontaneously or with low forceps. The blood loss associated with cesarean section places additional burdens on the woman, making it a less desirable method of delivery that is used only when absolutely necessary.

During and following delivery, careful efforts are made to prevent excessive blood loss, which would further tax her heart. Synthetic oxytocin rather than ergonovine is used, to avoid increases in blood pressure. Intravenous therapy is limited; if blood is needed, packed erythrocytes are used to reduce the amount of fluid introduced. Nurses should make sure that the mother receives a great deal of rest in the postpartum period. Visitors may need to be restricted and the environment manipulated so that rest is possible. The mother may need oxygen, and she may need to remain in Fowler's position to ensure adequate oxygenation. The woman should be ambulated early to prevent thromboembolic complications. Precautions should be taken to avoid exposing the mother to infection of any kind, particularly upper respiratory infection. Because of the severe complications that result from infection, prophylactic antibiotics are often given during labor or following delivery.

Women with class III cardiac disease may be hospitalized as they approach the peak circulatory stress near the end of the second trimester. Any woman with cardiac disease is hospitalized if she begins showing signs of impending or overt heart failure and usually remains hospitalized for the duration of the pregnancy. Heart failure in pregnancy is usually left-sided and is treated in the same way that it would be in the nonpregnant state. The woman receives digitalis, oxygen, sedatives, bedrest, diuretics, a low-sodium diet, and restricted fluids.

Cardiac surgery may be performed early in the pregnancy and may make childbearing safer for some women. The risk of surgery is not significantly greater during pregnancy than when the woman is not pregnant. However, even with surgery complications may still arise during pregnancy, and therapeutic abortion is the alternative chosen by some women.

ANEMIA

Approximately 95 percent of the women who develop anemia during their pregnancy do so because of iron deficiency. They have generally had a diet poor in iron prior to becoming pregnant; they may have had excessive menstrual bleeding; and often they have had a number of pregnancies in rapid succession. These women begin their pregnancy already anemic or with low iron reserves, and as pregnancy advances, anemia results from the additional iron demands created by pregnancy and by the needs of the fetus. This is a potentially dangerous condition, since there is some evidence that fetoplacental function is impaired in pregnancy anemias [4]. Hemoglobin concentrations of 10 grams per 100 milliliters or less and a hematocrit of 30 percent or less reflect an anemia significant enough to warrant evaluation and treatment.

The woman should receive diet counseling and iron supplements. Ferrous sulfate or gluconate is usually prescribed, and the woman usually takes 300 milligrams three times a day. If the iron is taken with meals, the woman avoids gastric irritation, which is often a problem. Diet counseling, emphasizing a well-balanced diet high in iron, should also stress the need for adequate fluids and roughage if the woman is receiving oral iron preparations. Roughage will decrease constipation, which often occurs as a side effect of iron therapy. The preparations are given throughout pregnancy and for about six months after delivery in order to restore normal hemoglobin and hematocrit levels and to replenish iron reserves. Women who are unable to tolerate oral iron preparations may be given intramuscular or parenteral preparations if the anemia must be corrected quickly, which is the case when a woman is severely anemic and close to term.

Folic acid and vitamin B_{12} deficiencies are also common causes of anemia during pregnancy. Because these substances are necessary for cell replication, it can easily be seen how important they are for the growing fetus. When the woman is deficient in these substances, replacement therapy is essential.

Less commonly, women experience anemia caused by abnormal hemoglobins. Sickle-cell anemia, which occurs predominately in blacks, is one example. Women who only have the sickling trait have no symptoms and their fetuses are at risk only from hypoxic stress, but women with sickle-cell disease experience chronic anemia and frequent infections, and have periodic crises marked by abdominal and joint pain. During pregnancy these women need close supervision. They must avoid infections and should have their hemoglobin levels checked frequently; their hemoglobin concentrations should be maintained at 7 grams per 100 milliliters, which is normal for them [17]. As term approaches, they may be given transfusions of whole blood or packed red cells in preparation for the stress of delivery and the accompanying blood loss. If the woman has a sickling crisis, which is common in late pregnancy, labor, and delivery, she is given oxygen and folic acid, and is placed on bed rest. During labor she is comfortably sedated and usually receives oxygen continuously. Women with sickle-cell disease have a 50 percent chance of delivering a live infant.

INFECTIONS

In general, pregnant women are no more susceptible to acute infectious disease than other women, but the consequences are serious if one is contracted. Frequently abortion results, the acute infection may become worse because of the stress of the pregnancy and labor, and the rate of maternal and fetal mortality increases.

Syphilis

Serological testing for syphilis is a part of routine early prenatal care, and the test is repeated in the third trimester to detect infection contracted during pregnancy. Administration of appropriate antibiotics prior to the eighteenth week of pregnancy is believed to prevent fetal infection, since it is felt that the organism does not cross the placenta before this time. Treatment of the mother later in pregnancy also treats the fetus, since penicillin crosses the placenta. Women with untreated syphilis generally experience premature labor.

Treatment consists of 2.4 million units of benzathine penicillin G intramuscularly or 4.8 million units of procaine penicillin G, divided into three doses given intramuscularly three days apart. If the woman is allergic to penicillin, she is treated with tetracycline or erythromycin. Following treatment the maternal serologic test may remain positive for eight months, and the newborn may have a positive test for up to three months.

Gonorrhea

Cervical cultures have become a routine part of prenatal care and have been useful in detecting dormant gonorrheal infections. A chronic infection is generally found localized in the urethra, in Skene's and Bartholin's glands, and in the cervix. It usually remains dormant until delivery, when it spreads and may produce endometritis, salpingitis, oophoritis, and/or pelvic peritonitis.

When acute gonorrhea is found during pregnancy, acute inflammation is found in the urethra, vulvar glands, and vaginal and vulvar epithelium. The woman has a greenish-yellow vaginal secretion and her vulva may be red, ulcerated, and covered with a grayish exudate or condylomas. Her cervix is usually swollen and eroded and may secrete a foul secretion in which the gonococci are found. Bed rest is highly recommended and intercourse is halted. Aqueous procaine penicillin G is given intramuscularly in a dose of 4.8 million units, 2.4 million units injected into each buttock. If the woman is allergic to penicillin, she is given tetracycline, kanamycin, or erythromycin. Further treatment using twice the initial dose may be necessary if the cultures remain positive. If the infant's eyes are contaminated with the gonococci during delivery, he develops the eye infection opthalmia neonatorum.

Urinary Tract Infections

Because of the physiological changes in pregnancy, urinary tract infections are common in pregnant women. In the second trimester, the renal pelves, calices, and ureters become dilated. The ureters also exhibit a decrease in peristalsis, and later in pregnancy the heavy uterus places pressure on them at the pelvic brim. All of these factors result in greatly increased collecting space within the urinary tract and urinary stasis, creating optimal conditions for infection. Kass [20] reports that between 5 and 10 percent of all pregnant women have significant bacteriuria, with *Escherichia coli* being the most commonly found organism. Many of these women are asymptomatic but approximately one-fourth of them will develop symptomatic urinary tract infections during pregnancy, most commonly acute pylonephritis. They usually have chills, a temperature around 39.4° C (103° F), frequent urination, and pain in the abdomen or flank area. Antibiotics, increased fluids (to 3000 milliliters daily), and heat to the flank are generally prescribed.

Tuberculosis

Tuberculosis is difficult to diagnose during pregnancy since diagnostic methods may take months and since the lung becomes compressed as the uterus raises the diaphragm. This compression may conceal the lung cavity. If tuberculosis is found, the usual treatment of isoniazid, para-aminosalicylic acid, and streptomycin is begun; these drugs do not seem to have an adverse effect on the fetus. The woman is hospitalized and restricted to bed, and her diet must be improved so that she gets increased protein, vitamins, and calories. Labor and delivery are carried out normally; however, the infant is isolated from his mother after birth to avoid his becoming infected. It is uncertain whether or not pregnancy aggravates the disease.

PSEUDOCYESIS

Pseudocyesis, or false pregnancy, is usually seen in young women with an intense desire to be pregnant or in women who are nearing menopause. They have many of the symptoms of pregnancy: irregular or absent menses, morning sickness, and increase in abdominal size, which may result from a rapid accumulation of abdominal fat, gas in the intestinal tract, or abdominal fluid. Sometimes their breasts will enlarge and show pigment changes. All of these symptoms may be due to endocrine disorders of the ovary, anterior pituitary, or hypothalamus. Contractions of the intestines or abdominal muscles may be misinterpreted as fetal movements. However, when a woman with pseudocyesis is examined, her uterus is found to be small. The most difficult part of her care is convincing her that she is not pregnant, a delusion that may be so strong that it persists for years [17].

REFERENCES

1. Ansari, A. New approach to amnioscopy. *Journal of the American Medical Association* 212:321, 1970.
2. Avery, M. E. Prenatal diagnosis and prevention of hyaline membrane disease. *New England Journal of Medicine* 292:157, 1975.
3. Bates, G. W. Management of gestational diabetes. *Postgraduate Medicine* 55:55, 1974.
4. Beischer, N. The effects of maternal anemia upon the fetus. *Journal of Reproductive Medicine* 6:21, 1971.
5. Brown, B., Gabert, H., and Stenchever, M. Respiratory distress syndrome, surfactant biochemistry, and acceleration of fetal lung maturity: A review. *Obstetrical and Gynecological Survey* 30:71, 1975.
6. Churchill, J. A., Berendes, H. W., and Nemore, J. Neuropsychological deficits in children of diabetic mothers. *American Journal of Obstetrics and Gynecology* 105:257, 1969.
7. Cruz, A. C., Buhi, W. C., and Spellary, W. N. Comparison of fetogram and L/S ratio for fetal maturity. *Obstetrics and Gynecology* 45:147, 1975.
8. Daughter's cancers linked to mother's use of estrogen. *Journal of the American Medical Association* 220:653, 1972.
9. Davidson, O. Hemoglobin F in newborn infants of diabetic mothers. *Acta Endocrinologica* 181 (Supplement):73, 1974.
10. Droegemueller, W., Jackson, C., Makowski, E. L., and Battaglia, F. C. Amniotic fluid examination as an aid in assessment of gestational age. *American Journal of Obstetrics and Gynecology* 104:424, 1969.
11. Duhring, J. L. The high risk fetus. *Hospital Medicine* 10:77, 1974.
12. Fencl, M., and Tulchinsky, D. Total cortisol in amniotic fluid and fetal lung maturation. *New England Journal of Medicine* 292:133, 1975.
13. Gallup, D., and Lucas, W. Heparin treatment of consumption coagulopathy associated with intrauterine fetal death. *Obstetrics and Gynecology* 35:690, 1970.
14. Golditch, I., and Boyce, N. E. Management of abruptio placentae. *Journal of the American Medical Association* 212:288, 1970.
15. Greenhill, J. P., and Friedman, E. A. *Biological Principles and Modern Practice of Obstetrics.* Philadelphia: Saunders, 1974.
16. Hafez, E. S. Physiology of multiple pregnancy. *Journal of Reproductive Medicine* 12:88, 1974.
17. Hellman, L. M., and Pritchard, J. A. *William's Obstetrics* (14th ed.). New York: Appleton-Century-Crofts, 1971.
18. Huber, C. P., Melin, J. R., and Vellios, F. Changes in chorionic tissue of aborted pregnancy. *American Journal of Obstetrics and Gynecology* 73:569, 1957.
19. Hyde, E., Joyce, D., Gurewich, V., Flute, P., and Barrera, S. Intravascular coagulation during pregnancy and the puerperium. *Journal of Obstetrics and Gynecology of the British Commonwealth* 80:1059, 1973.
20. Kass, E. H. Symposium on the newer aspects of antibiotics: Chemotherapeutic and antibiotic drugs in the management of infections of the urinary tract. *American Journal of Medicine* 18:764, 1955.
21. Khojandi, M., Tsai, A., and Tyson, J. Gestational diabetes: The dilemma of delivery. *Obstetrics and Gynecology* 43:1, 1974.
22. Kilker, R., and Wilkerson, B. Nursing care in placenta previa and abruptio placentae. *Nursing Clinics of North America* 8:479, 1973.
23. Milunsky, A., and Alpert, E. The value of alpha-fetoprotein in the prenatal diagnosis of neural tube defects. *Journal of Pediatrics* 84:889, 1974.
24. Molar pregnancy. *OB World* 3:1, July-August 1974.
25. Myers, J., Harrell, M. J., and Hill, F. Fetal maturity: Biochemical analysis of amniotic fluid. *American Journal of Obstetrics and Gynecology* 121:961, 1975.
26. Oakes, G., Chez, R., and Morelli, I. Diet in pregnancy: Meddling with the normal or preventing toxemia. *American Journal of Nursing* 75:1135, 1975.
27. Panayotou, P., Kaskarelis, D., Miettinen, O., Trichopoulos, D., and Kalandidi, A. Induced abortion and ectopic pregnancy. *American Journal of Obstetrics and Gynecology* 114:507, 1972.
28. Reid, D., Ryan, K., and Benirschke, K. *Principles and Management of Human Reproduction.* Philadelphia: Saunders, 1972.

29. Seppala, M., and Ruoslahti, E.   Alpha-fetoprotein in Rh-immunized pregnancies. *Obstetrics and Gynecology* 42:701, 1973.
30. Spellacy, W. N., Buhi, W. C., and Birk, S. A.   The effectiveness of human placental lactogen measurements as an adjunct in decreasing perinatal deaths. *American Journal of Obstetrics and Gynecology* 121:835, 1975.
31. Spontaneous abortion's cause studied with fetal tissues. *Journal of the American Medical Association* 197:41, 1966.
32. Stocker, J., and Mawad, R., Deleon, A., and Desjardins, P.   Ultrasonic cephalometry. *Obstetrics and Gynecology* 45:275, 1975.
33. Tapia, H., Johnson, C., and Strong, C.   Renin-angiotensin system in normal and in hypertensive disease of pregnancy. *Lancet* 2:847, 1972.
34. Thompson, H. E.   The clinical use of pulsed echo ultrasound in obstetrics and gynecology. *Obstetrical and Gynecological Survey* 23:903, 1968.
35. Tsudaka, T., Bloch, D., and Wolf, P.   An automated profile of amniotic fluid. *Laboratory Medicine* 2:32, 1971.
36. Ueland, K., Novy, M., and Metcalfe, J.   Hemodynamic responses of patients with heart disease to pregnancy and exercise. *American Journal of Obstetrics and Gynecology* 113:47, 1972.
37. Weir, R., Fraser, R., Lever, A., Morton, J., Brown, J., Kraszewski, A., McIlwaine, G., Robertson, J., and Tree, M.   Plasma renin, renin sudstrate, angiotensin II, and aldosterone in hypertensive disease of pregnancy. *Lancet* 1:291, 1973.
38. When are identical twins not identical? *Emergency Medicine* 2:39, 1970.
39. Williams, S. R.   *Essentials of Nutrition and Diet Therapy.* St. Louis: Mosby, 1974.

FURTHER READING

Abramson, J., Sacks, T., Flug, D., Elishkowsky, R., and Cohen, R.   Bacteriuria and hemoglobin levels in pregnancy. *Journal of the American Medical Association* 215:1631, 1971.
Arehart, J.   Sounding out the womb. *Science News* 100:424, 1971.
Cabaniss, C. D.   Management of heart disease in pregnancy. *Journal of Reproductive Medicine* 8:61, 1972.
Cahill, J., Cohen, H., and Starkovsky, N.   A rapid screening test for detection of alpha-1 fetoprotein as an indicator of fetal distress. *American Journal of Obstetrics and Gynecology* 119:1095, 1974.
Cohen, E., Belleville, J. W., and Brown, B.   Anesthesia, pregnancy, and miscarriage: A study of operating room nurses and anesthesiologists. *Anesthesiology* 35:343, 1971.
Essex, N., Pyke, D. A., Watkins, P. J., Brudenell, J. M., and Gamsu, H. R.   Diabetic pregnancy. *British Medical Journal* 4:89, 1973.
Goebelsmann, U., Freeman, R., Mestman, J., Nakamura, R., and Woodling, B.   Estriol in pregnancy. *American Journal of Obstetrics and Gynecology* 115:795, 1973.
Herbst, A., Poskanzer, D., Robboy, S., Friedlander, L., and Scully, R.   Prenatal exposure to stilbestrol. *New England Journal of Medicine* 292:334, 1975.
Horger, E., Miller, M. C., and Connor, E.   Relation of large birthweight to maternal diabetes mellitus. *Obstetrics and Gynecology* 45:150, 1975.
Human fetus is successfully treated. *Science News* 108:121, 1975.
Leon, J.   High-risk pregnancy: Graphic representation of the maternal and fetal risks. *American Journal of Obstetrics and Gynecology* 117:497, 1973.
Lockwood, G., and Newman, R.   Estriol determinations in gestational diabetes. *Obstetrics and Gynecology* 44:642, 1974.
Milunsky, A., and Atkins, L.   Prenatal diagnosis of genetic disorders: an analysis of experience with 600 cases. *Journal of the American Medical Association* 230:181, 1974.
Murata, Y., and Martin, C.   Growth of the biparietal diameter of the fetal head in diabetic pregnancy. *American Journal of Obstetrics and Gynecology* 115:252, 1973.
Oparil, S., and Swartout, J.   Heart disease in pregnancy. *Journal of Reproductive Medicine* 11:2, 1973.
O'Sullivan, J., Mahan, C., Charles, D., and Dandrow, R.   Medical treatment of the gestational diabetic. *Obstetrics and Gynecology* 43:817, 1974.
Peckham, C.   Uterine bleeding during pregnancy. *Obstetrics and Gynecology* 35:937, 1970.

Prenatal diagnosis of Cooley's anemia. *Science News* 107:352, 1975.

Prenatal diagnosis: Problems and outlook. *Journal of the American Medical Association* 222:132, 1972.

Reproductive tract lesions in male mice exposed prenatally to diethylstilbestrol. *Science* 190:991, 1975.

Santos-Ramos, R., and Duenhoelter, J.   Diagnosis of congenital fetal abnormalities by sonography. *Obstetrics and Gynecology* 45:279, 1975.

Schwarz, R.   Antenatal diagnosis of congenital disorders. *Pennsylvania Medicine* 75:47, 1972.

Schwarz, R., Fields, G., and Kyle, G. C.   Timing of delivery in the pregnant diabetic patient. *Obstetrics and Gynecology* 34:787, 1969.

Stallone, L., and Ziel, H.   Management of gestational diabetes. *American Journal of Obstetrics and Gynecology* 119:1091, 1974.

Stitt, A.   The rheumatic heart in pregnancy. *Emergency Medicine* 3:123, 1971.

Wallace, W., Harken, D., and Ellis, L.   Pregnancy following closed mitral valvuloplasty. *Journal of the American Medical Association* 217:279, 1971.

Chapter 15 Complications of Labor

PREMATURE LABOR

Premature labor (labor prior to 38 weeks' gestation) may end with delivery of a preterm infant too immature to survive. When this circumstance arises, steps are taken to stop labor. The woman is placed on absolute bed rest and is sedated. No vaginal examinations are performed. Some physicians prefer to use an intravenous infusion of alcohol in which 100 milliliters of 95% ethanol is added to 900 milliliters of 5% dextrose in water. The alcohol will inhibit oxytocin release from the posterior pituitary, thus halting the labor. Alcohol will not stop labor if the membranes already have ruptured or if the cervix is incompetent.

The woman receiving intravenous alcohol may experience vomiting and may act inebriated; she may act in ways or say things that later cause her embarrassment. The nurse caring for this patient must remember that the woman must not be made to feel guilty in any way for her actions and must be reassured that her actions are expected in this type of therapy.

Beta-adrenergic drugs such as isoxsuprine, ritodrine, and diazoxide are currently being used to halt labor by inhibiting uterine contractions. However, they have side effects, including maternal hypotension, tachycardia, and syncope.

While attempts are being made to halt labor, the amniotic fluid is likely to be tested to assess fetal maturity. The woman may also receive betamethasone or dexamethasone to accelerate fetal lung maturation.

INDUCTION OF LABOR

It has become common for women to have labor initiated artificially at or near term for a variety of reasons. Most often, labor is induced for the convenience of the woman and her physician. The advantages of induction are that the mother is well rested, has time to organize her family for her absence, and is psychologically ready for labor. In addition, it can be assured that her bowel, bladder, and stomach are empty, and the risk of excessively rapid labor and possible delivery en route to the hospital is avoided. This method ensures that the physician can be present, and provides for labor and delivery when adequate personnel are available. Induction of labor also may be necessary to terminate pregnancy if the woman's life is in danger or if the fetus may be compromised. This often is the case when the woman has hypertensive disease, diabetes, or a renal disorder; when the fetus has erythroblastosis; and in prolonged pregnancy with associated placental insufficiency.

For labor to be induced, the woman must be near term, with a mature fetus. Her cervix must be soft with a moderate amount of effacement and dilatation (a ripe cervix). The fetal head must be fixed in the pelvic inlet, and there must be no cephalopelvic disproportion. Women with cephalopelvic disproportion, previous uterine surgery including cesarean section, malpresentation, placenta previa, or uterine overdistention should not have induced labor. Complications of induction are those associated with uterine overstimulation. They include tetanic contractions, uterine rupture, abruptio placentae, postpartum hemorrhage, fetal distress, birth injuries, and cervical lacerations.

One of the most popular methods of inducing labor is by artificial rupture of the membranes, or amniotomy. The perineum and vulva are washed with antiseptic solution. Using sterile gloves, the physician inserts two fingers into the vagina and into the cervix and separates the membranes from the lower uterine segment. He then ruptures the membranes with an amnihook, toothed forceps, or stylet. The nurse should take the fetal heart sounds immediately prior to rupture and immediately afterward to determine what effect the procedure has had on fetal oxygenation. If the cord has washed down with the amniotic fluid or has become compressed between the bony pelvis and the presenting part, a fetal bradycardia can be detected promptly and appropriate intervention begun. The color and amount of amniotic fluid expelled should also be noted and recorded.

If the cervix is effaced and partially dilated and the fetal head is deep in the pelvis, labor usually will begin. The procedure is most successful if performed within two weeks prior to the woman's expected date of confinement. If labor must be induced before this time for medical reasons, amniotomy is preceded by stripping of the membranes and is followed by oxytocin induction. With amniotomy, failure rates of 10 percent have been reported [2]. If the woman does not go into labor after the procedure, she may become infected by an ascending amnionitis. This woman, like the woman whose membranes rupture prematurely during the latter weeks of pregnancy, may be placed on antibiotic therapy and delivered within a few days if the fetus is mature. The incidence of infection increases significantly if the membranes have been ruptured for over 24 hours.

Stripping the membranes from the lower uterine segment without rupturing them is another method used to induce labor. When the membranes are separated as described previously, labor is possibly initiated by the release of oxytocin in response to the cervical manipulation that occurs. The loosened membranes also act as a wedge in dilating the cervix. This method does not always work. It may increase the incidence of infection and may result in accidental rupture of the membranes. The method is also not effective if the presenting part of the fetus is high in the woman's pelvis. This procedure may be more painful than amniotomy for some women.

Another widely used method of inducing labor is by the administration of oxytocin. A solution of 5 international units of oxytocin is added to 500 milliliters of 5% dextrose in water. The solution is given intravenously at 6–8 drops per minute, and the woman is observed carefully. Her blood pressure, pulse rate, and fetal heart tones are recorded every 15 minutes, and she is observed closely for the beginning of uterine contractions. The rate of infusion is increased carefully; Greenhill and Friedman [2] suggest increasing it at a rate of 4 drops every 15 minutes. The rate is increased until the contractions reach moderate to severe intensity, lasting 45–60 seconds at intervals of 2–3 minutes. Some authorities suggest that the infusion not be above 60 drops per minute [3]. The intravenous infusion rarely is continued for more than 8 hours; the woman becomes exhausted if it is continued any longer. At that point, it is discontinued and induction may be attempted the following day.

If the fetal heart rate indicates distress or if contractions last 90 seconds or more (tetanic contractions), the intravenous solution is discontinued immediately. If tetanic contractions result (hypersensitivity), they will usually occur within the first five contractions. The nurse should immediately monitor fetal heart tones, and if they are slow, administer oxygen to the woman. While blood pressure elevation rarely occurs with the use of synthetic oxytocin, the woman's blood pressure never-theless should be monitored carefully for any changes.

Induction of labor with intramuscular, intranasal, or sublingual administration of oxytocin is not commonly used because of problems in controlling the rate of absorption via these routes.

Some clinicians have objected to the frequency of elective induction of labor and its possible effects on the fetus. The main hazard associated with artificial induction is premature delivery. While one study [4] of almost 3000 elective inductions found only 0.7 percent of the perinatal deaths to be related to the induction, Schwarcz and colleagues [8] reported an increased incidence of type I dips and increased intensity of uterine contractions in women with induced labor. They question the effect this will have on the child's future growth and development.

DYSTOCIA

The term *dystocia* refers to a labor that is difficult because of mechanical or func-tional factors, or both. Mechanical causes of dystocia include maternal elements, such as a contracted pelvis (passage). Fetal (passenger) causes of mechanical dys-tocia include failure to rotate from an occiput transverse or posterior position, malpresentation, malformation such as hydrocephalus, and excessive size.

Functional Dystocia

Functional dystocia (or dysfunctional labor) results from contractions that deviate from normal. These contractions may be extremely forceful, with a rapid and trau-matic labor and precipitate delivery. More commonly, the contractions are ineffec-tual. In the majority of cases there is no apparent cause, although contributing conditions include uterine anomalies, overdistention such as is found in multiple pregnancy or hydramnios, delayed labor or postmaturity, cervical scar tissue from previous surgery, or chronic disease. Cervical resistance may be an important con-tributing factor, although this is usually restricted to first labors. Once the cervix has been dilated, it is no longer that resistant.

The contractions of functional dystocia may differ in quality and synchroniza-tion of activity. They may be localized to one portion of the uterus rather than involving the entire organ. They may be stronger in the lower uterine segment than in the upper uterine segment or may move upward over the uterus rather than downward. On the other hand, they may be properly synchronized and have a normal pattern but may exert so little pressure on the cervix that it does not dilate.

Desultory or prolonged labor may be evident within 6–8 hours after the onset of labor, particularly if the woman's progress is plotted on a graph that features a normal labor curve for comparison (Figure 15-1). Once labor begins, its progress should be definite and sustained until the baby is successfully delivered within the period of time defined for normal labor—20 hours. If it goes beyond that time, there is a resulting increase in fetal and maternal morbidity and mortality. In order to avoid these misfortunes supportive measures and uterine stimulation are used if the pattern of labor becomes abnormal.

For functional dystocia labor is stimulated by the common methods used for artificial induction. Amniotomy is chosen with the knowledge that delivery should occur within 24 hours if increased fetal and maternal morbidity is to be avoided. Oxytocin also is frequently used to prevent and treat functional dystocia by producing uterine contractions that are strong enough to dilate the cervix and by demonstrating over a short time whether or not the uterus will contract effectively to complete at least the first stage of labor. Usually progress is evident in 3–4 hours; if none occurs, the oxytocin stimulation process is abandoned, since an increase in fetal morbidity is likely to follow. Although the use of a specialized pump, such as a Harvard pump, in the administration of intravenous oxytocin does not eliminate the associated hazards or add to the efficiency of the medication [7], the drug can be titrated more accurately and controlled more readily with a pump. Since tetanic contractions may occur, with the resulting hazards of uterine rupture or fetal asphyxia, the woman must be observed constantly while she is receiving the drug.

Decisions regarding delivery for a woman with functional dystocia depend on the

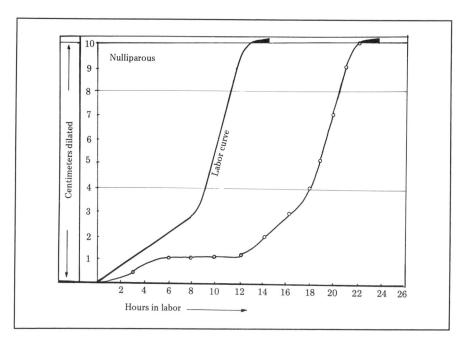

Figure 15-1. Abnormal labor can be detected early when plotted against a normal labor curve. This graph shows a prolonged latent phase.

degree of cervical dilatation and the station of the fetal presenting part. If the woman's cervix is more than half dilated, if the presenting part is near her pelvic floor, and if her outlet is ample, vaginal delivery may be possible. Otherwise, a cesarean section is less traumatic and far safer.

LATENT PHASE

Functional causes of labor abnormalities may be divided into three types according to the phase of labor affected—latent, active, or deceleration. The latent phase of dilatation is prolonged if it lasts over 20 hours in a nullipara and over 14 hours in a multipara. Almost half of the time prolonged labor during this phase is due to excessive or untimely sedation or anesthesia. About 20 percent of the time a thick, uneffaced, undilated, and unyielding cervix is the cause. In another 10 percent of cases false labor is diagnosed in retrospect, and in an additional 10 percent of women the cervix just dilates very slowly [2].

The uterine contractions that occur when the latent phase is prolonged are often hypertonic and uncoordinated, with an improper gradient and transmission over the uterus. The woman becomes exhausted, emotionally discouraged, and anxious, since these contractions can be very painful and can result in little progress of labor. The usual treatment involves giving the woman a significant period of rest and suspending labor temporarily by the use of a narcotic such as morphine. When the effects of the narcotic wear off and contractions resume, they are almost always likely to be of normal quality; in addition, the woman is usually well rested, emotionally rejuvenated, and better able to cope with the labor ahead of her. In the few cases in which the contractions do not resume normally, intravenous administration of oxytocin is usually helpful.

ACTIVE PHASE

When labor is prolonged in the active phase, there are abnormally slow rates of cervical dilation and descent of the fetus. The cervix dilates at a rate of less than 1.2 centimeters per hour in nulliparas and less than 1.5 centimeters per hour in multiparas. Such small degrees of dilation are impossible to determine at each individual examination, of course, but over a period of time they may be determined in retrospect, and plotting the mother's progress of labor on a graph will facilitate keeping track of these changes. Labor is also considered to be prolonged in the active phase if descent of the fetus occurs at a rate of less than 1 centimeter per hour in nulliparas and less than 2 centimeters per hour in multiparas.

The underlying pathogenesis for prolonged labor in the active phase is essentially unknown. Associated factors include minor fetal malposition, excessive sedation, or conduction anesthesia given at a high level or administered too early. Cephalopelvic disproportion is a contributory factor in about one-fourth of the cases.

The contractions associated with this type of dysfunctional labor are likely to be hypotonic, exerting less than the pressure of 15 millimeters of mercury necessary for progress to occur. The woman becomes exhausted, and there is a substantial risk of ascending infection, since it is likely that the membranes ruptured previously. Maintenance of the woman's fluid and electrolyte balance is a special consideration.

Following a careful evaluation of the fetopelvic relationship, oxytocin is usually administered. Most of these women can then deliver vaginally. If there is fetopelvic disproportion or if progress in labor does not result from the oxytocin administration, a cesarean is performed to decrease fetal and maternal risks.

DECELERATION PHASE (TRANSITION)

Labor can also be prolonged in the deceleration phase of the first stage of labor, or cervical dilation and/or descent of the fetus may come to a standstill at this time. The deceleration phase is prolonged if it lasts over 3 hours in nulliparas and over 1 hour in multiparas. Dilation is said to be arrested when expected progress ceases for at least 2 hours. Arrested descent exists when descent is interrupted for at least 1 hour; it usually occurs in the second stage. When arrest develops, a cesarean section becomes a likely possibility, although about 60 percent of women can deliver vaginally if given the opportunity [2]. The most ominous cause of arrested dilation or descent is cephalopelvic disproportion, occurring in about 40 percent of cases and necessitating, of course, a cesarean section. Other causes of arrested dilation or descent include minor malpositions, excessive sedation, or conduction anesthesia. Needless to say, before any therapy for functional dystocia is instituted, x-ray pelvimetry should be done to rule out cephalopelvic disproportion. If the cause of the difficulty is excessive sedation or anesthesia, normal labor is likely to ensue when the effects wear off. If the woman needs to be given oxytocin stimulation, she will probably respond with additional progress in dilation and descent in less than 3 hours. The earlier the diagnosis and the more careful the treatment, the less likely the woman and fetus are to suffer serious consequences.

When caring for women with functional dystocia, the nurse should be particularly aware of their general physical and emotional status, paying careful attention to the intensity of contractions, signs of fetal distress, and signs of maternal distress, such as a rising temperature with prolonged rupture of membranes, exhaustion, or dehydration. Since patterns of dysfunctional labor are very discouraging to parents and usually increase their levels of anxiety and tension, nursing care should include careful explanations of the treatment and words of reassurance and encouragement. It is important to promote the woman's relaxation and make her as comfortable as possible so she can conserve her strength. Nursing actions may include giving her a sponge bath, changing her position, rubbing her back, and keeping her clean and dry. She may also find some diversionary activity helpful. Since a full bladder or rectum can block labor's progress or may be traumatized during the labor and delivery process, it is essential to provide for adequate elimination.

Probably one of the most important elements in helping parents to cope with the crisis situation of abnormal labor is the constant presence of a calm, knowledgeable, and supportive nurse—one who also provides for continuity of care by informing postpartum and nursery personnel about the particular stresses that the couple has already encountered.

Dysfunction of Abdominal Muscles.   In order for the second stage of labor to progress normally, some voluntary pushing by the woman, using her abdominal muscles, is usually required. Sometimes the second stage is prolonged if, for some reason, the mother is unable to push effectively. Possible causes of this inability are relaxed abdominal musculature (in the multipara), an anesthesia-blocked perineal reflex, weakness from exhaustion, or the woman's refusal to push if her discomfort is severe. Forceps are commonly used to shorten the second stage of labor.

Mechanical Dystocia

MATERNAL PELVIC CONTRACTION

In 75 percent of nulliparas with a vertex presentation, engagement has occurred by the thirty-eighth week of gestation; in 95 percent, by the onset of labor. If the vertex is engaged at the onset of labor, a vaginal delivery can be anticipated in 99 percent of pregnant women; if the vertex is not engaged at the onset of labor, the need for a cesarean section can be anticipated in 36 percent.

A contracted pelvis may be the cause of nonengagement of the vertex at the onset of labor. The definition of a contracted pelvis is somewhat arbitrary, since the type of pelvis in the individual woman is an important consideration. Enlargement in one pelvic diameter may compensate for narrowing in another and may actually permit vaginal delivery. Other factors that affect pelvic adequacy are the size of the fetus, the hardness and moldability of the head, the presentation, position, and attitude. It is possible for all three planes of the pelvis to be contracted, either singly or in combination.

Inlet.   Contraction of the pelvic inlet is suspected when the anterior-posterior diameter (diagonal conjugate) is less than 11 centimeters (average, 12.5 centimeters). The contracted conjugate vera is generally considered to be below 10 centimeters (average, 11 centimeters), although a nullipara with a conjugate vera of 9.0–9.5 centimeters is usually permitted a trial labor, especially if the fetus is not large.

If there are consistently strong labor contractions but no descent of the fetal head through the pelvis, the head will develop large caput succedaneum; in addition, there may be placental insufficiency, fetal cerebral injury and hemorrhage, or a ruptured uterus. Hopefully the contracted pelvis is usually suspected and diagnosed, and a cesarean section is done before the mother or infant suffers such consequences.

Midpelvis.   The average bispinous diameter of the midpelvis is 10.5 centimeters. A measurement of less than 9.5 centimeters between the ischial spines usually results in a contracted pelvis. This measurement is one that can be accurately obtained only by x-ray pelvimetry.

Outlet.   The pelvic outlet has an average bituberous diameter of 10.5 centimeters; it is usually contracted when the diameter is less than 8.5 centimeters. Ordinarily the coccyx can be forced back 2.5 centimeters or more during delivery, adding to the available outlet space. When the sacrococcygeal joint is healthy, no problems result. If it is ankylotic, the bone may be fractured or the joint may break open. Chronic arthritis may develop as a result.

The mother who has a fractured coccyx may be unable to sit comfortably. She may complain of pain running up her back and down her thighs and of difficulty in walking. The fracture usually heals by itself within six months. The application of heat or the injection of procaine around the joint and nerve supply will probably relieve the associated discomfort. Rarely will the mother need to have the bone excised.

Although the pelvic planes are described separately, the midpelvis and outlet are usually considered together in evaluating pelvic adequacy. Their contraction may actually be more dangerous than a contracted inlet, since it may not be discovered until late in labor or when an attempt is made to deliver the baby vaginally. This problem is commonly associated with android pelves. Contractures are less often seen with the anthropoid type, and the low incidence of platypelloid (flat) pelves makes pelvic contraction associated with this type relatively rare. In general, the most common problem seen clinically is that of pelvic inlet contraction.

A pelvic contraction is diagnosed when labor is not progressing normally, when the presenting part of the fetus is high and undescending, or when a dysfunctional labor pattern develops. X-ray pelvimentry is used to confirm the diagnosis. This procedure involves a small amount of radiation but not enough to discourage its use for this purpose, for placentography, or to determine fetal position; however, if possible, it should not be repeated.

Abnormal fetal presentations are four times as frequent with contracted pelves as with normal ones. Prolapse of the fetal arm, foot, and cord are therefore relatively common, and at the beginning of labor the fetal head is likely to be high and not engaged. Since a contracted pelvis often causes a large caput succedaneum to form, it may be wrongly surmised that the head is actually engaged when in reality it is still high. Caput often obscures the landmarks of the head and makes accurate diagnosis of its position difficult. Because the head may not fill the lower uterine segment normally, the membranes over the cervical os may be exposed to the full force of the uterine contractions. As a result, they may rupture prematurely, predisposing the fetus to prolapsed cord and the mother to uterine infection. Sometimes the cervix is compressed between the bony surface of the fetal head and the maternal pelvis and becomes edematous.

If the pelvic contraction is a serious one, the fetal prognosis is actually better since the abnormality is likely to be recognized early and a cesarean section can be performed before the fetus is distressed. If the contraction is very slight, usually the woman will deliver spontaneously, provided the fetus is of moderate size, fetal presentation and position are normal, and uterine contractions are strong.

Any problem that causes a delay in the progress of labor increases the parents' anxiety level; therefore, careful explanations of the procedures involved in the diagnosis and of the alternative methods of treatment to ensure maternal and fetal safety are reassuring.

TRIAL LABOR

As already mentioned, when the adequacy of a woman's pelvis is borderline or functional dystocia is diagnosed, she may be permitted a trial labor. Trial labor usually is a period of 6–12 hours, during which the obstetrician concludes that the woman can be safely delivered vaginally or that she must have a cesarean section.

It is rare that cephalopelvic disproportion is absolute, given the fact that the pelvis does expand somewhat during the process of labor. In addition, if the woman is permitted to have a trial labor, the obstetrician can be more certain that the labor has progressed as long as possible and that a cesarean section is not done unnecessarily.

A trial labor is probably most anxiety-producing in the primigravida who wishes to avoid a primary cesarean section in light of future childbearing. The constant presence of a supporting nurse is helpful. In order to ensure maximum pelvic space, it is important that the woman's bladder and bowel remain as empty as possible.

Soft Tissue Dystocia

While a narrow bony pelvis can be a serious cause of dystocia, another possible cause is an anomaly of the maternal soft parts. Sometimes the woman's cervix is very rigid. This may be caused by chronic cervicitis, deep cauterizations, or previous surgical procedures. Digital dilation or softening with intravenous oxytocin stimulation may be the clinician's choice of treatment. Sometimes a cesarean section is necessary.

Tumors, congenital deformities, edema, scars, or hematomas may contribute to vulvar or vaginal stenosis. Usually the obstruction clears spontaneously as the tissues soften during pregnancy and labor. An episiotomy often solves the problem. Rarely, a cesarean section becomes necessary.

Fetal Causes of Mechanical Dystocia

PERSISTENT OCCIPUT POSTERIOR

A common cause of arrested labor is the failure of the fetal occiput to rotate anteriorly, so that it remains posterior or transverse. Generally, this occurs in pelves other than the gynecoid type. If the occiput is posterior, the fetal head meets resistance at the sacrococcygeal platform and the ischial spines and becomes deflexed. Complete descent is prevented, so that the head is arrested between the spines and the perineum. If the head is deflexed, the cervix may fail to dilate completely and may become edematous from being pressed between the presenting part and the symphysis pubis. The progress of labor will slow as a result, especially in the deceleration phase of the first stage and in the second stage. As a rule, if delivery does not occur within an hour, the vertex will only extend further and the cervix will become more edematous.

Generally, the persistent occiput rotates spontaneously once it reaches the slinglike musculature of the pelvic floor. If this does not happen, there is less risk of maternal soft tissue damage if the vertex can be rotated and delivered in an anterior position. In addition, the amount of force necessary for delivery is three times less if the occiput is anterior. Rotation of the fetal head can be accomplished either manually or by forceps. Manual rotation is often possible and results in fewer vaginal lacerations. If manual rotation is not possible, rotation by forceps is necessary. (Rotation of the fetal head by forceps and application of another set of forceps for delivery is referred to as the *Scanzoni maneuver*.)

If the head presents posteriorly, spontaneous delivery requires more uterine and abdominal effort than if the head presents anteriorly. The sinciput passes well below the inferior aspect of the symphysis pubis, and the vertex is delivered face up by flexion. In the posterior position, the larger occipitofrontal diameter (11.5 centimeters or more) of the vertex appears at the outlet rather than the suboccipitobregmatic diameter, a difference of 2.5–3 centimeters, causing the woman's perineum to become greatly distended. The underlying endopelvic fascia often separates despite an extensive mediolateral episiotomy unless the outlet is exceptionally large. Thus, rather severe perineal lacerations commonly occur unless the fetus is small or the woman is a multipara. Since a large caput succedaneum generally forms, there may be fetal head damage as well.

The woman who is carrying a fetus in the posterior position often has severe pain in her back with contractions, as the fetal head presses against her sacrum. Back rubs and position changes are sometimes helpful. In this presentation, fetal heart tones are heard best deep in the mother's flank. Her labor contractions commonly follow a pattern of alternating large and small contractions.

Occiput posterior fetal positions per se do not increase maternal morbidity or infant mortality; however, they are commonly associated with prolonged labor, arrested descent, or operative deliveries and thus can be contributing factors.

SINCIPUT PRESENTATION

If the amount of head deflexion is only slight, the fetus' sinciput will present (Figure 15-2). In this presentation the woman's labor and her treatment are like that for the occiput posterior presentation. The occiput still remains the point of reference. Usually, when the fetal head reaches the pelvic floor, contractions improve, the head flexes, and the child is born without further difficulty.

PERSISTENT OCCIPUT TRANSVERSE

Transverse arrest occurs when the occiput, which is originally in a transverse position, fails to rotate. This is usually no problem if the woman's pelvis is gynecoid, since rotation to the anterior position is easily accomplished and forceps extraction of the head is not difficult. If her pelvis is android, or possibly if her midpelvis and outlet are contracted, a cesarean section is usually done to avoid traumatizing the fetus or the woman's soft tissues. Severe vaginal lacerations may follow the use of forceps in the case of persistent occiput transverse.

BREECH PRESENTATION

Since vertex presentations of the fetal head constitute 95 percent of all deliveries, any other presentation—breech, face, brow, shoulder—is considered a deviation from normal. In about 3–4 percent of all deliveries, the breech will be the presenting part, with the fetal head in the woman's fundus and the buttocks in her lower uterine segment. The point of reference is the sacrum. The most common breech positions are left sacroanterior (LSA) and right sacroposterior (RSP).

The fetus does not necessarily assume the final presentation and position in the

Figure 15-2. Sinciput presentation with slight head flexion, forcing a larger fetal head diameter to present.

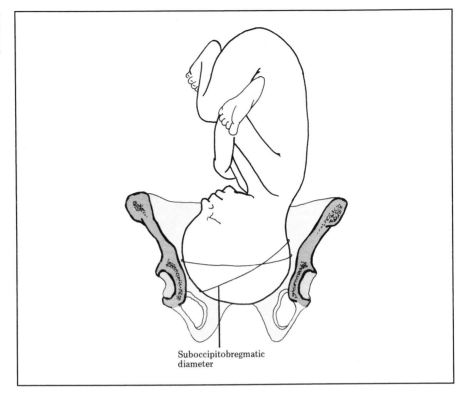

Suboccipitobregmatic
diameter

uterus until the last weeks of pregnancy, when it must accommodate itself to available space. Therefore, breech presentations are more common in premature labor than in full-term labor, since the law of accommodation is not operative yet. They are also more common in hydramnios or multiple pregnancy, in which excessive distention of the uterine cavity or the presence of another fetus can interfere with the development of normal uterine polarity. Anencephalic or hydrocephalic fetuses commonly present in the breech position, often with accompanying hydramnios. Breech presentations are also linked with placenta previa, which occupies space in the lower uterine segment, although transverse lie is probably more common in association with this disorder.

There are three varieties of breech presentations. In the frank breech, the fetus' thighs are flexed on the abdomen and the legs are extended in such a way that the feet are at the level of the thorax or shoulders. The buttocks are in the woman's lower uterine segment. The frank breech provides a better dilating wedge than the complete breech.

The complete or full breech has almost the same attitude as a vertex presentation but with reversed polarity. The fetus' thighs are flexed on the abdomen and the lower legs are on the thighs. The feet appear in the woman's birth canal at the same level as the buttocks. This presentation is considered more satisfactory for immediate delivery, since one of the feet may be brought down readily for traction, if necessary.

If the infant is in a footling breech presentation, one leg is extended and the foot is in the woman's birth canal before the buttocks. If both legs are extended, it is a double footling breech.

Breech presentations are diagnosed by abdominal palpation and vaginal examination in the later weeks of pregnancy, and the diagnosis is verified by x-ray studies. With Leopold's maneuvers, the round fetal head is found in the woman's fundus, the back is felt on either side, and the irregular breech is usually well above the pelvic brim, but occasionally it is fixed in the inlet. Fetal heart tones are heard at or above the woman's umbilicus.

If the membranes are ruptured, the fetal landmarks are more distinguishable on vaginal examination. The gluteal cleft and anus are palpable, with the two ischial tuberosities on either side. Sometimes the gluteal cleft is mistaken for the mouth, and a face presentation is wrongly diagnosed. Exact differentiation of genitalia by palpation may be obscured by compression and edema (although the examiner is often tempted to predict the sex of the infant). After birth, genitalia may be ecchymotic. If one of the fetus' legs has been in the woman's birth canal, it may be swollen and ecchymotic. All of these sequelae disappear within a week.

Usually the breech does not enter the pelvis until labor begins. Descent may be slow since the breech is not as firm a dilating wedge as the head, but the overall time of labor is not appreciably longer than in a vertex presentation [1]. After the largest diameter of the breech (bitrochanteric—9 centimeters) clears the pelvic outlet, the fetus is easily born to the umbilicus. Usually the legs slip out of the birth canal spontaneously and the fetal sacrum then normally rotates 45 degrees or more anteriorly, thus favoring anterior rotation of the occiput of the aftercoming head. The shoulders are usually delivered with the widest diameter (bisacromial—12 centimeters) passing through the anterior-posterior dimension of the pelvic outlet by lateral flexion. This diameter can be shortened a bit by compression and by the range of mobility of the shoulder girdle. The anterior shoulder appears beneath the pubic arch, and the posterior shoulder then passes over the perineum.

If the infant's arms remain flexed on his chest, they are beside the thorax as it emerges. It is possible for one or both of the arms to become extended above the shoulders, especially if the woman's pelvis is contracted. This situation demands the assistance of the obstetrician; otherwise, the fetus is subjected to increasing hypoxia from compression of the umbilical cord after the umbilicus has passed through the woman's pelvic outlet.

Normal engagement of the aftercoming head takes place with the occiput in the anterior position. As descent occurs, the fetus' cervical spine, the region of maximum flexibility, is brought into the curve of the lower birth canal. The suboccipital region of the head is the fulcrum around which the chin, mouth, face, vertex, and finally the occiput pass over the woman's perineum. Usually a deep episiotomy is performed to avoid delay in delivering the fetal head and shoulders and to prevent severe maternal perineal lacerations. Sometimes Piper forceps are used to facilitate the head's delivery (Figure 15-3).

In general, maternal morbidity is higher in breech presentations than in vertex. The associated perinatal loss is between 12 and 15 percent. The breech does not fill the lower uterine segment as completely as the vertex; therefore, there is greater

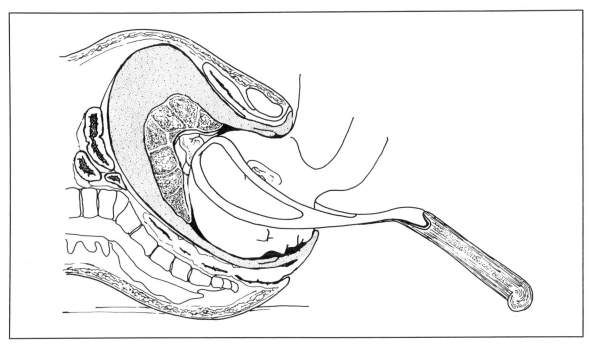

Figure 15-3. Fetal head delivered with Piper forceps in breech delivery.

opportunity for the umbilical cord to prolapse when the membranes rupture. Premature rupture of the membranes is frequent in breech presentation, and amniotic fluid may be stained with meconium. The latter is a rather insignificant fact of breech presentation, however, since meconium may be pressed out naturally by the increased intrauterine pressure on the breech during a contraction.

During the usual delivery process in a breech presentation, the umbilical cord is subjected to greater degrees of pressure, leading to fetal hypoxia. The fetal prognosis is also more hazardous in breech presentations because cephalopelvic disproportion may become apparent only after delivery of the breech and shoulders, leaving the head remaining in the birth canal; attempts to extract the head are usually traumatizing to the fetus. Also, after the delivery of the hips and shoulders the uterus decreases in size, and this may facilitate placental release while the head is still in the birth canal.

For all of the previously mentioned reasons, the fetal heart tones are constantly monitored during labor and delivery. Fetal complications include anoxia, intracranial damage from rupture of the tentorium with or without associated hemorrhage, and traumatic injury of the spinal cord. Fractures of the infant's clavicle or extremities may occur. A cesarean section may be the delivery of choice if the breech infant is large or if the woman's pelvis is small.

It is common for a breech presentation to convert to a vertex presentation spontaneously. If this does not happen, sometimes the obstetrician will attempt an external cephalic version [6]. In order for this to be done, there should be an accurate diagnosis of presentation and position, a nonirritable uterus, an unengaged breech, and enough amniotic fluid to allow the fetus to be turned. Before the version is attempted, the fetal heart rate and rhythm are carefully noted. The obstetrician grasps the fetal caudal pole and cephalic pole through the woman's abdominal wall and turns them slowly and intermittently. The fetal heart tones are checked frequently throughout the procedure, since the change in fetal position may place tension on the umbilical cord or compress it between the fetus and the uterine wall. If the heart tones decrease or become irregular, the fetus is reconverted to a breech presentation.

The best time for attempting an external cephalic version is between 34 and 35 weeks' gestation. At that time the fetus can be turned with a minimum amount of force, and there is less chance that it will spontaneously reconvert to a breech presentation, since the woman's abdominal wall is comparatively relaxed. If the version is done later in pregnancy, there is greater likelihood of trauma to the umbilical cord and placenta and a chance that premature labor might be initiated. However, if rupture of the membranes accidently occurs, the fetus is more likely to be mature enough to survive. Conversion at 34–35 weeks' gestation is more likely to be successful in the multigravida who has relaxed abdominal walls and a large amount of amniotic fluid [7].

Since expectant parents may be aware of the complications involved in breech presentations or may be alerted to the fact that something is unusual based on the extra-careful monitoring of the woman's condition, their anxiety level will be high. Frequent explanations and reassurance regarding the status of the fetus and the woman are important psychological elements of a nurse's actions in this situation.

BROW AND FACE PRESENTATIONS

Generally, brow and face presentations have the same etiology and are diagnosed by the same methods. Pelvic contracture, fetal abnormalities, or a very large maternal pelvis are contributing factors. These presentations are two to three times as frequent in multiparas as in nulliparas, probably due to the multipara's decreased abdominal and pelvic muscle tone. A fetus with excessive muscle tone in the extensor muscles of the back and neck can also be a cause of brow and face presentations.

Deflexion to the greatest degree results in a face presentation, and anencephaly accounts for 5 percent of these cases. The chin, or mentum, is the point of reference. Early diagnosis of the extended vertex depends on abdominal palpation, and a brow or face presentation is suspected when the most prominent portion of the vertex is on the same side as the fetal back or opposite the fetal small parts. X-ray or vaginal examination, or both, confirms the diagnosis.

If the woman's pelvis is normal and the membranes are intact, her labor progress is observed carefully, with no specific intervention, since spontaneous conversion of a brow presentation to a face presentation or flexion to a more desirable vertex presentation may occur. The obstetrician may attempt to flex the fetal head manually, with the woman under anesthesia, but extension frequently recurs. With more manipulation, cord prolapse becomes more of a possibility. Usually the delivery of the infant is accomplished with the aid of forceps and a deep episiotomy to minimize maternal and fetal injuries. In about 30 percent of cases, either the membranes rupture early or progress is unsatisfactory, and a cesarean section becomes a necessity.

Needless to say, in brow and face presentations the baby's head becomes molded and a large caput succedaneum develops. Fetal morbidity and mortality are high due to hypoxia, cranial compression with tentorial or falx tears, compression of the neck against the mother's pubis, and fractures of the trachea and larynx. Maternal mortality is also increased because of a longer labor, a greater danger of infection, and the increased frequency of a contracted pelvis and need for operative procedures.

After birth the baby's face is often disfigured and bruised, especially if the labor has been prolonged and the mother's membranes have been ruptured. There may be edema over his cheek and eye. His eyes may bulge, may have a mucoserous discharge, and may be swollen. The baby often lies on his side with his head extended and his back straight. Parents should be reassured that their infant's features will regain a normal appearance within two weeks.

TRANSVERSE LIE

If the fetus is in a transverse lie, the acromial process of the shoulder is commonly the presenting part (Figure 15-4). The etiology of this presentation is any condition that prevents engagement of the fetal head in the mother's pelvis or that permits the fetus to be very mobile. Placenta previa is a contributing factor in about 27 percent

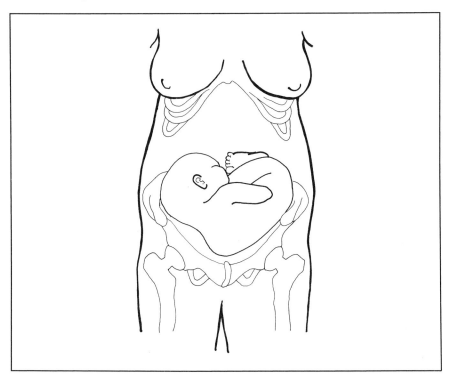

Figure 15-4. Transverse lie with shoulder presenting.

of the cases, and other factors are the same as those contributing to the face and brow presentations.

With the fetus in a transverse lie, the uterus is a transverse ovoid. Nothing is felt over the inlet and nothing is in the inlet. X-ray or ultrasound studies verify the diagnosis and often reveal the prolapse of a fetal arm or elbow. External version is often attempted to convert either one of the fetal poles to the inlet, but the fetus often reverts to the transverse position and a cesarean section must be performed.

The prognosis for the mother and fetus is good if the transverse lie is diagnosed early. Unfortunately, it is too frequently discovered late in labor, and the prognosis for both is then considerably worse. It is improved if a cesarean section is done, and the classic incision is the one of choice.

COMPOUND PRESENTATION

On rare occasions one of the fetal extremities prolapses alongside the presenting part so that both enter the pelvic cavity at the same time, resulting in a compound presentation. Associated factors that contribute to compound presentation include twinning, prematurity, and an unengaged or persistently high presenting part, with ruptured membranes.

If a hand presents with the vertex, it will usually slip back as the cervix dilates and the fetal head descends. If the head is engaged with the arm down, nothing particular is done, since there is obviously enough room for both. The labor is longer, however, and the mechanisms of descent and rotation may be abnormal.

OVERSIZE INFANT

Fetal morbidity and mortality are increased significantly in vaginal deliveries when the fetus weighs more than 4500 grams (10 pounds). During pregnancy the woman's abdomen is usually overdistended, and once her labor begins, it progresses very slowly. The fetal head, which may be more ossified than usual, is less moldable and does not readily engage.

If the fetus' shoulders are very large, the dystocia is apparent immediately after the head is delivered. The woman must bear down strongly, and the excessive abdominal, uterine, and suprasymphyseal pressure applied to deliver the shoulders may cause the rupture of her lower uterine segment. In addition, excessive traction on the infant's neck may result in permanent damage to his brachial plexus, Erb's palsy, the dislocation of his cervical vertebrae, spinal cord damage, or even death. His humerus or clavicle may be fractured (sometimes intentionally) in order to reduce the size of his shoulder girdle. Healing occurs readily.

HYDROCEPHALUS

The skull of the hydrocephalic fetus may hold several liters of cerebrospinal fluid. This condition is commonly diagnosed when the fetal head overrides the pelvis, and it is confirmed by x-ray or ultrasound studies. The large head provides a mechanical obstruction to labor, and as the overdistended lower uterine segment thins, the uterus may rupture. A cesarean section is usually done since the large head often makes vaginal delivery impossible. Postpartum hemorrhage from atony or lacerations frequently occurs.

PATHOLOGICAL RETRACTION RING (BANDL'S RING)

If a prolonged labor is neglected, a palpable ring may develop at the point where the upper and lower uterine segments meet, and the woman's uterus may develop an hourglass shape and is in danger of imminent rupture. As a rule, a cesarean section is less hazardous than a vaginal delivery in such cases, and anesthesia is used to provide maximum uterine relaxation.

The woman whose labor reaches this point is understandably exhausted and extremely apprehensive. Her lack of progress contributes to her loss of morale. The fact that she is predisposed to develop a uterine infection from prolonged rupture of membranes, or an electrolyte imbalance from dehydration, should be considered when her care is being planned.

Since fetal morbidity and mortality are increased with this condition, it is fortunate that it occurs infrequently in current obstetrical practice.

PRECIPITATE LABOR

A precipitate labor is one that lasts 4 hours or less or one in which cervical dilatation in the active phase is greater than 5 centimeters per hour in nulliparas or greater than 10 centimeters per hour in multiparas. Obviously, it is abnormally fast and tumultuous. When the maternal soft tissues offer little resistance and the uterus contracts strongly and frequently, both fetal and maternal trauma may result. Since the uterus relaxes for only a short time between contractions, the intervillous blood flow may be impaired enough to cause fetal hypoxia. Rapid passage of the fetal head through the birth canal may result in gross intracranial hemorrhage. Because a precipitate labor may be unexpected and thus the delivery may be unattended, the baby may not receive necessary resuscitation. The woman may have cervical and vaginal lacerations as well as rupture of her lower uterine segment. In most instances, however, the trauma is restricted to her perineum, labia minora, urethra, and clitoris. As a result of excessively strong contractions, she may develop an amniotic fluid embolism.

Women with a history of precipitate labor are often induced electively so that their labor may be somewhat controlled. Amniotomy is commonly done to initiate contractions, which are then carefully monitored along with the fetal heart rate. Because these contractions can be very stressful and because the woman's condition may change very rapidly, she should not be left alone. Sometimes anesthesia (e. g., pudendal block) is administered to decrease the strength of contractions or to abolish the woman's perineal reflex, thus preventing her from pushing with her abdominal muscles at delivery. No attempt should ever be made to hold back the fetal head, such as holding the woman's legs together or having her sit up, since intracranial damage is likely to result.

Because the passage through the birth canal is so rapid and stressful, the baby should be evaluated very carefully for any injury immediately after birth, and nursery personnel should be informed of the stresses the infant has undergone. The mother should also be observed carefully for signs of hemorrhage from unrepaired lacerations.

POSTPARTUM HEMORRHAGE

Postpartum hemorrhage is the loss of more than 500 milliliters of blood, either measured or estimated [7]. It occurs in about 10 percent of all deliveries and is a major cause of maternal mortality. Whether the blood flows freely or seeps slowly, the blood loss may be great. In fact, it is more often fatal when it occurs slowly, since it tends to be neglected.

Factors predisposing a woman to immediate postpartum hemorrhage are high parity, previous obstetrical trauma, third-stage complications of labor, and coagulation disorders. The three most common causes are lacerations of the birth canal, uterine atony, and retention of placental fragments.

Lacerations of the birth canal commonly follow operative deliveries, especially when forceps have been improperly applied. The vaults or lateral fornices of the vagina and the vaginal wall behind the pubic arch and lateral to the urethra are frequently involved. Perineal and cervical lacerations also occur. Lacerations of the birth canal are suspected when the woman's uterine tone is good but she still has bright red bleeding. The lacerations must be located and repaired to stop the blood loss.

Uterine atony occurs when the myometrium fails to constrict the endometrial blood vessels. It is often precipitated by failure of the placenta to separate normally and be completely expelled. Other contributing factors include deep inhalation anesthesia, prolonged labor, marked distention of the uterus, the presence of fibroid tumors, and hypotension.

If the woman is losing an abnormal amount of blood, the nurse should massage her fundus frequently and palpate it deeply to express blood and clots. This can be a painful, disturbing procedure which can increase the woman's anxiety. The nurse should make the necessary observations of uterine size, position and blood loss as quickly and as efficiently as possible. The couple's concern can be somewhat allayed by appropriate explanations of what is being done and why. Vital signs are taken every 5 or 10 minutes, but it should be remembered that marked fluctuations in blood pressure and pulse will not occur until the woman has lost a large amount of blood. Charting also includes a pad count and saturation description. (It has been estimated that a blood loss of 500 milliliters will fully saturate six surgical towels or partially saturate 10 of them.) Generally the intravenous fluids will already contain an oxytocic drug, so the rate of flow should be speeded up, or she may receive an additional dose of oxytocin, usually ergonovine, intramuscularly. As mentioned in Chapter 11, she should be taught how to palpate and massage her own fundus before she leaves the recovery room area.

LATE POSTPARTUM HEMORRHAGE

Postpartum hemorrhage can also occur after the first 24 hours, even as late as the fifth month post partum. Secondary bleeding may result on or about the tenth postpartum day from lacerations of the birth canal, coinciding with absorption of sutures used to control a primary hemorrhage.

If placental tissue has been retained, the hemorrhage usually occurs about the tenth day post partum, when the decidua of the placental site undergoes maximum slough, or even weeks or months later. A curettage is usually curative.

In the case of placental subinvolution, due perhaps to a low-grade endometritis, some of the thrombosed portions of the decidual blood vessels slough away, leaving the ends of the spiral arteries open. Profuse bleeding may occur suddenly around the sixth to tenth week post partum. Again, as in the case of retained placental tissue, a curettage is usually curative.

Anxiety may be at a high level for the couple, since the situation presents as an emergency and arrangements must be made for care of the infant and other family members. The mother should receive counseling about the importance of getting adequate rest when she returns home.

In the treatment of hemorrhage, recognition of the cause and restoration of the blood volume to normal are very important. Adequate inspection of the placenta for completeness upon delivery can often prevent hemorrhagic problems due to retention of placental fragments by indicating the need for a curettage. The value of uterine packing in the control of blood loss is a controversial issue; presently, packing is not often used.

UTERINE RUPTURE

Uterine rupture is also a serious cause of hemorrhage. It rarely occurs during pregnancy but may happen during labor, when it may be spontaneous or traumatic, in an intact uterus or in one previously incised. Uterine rupture occurs eight or nine times as often in multiparas as in nulliparas.

In the past 20 years the overall incidence of uterine rupture has remained relatively constant, while its causes have changed. There has been a decrease in those caused by obstetrical trauma, since procedures such as x-ray pelvimetry have indicated a sound basis for not allowing an unproductive labor to continue. In sophisticated obstetrical practice today, many hazardous maneuvers, such as manual dilation of the cervix and internal podalic version, have been largely eliminated. As a result, the number of cesarean sections being performed has increased, so that a previous cesarean section scar is becoming a more frequent cause of uterine rupture.

The most frequent cause of spontaneous rupture of an intact uterus is labor that is obstructed by any of the conditions discussed previously. Another cause of uterine rupture is the use of oxytocin, which may stimulate violent uterine contractions, causing rupture at a point where the uterine wall happens to be weak. Traumatic rupture of the uterus may be caused by internal podalic version, application of forceps and extraction of the fetus before the cervical os is completely dilated, or excessive fundal pressure to deliver a large baby.

Spontaneous uterine rupture is likely to begin in the lower uterine segment and extend into the body. The onset is usually sudden and without warning, although in prolonged or obstructed labor the woman experiences increasing tenderness over her lower uterus. Her contractions may be tetanic, and she may reflexively support her uterus with her hand during each contraction. Her mouth may be dry and she may have the desire to void frequently. Her respirations and pulse will be rapid. When the uterus ruptures, she will have a sudden, stabbing abdominal pain, with the sensation of something giving way. She may or may not have vaginal bleeding, but she will begin to appear to be in shock due to intraperitoneal hemorrhage. Contractions and pain cease when the uterus ruptures; the fetal heart tones disappear, and the fetus may become palpable in the abdominal cavity if the rupture is complete. If the rupture is incomplete, the uterine muscle is torn but the peritoneum remains intact and a hematoma develops.

Uterine rupture can be prevented by careful evaluation of the woman's pelvis before labor and by avoiding a prolonged labor once it begins. Once the uterus has ruptured, it may be repaired or an immediate abdominal hysterectomy may be necessary, depending on the extent of the tear.

Fetal prognosis is very poor unless delivery can be accomplished immediately. Maternal prognosis is grave, especially if the rupture is traumatic. Although associated maternal mortality used to be close to 25 percent, it is now about 5–10 percent. This improvement is due to more sophisticated obstetrical practice, antibiotics, blood transfusions, and earlier recognition and treatment.

INJURIES TO THE BIRTH CANAL

Vulvar lacerations occur commonly in almost all nulliparas and in many multiparas. They appear most frequently around the vulvar orifice, in the vagina, and around the urethra but are seldom deep enough to cause serious problems.

Some lacerations of the perineal body occur in most first deliveries, but these are less important than deeper tears of the pelvic floor (levator ani and its fascia). If they are unrepaired or improperly repaired, the woman's pelvic supports will not be as strong, leading to the development of a rectocele or cystocele, which will require surgical repair at a later date. When these deeper structures are torn, the skin often remains intact, thus giving the clinician a false sense of security.

The cervix undergoes some injury during almost every labor. This can result from too rapid or forceful dilation or from very large fetal diameters. Many times cervical lacerations are not discovered until after delivery, when an unusual amount of bright red blood is noticed. Repair of the lacerations prevents further blood loss.

AMNIOTIC FLUID EMBOLISM

Amniotic fluid embolism is a major cause of the few maternal deaths that occur during labor. Predisposing factors include tetanic uterine contractions and multiparity, especially if the fetus is very large. Sudden dyspnea and cyanosis are the initial signs and symptoms, and the woman may die within 30 minutes after the symptoms appear. If she survives the initial shock, she may still die from postpartum hemorrhage.

It is believed that the particulate matter in amniotic fluid causes embolization of the pulmonary arterioles and capillaries. In addition, since amniotic fluid has thromboplastic qualities, death may result from extensive disseminated intravascular clotting (DIC) and subsequent postpartum hemorrhage.

Amniotic fluid embolism occurs, by amniotic fluid's entering the woman's circulation. The generally accepted route is rupture of membranes in the upper uterine segment, with escape of the fluid through the vessels of the placental site. This process can be accentuated if the uterine contractions are especially forceful and if conditions exist in which the myometrial vessels are exposed, such as marginal placental separation, uterine rupture, or hysterotomy.

The amniotic fluid may also enter the maternal circulation through the endocervical veins, which are normally torn in labor as the cervix dilates. Probably the most significant contributing factor is a very forceful and rapid labor; the improper administration of oxytocic medications may be responsible for this. Vigorous and immediate treatment will help some mothers to survive by relieving their respiratory distress, preventing the development of a coagulation problem, and maintaining their normal blood volume. The fetus is in great danger, and should be delivered as soon as possible.

INVERSION OF THE UTERUS

Inversion of the uterus is a very rare complication of the third stage of labor. In this condition the corpus virtually turns inside out. It usually occurs after the distended uterus empties very suddenly and some forceful pressure or traction is placed on the uncontracted fundus, such as from improper placental expression or traction on the umbilical cord. Maternal symptoms of shock and profuse hemorrhage are readily apparent. Generally, manual replacement of the uterus is successful if the inversion is recognized at the time it occurs; an intravenous drip of oxytocin helps to keep the uterus well contracted and in position.

CORD PRESENTATION

In approximately 1 of every 200 deliveries, the umbilical cord prolapses in front of or alongside the presenting part (funic presentation). The presentation may be occult (at or near the mother's pelvis but not reachable on vaginal examination), forelying (palpable through the cervical os but within the intact membranes), or prolapsed (in the vagina or even outside the vulva following membrane rupture).

Anything that favors an abnormal adaptation of the presenting part to the lower uterine segment or prevents head engagement will contribute to the incidence of funic presentations. These factors include a contracted pelvis, placenta previa, an unusually long cord, multiple pregnancy, hydramnios, or breech presentation.

The actual course of the woman's labor is not affected by cord presentations. However, for the fetus the situation is life-threatening; about one-sixth of them do not survive. Compression of the cord between the presenting part and the bony pelvis greatly restricts the flow of oxygen to the fetus. If the cord is exposed to cold room air, there may be a reflex constriction of umbilical blood vessels with the same end result.

Many times cord presentations are diagnosed by an irregular fetal heart rate pattern, with periodic bradycardia of *variable* duration and *variable* association with maternal contractions.

If the woman's pelvis is contracted or if an immediate vaginal delivery is impossible, an immediate cesarean section is done. While preparations are being made, the woman is given oxygen and is placed in the Trendelenburg, elevated Sims', or knee-chest position. If the cord is outside the vulva and the fetus is alive and viable, the fetal head may be held up out of the woman's pelvis by the clinician's hand in her vagina. Attempts to replace the cord are of questionable value, since handling the cord may cause spasm of the umbilical vessels.

It is easy to understand that this can be a very frightening experience for the prospective parents. The nurse who remains by the couple's side, calmly and efficiently providing the care necessary for their baby's safety, can reassure them that everything is being done to ensure a favorable outcome.

It is interesting to note that formerly, when a woman's membranes ruptured early and the fetal presenting part was high, she was always kept prone in the belief that the upright position would predispose the cord to prolapse. With the woman in the standing position, however, the presenting part actually dips further below the pelvic inlet than when she is recumbent; theoretically, then, this leaves less room for the cord to prolapse. It would seem that the more rational approach would be to encourage ambulation in such a woman, providing she does not have a shoulder presentation or true cephalopelvic disproportion.

OPERATIVE OBSTETRICS

Cesarean Section

Legend holds that Julius Caesar was born by cesarean section. In his time, however, and as late as the seventeenth century, the operation is believed to have been invariably fatal to the mother, even though Caesar's mother lived for many years after his birth. As described in ancient mythology, birth in this extraordinary manner was believed to confer supernatural powers and elevate those so born above the ordinary level of humanity to the heroic level.

The extraordinary maternal mortality (85 percent in 1865) continued until Max Sanger, in 1882, introduced the technique of suturing the uterine wall. This reduced the death rate due to hemorrhage, but generalized peritonitis remained a major cause of maternal death. Today, for cesarian sections performed by competent practitioners the maternal mortality is 0.2 percent or less [3]. Repeat abdominal deliveries are common, and women who have undergone four, five, or six cesarean sections are seen.

The delivery of a fetus through an incision in the abdominal and uterine wall is a major surgical procedure. It is performed when a woman cannot deliver vaginally without seriously jeopardizing her life or health or that of the fetus. Cesarean section is also usually done if a woman has had a previous cesarian section or other extensive uterine or vaginal surgery. It is also necessary in cases of cephalopelvic disproportion, fetal distress, malpresentation, obstructive tumors, and certain chronic disorders, such as diabetes or hypertension.

While previous cesarian section is the most common indication for cesarian section, not all women who have had a previous section have deliveries this way. The baby may be delivered vaginally if the reason for the original cesarean section no longer exists (e.g., an abruptio placentae) and if she is monitored very carefully during labor, with standby facilities for an emergency operation if it becomes necessary. Cesarean section is avoided if the fetus is dead or if the woman has a full stomach or an upper respiratory infection, is in ketoacidosis or cardiac decompensation, or has convulsed recently.

There are four types of cesarian section: classic cesarian, low-segment cesarian, extraperitoneal cesarian, and cesarian hysterectomy (Figure 15-5). The low-segment cesarian section is the one most commonly performed. The incision is made either transversely or vertically in the lower uterine segment; since this is a fibrous rather than a muscular area, there is less chance of hemorrhage, subsequent rupture, or postpartum adhesion formation. The surgery takes longer than the classic cesarian, however.

Speed is the main advantage of the classic approach, in which a vertical incision is made into the upper portion of the uterus. Since this is a muscular part of the uterus, there is a greater chance of hemorrhage, rupture, hematoma, adhesion formation, poor healing, and febrile morbidity. This method may be used in emergencies, in which rapidity is important, or in cases in which the lower uterine segment has tumors, adhesions, or a low-lying placenta.

The incision for the extraperitoneal cesarian section is in the lower uterine segment, after the peritoneum has been dissected away from the uterine wall. The peritoneum is not incised. This method has been used in the past to prevent infection in the uterus from being introduced into the peritoneal cavity. It is a difficult procedure, that often results in bladder or ureteral injury and is not commonly used today.

Cesarean hysterectomy may be performed as a method of sterilization after a woman has had several cesarean sections. It also may be performed if the uterus fails to contract, as with a Couvelaire uterus, or in placenta previa, when bleeding is uncontrolled. After delivery of the baby and the placenta, the uterus is removed.

Preparation of the woman for cesarean section includes skin preparation, blood type and crossmatch, hemoglobin and hematocrit determinations, and urinalysis. Preoperative medication usually includes atropine, but no narcotic is given, since it would cause depression in the infant. Spinal or epidural anesthesia is used most commonly, and the woman may be given oxygen by face mask during surgery to increase the fetus' oxygen levels. As in all pelvic surgery, a Foley catheter is inserted prior to surgery to keep the bladder deflated. When the surgery is imminent, the woman's pediatrician should be notified so that he or she may be present to

*Figure 15-5. A. Low-
segment cesarian section
with transverse uterine
incision into lower uterine
segment. B. Classic
cesarian section with
vertical uterine incision
into upper, more muscular
portion of the uterus.
C. Extraperitoneal
cesarian section with
vertical uterine incision.
Surgeon's fingers separate
peritoneum and bladder
from uterus.*

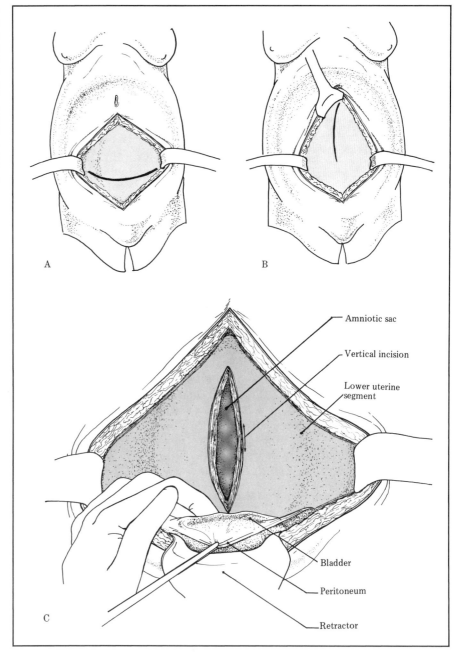

resuscitate the baby if it becomes necessary. The nursery also should be notified so that it is prepared for the infant's arrival.

Following the surgery and the delivery of the infant, the woman is given oxytocin to keep her uterus contracted, her vital signs are monitored until they are stable, she receives intravenous fluids, and her urine output is observed for volume and for any bleeding that might indicate bladder trauma during surgery. The nurse should encourage her to get out of bed the following day. This improves her circulation, the aeration of her lungs, and her muscle tone as well as lochial drainage. The mother should be taken to see her infant and to hold and feed him as soon as possible.

The incidence of respiratory distress is higher in infants born by cesarian section than in those delivered vaginally. This may be because of the need to deliver the infant prior to term, or because the thorax is not compressed during delivery and therefore the respiratory tract is not drained of fluids prior to birth. More recently, it has been noted that delivery by cesarian section eliminates the stress of labor to the infant; thus, his cortisol levels are not raised as are those of infants born vaginally, and the lower cortisol levels may make the infant's lungs less ready to aerate at birth [5].

Forceps Deliveries

Forceps are used in instances in which the life or well-being of the woman or fetus may be compromised, and when the danger may be relieved by more rapid delivery. This occurs in cases of uterine dysfunction in which oxytocin has been ineffective and the fetal head is well down in the pelvis. It may also be indicated in eclampsia, heart disease, acute pulmonary edema, hemorrhage from placental abruption, maternal exhaustion, and intrapartum infection. Excessive analgesics and certain types of anesthesia interfere with the woman's voluntary expulsive efforts, increasing the number of forceps deliveries. Forceps deliveries also are performed for fetal indications, including cord prolapse, abruptio placentae, excess pressure on the fetal head from arrested descent, and fetal distress.

Forceps are designed for extracting or rotating the fetal head. They consist of two pieces: a right blade, which is slipped into the right side of the mother's pelvis, and a left blade, which is slipped into the left side. Each piece consists of a blade, handle, shank, and lock. The blades have two curves: that on the outer edge conforms to the curve of the birth canal (pelvic curve), while the inside of the blade conforms to the curve of the fetal head (cephalic curve). The blade may be solid or have a window; the latter type is referred to as *fenestrated*. The two blades articulate at the lock, which is designed to prevent excessive pressure on the fetal head.

While there are more than 600 types of forceps, there are only two major classifications of classic forceps (Figure 15-6). The Simpson type has separated shanks and is used to extract fetuses with elongated, molded heads. This type is used commonly with nulliparas who have long labors; the DeLee forceps is an example. The second major type is the Elliot forceps, which has overlapping shanks and is used to deliver infants with unmolded, rounder heads. This type is used commonly with multiparas who have briefer labors; the Tucker-McLean forceps is an example. In addition to these major types, there are also special forceps. The Piper forceps is used to deliver the aftercoming head in a breech presentation. Kielland and Barton forceps are used to rotate the head from a transverse or occipital position to an anterior position. Kielland forceps commonly are used to deliver women with anthropoid pelves, while Barton forceps are designed to be used in women with flat pelves with the fetal head in a transverse position.

Prior to forceps delivery, the fetal head must be engaged; the fetus have a vertex

*Figure 15-6. The classic
types of forceps.
A. Simpson forceps.
B. Elliot forceps.
C. Forceps blade, at angle
to show fenestration.*

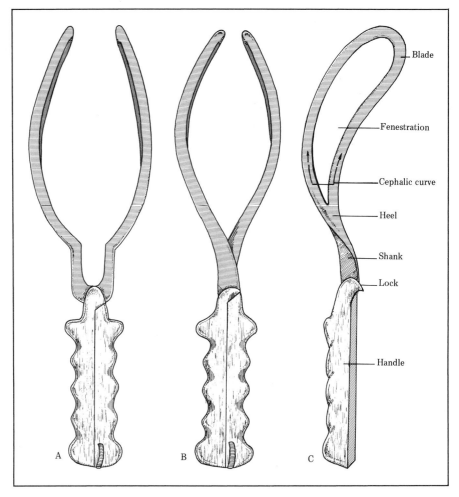

presentation or a face presentation with the chin anterior; the position of the head must be known; there must be no cephalopelvic disproportion; the cervix must be completely dilated and the membranes ruptured; and the mother's bladder and preferably also her rectum should be empty. Anesthesia is required. When these criteria are met, a low or midforceps delivery may be effected; high forceps deliveries are no longer used today.

The extraction is classified as low or midforceps according to the level and position of the fetal head when the blades are applied. In a low forceps delivery, the forceps are applied after the fetal head has reached the perineal floor, with the sagittal suture in the anterior-posterior diameter of the outlet. When the head is on the perineal floor, a low forceps delivery, preceded by episiotomy, is a simple, safe procedure, requiring only gentle traction. It is usually performed when the mother has insufficient expulsive forces or abnormally great perineal resistance.

In midforceps deliveries, the forceps are used to grasp the fetal head after engagement has taken place but before the head reaches the perineal floor. Any forceps delivery requiring rotation, regardless of the station, is considered a midforceps delivery. Since the fetal head is higher in the pelvis before rotation takes place, greater traction is required.

Some compression of the fetal head is inevitable. The widest dimension between the two blades of the forceps when they are articulated is 7.5 centimeters, while the biparietal diameter of the average term infant's head is 9.5 centimeters. Compression can be harmful since circulation may be impaired, causing asphyxia and hemorrhage, in addition to possible direct injury to the cranial bones, tentorium, falx, vessels, and brain. It should be remembered that the diameters of the fetal head are reduced during forceps delivery and during spontaneous delivery by overriding of the cranial bones. Fetuses vary in their ability to withstand compression, full-term infants being able to withstand greater compression than preterm infants. The physician avoids compression by placing a finger between the handles of the forceps.

In high forceps applications, the forceps are applied to the fetal head before engagement has occurred. This procedure had a place when cesarean section was dangerous, but it is not used today.

When a forceps delivery has been decided on, the forceps are slipped into the right and left sides of the woman's pelvis. The physician then slides two fingers along the forceps blades to examine the application and to ensure that no cervical tissue has been grasped. When the blades are on correctly, the handles are held in one hand and gentle, intermittent, horizontal traction is exerted with each contraction until the perineum begins to bulge. As soon as the vulva is distended by the occiput, the handles are gradually elevated, eventually pointing upward as the parietal bones emerge.

Occasionally, the Scanzoni maneuver is used for posterior presentation. The fetal head is rotated anteriorly with forceps. Then, since the position of the forceps is not one in which the fetal head could be extracted, the forceps are removed and another pair is applied for extraction.

Important factors in the overall incidence of forceps deliveries are the attitudes of the hospital staff and of the population served. The perinatal mortality associated with forceps delivery depends on the condition of the fetus and on the station of the head during delivery. There usually is no mortality when the head is at or very near the perineum. Use of forceps at higher stations of the head is attended by perinatal loss or damage in direct proportion to the height of the skull. The fetus may sustain injuries to the face, eyes, and skull. The woman may also sustain injuries from a difficult forceps delivery, including cervical laceration and injury to the bladder, rectum, or vagina. She may experience hemorrhage or infection as a result of the trauma. There are usually few complications following low forceps delivery.

Vacuum Extraction

With the use of a vacuum extractor, suction applied to the fetal head creates an artificial caput within the suction cup if it holds firmly and allows adequate traction, which it should (Figure 15-7). This method is used mainly in dysfunctional labor accompanied by minor cephalopelvic disproportion. It has the advantage over forceps of avoiding the use of an instrument that would occupy space between the

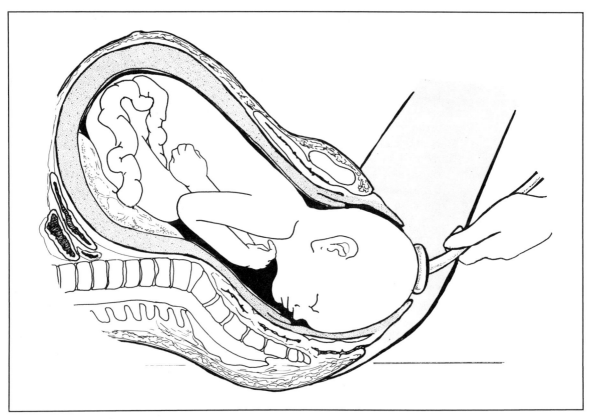

Figure 15-7. Delivery using the vacuum extractor.

fetal head and maternal pelvis; in addition, it carries less risk of potential damage to the infant.

This method is not used extensively in the United States, partly because of numerous reports of fetal damage, including lacerations of the scalp, cephalhematomas, intracranial hemorrhage, and infant mortality. In Europe the vacuum extractor is more widely used and is felt to be superior to forceps delivery in regard to perinatal mortality and morbidity of infants and mothers.

REFERENCES

1. Friedman, E. A., and Kroll, B. Computer analysis of labor progression v. effect of fetal presentation and position. *Journal of Reproductive Medicine* 8:117, 1972.
2. Greenhill, J. P., and Friedman, E. A. *Biological Principles and Modern Practice of Obstetrics*. Philadelphia: Saunders, 1974.
3. Hellman, L. M., and Pritchard, J. A. *Williams Obstetrics* (14th ed.). New York: Appleton-Century-Crofts, 1971.
4. Niswander, K. R., and Patterson, R. J. Hazards of elective induction of labor. *Obstetrics and Gynecology* 22:228, 1963.
5. Pokoly, T. B. The role of cortisol in human parturition. *American Journal of Obstetrics and Gynecology* 117:549, 1973.

6. Ranney, B. The gentle art of external cephalic version. *American Journal of Obstetrics and Gynecology* 116:239, 1973.

7. Reid, D., Ryan, K., and Benirschke, K. *Principles and Management of Human Reproduction.* Philadelphia: Saunders, 1972.

8. Schwarcz, R., Beliyan, J., Cifuentes, J., Cuadro, J., Marques, M., and Caldeyro-Barcia, R. Fetal and maternal monitoring in spontaneous labors and in elective inductions. *American Journal of Obstetrics and Gynecology* 120:356, 1974.

FURTHER READING

Avery, M. E. Prenatal diagnosis and prevention of hyaline membrane disease. *New England Journal of Medicine* 292:157, 1975.

Hochberg, H. M. *Clinical Interpretation of Fetal Monitoring Records.* Cranbury, New Jersey: Hoffmann-LaRoche, 1974.

Klavan, M., and Boscola, M. A. *A Guide to Fetal Monitoring.* Chester, Pennsylvania: Crozer-Chester Medical Center, 1973.

Larsen, J., Goldkrand, J., Hanson, T., and Miller, C. Intrauterine infection on an obstetric service. *Obstetrics and Gynecology* 43:838, 1974.

Lynn, J. Intravenous alcohol infusion for premature labor. *Journal of the American Osteopathy Association* 70:167, 1970.

More oxygen during cesarean section results in healthier neonates. *Journal of the American Medical Association* 214:1634, 1970.

Schifrin, B. S. Fetal heart rate monitoring during labor. *Journal of the American Medical Association* 222:196, 1972.

Schifrin, B. S., and Dame, L. Fetal heart rate patterns. *Journal of the American Medical Association* 219:1322, 1972.

Chapter 16 Complications During the Postpartum Period

When postpartum complications arise, the family faces stress from a number of sources. The mother has recently experienced the stress of delivery and now faces an increased physical and emotional burden. The father, who is generally shouldering more responsibility in the home during the mother's hospitalization, faces the possibility of doing so over a longer period in addition to his concern with her condition. There is an added financial burden and the possibility that the newborn may be discharged before his wife. The mother in this situation may not be able to interact with the newborn or to establish a relationship with him. Other young children the couple may have will wonder why "mommy" is not coming home and may be particularly upset if "daddy" spends much time away from the home to be with his wife.

Nurses in this situation can be invaluable. They should start by acknowledging to the parents that this is often a difficult time for couples. They might mention that many couples find that in addition to worry created by the mother's condition, the home responsibilities can be very demanding and other children at home often become concerned. This approach opens the door for the parents to share their feelings and possible anxiety. The nurse can then assess the couple's response to the woman's state of health, the father's ability to cope with the home situation, and the response of other children at home. If the father needs additional help, it is advisable to discuss with the couple the possibility of friends or relatives helping out, or to explain the services available from agencies in the community. This is particularly important if the newborn is to be discharged before the mother. Such planning should be done well in advance of the discharge so the family is spared the added stress of last-minute crisis arrangements.

While the newborn is in the hospital, nurses can do much to support his incorporation into the family unit. The mother should see him as much as possible. Whenever feasible she should be wheeled to the nursery not only to see him, but, as soon as permitted, to hold and feed him. If she is confined to her room, nurses caring for the infant should give her daily reports on his progress, including personal characteristics that make him unique. When the father visits he also should be encouraged to hold and feed his child and should be told of the baby's progress.

When there are other young children in the home, the mother can maintain contact with them by phone. Small gifts such as a pack of gum or a lollipop from "mommy" help a great deal. The children can be encouraged to draw pictures or write her a note that "daddy" can deliver. When she is able, the mother should be taken to an area of the hospital where she can visit with the children. In short, the nurse should support the family in any activity that helps them to maintain their unity.

PUERPERAL INFECTION

A puerperal infection is an infection of the genital tract that appears in the postpartum period, although the invasion of organisms may have occurred during labor. It remains a serious problem today despite the use of antibiotics and is currently one of the three major causes of maternal death. Clinicians and researchers attribute the problem to the evolution of resistant organisms, the sensitivity that some women have developed to antibiotic drugs, and a periodic relaxation of aseptic technique and preventive care by health care workers who have come to rely too heavily on antibiotics to combat the organisms; historically this cavalier attitude has been one of the major contributing factors in puerperal infection.

Prior to the mid-nineteenth century, it was commonplace for medical students and physicians returning from cadaver dissection to attend women in labor without so much as washing their hands. No precautions were taken when examining more than one woman in labor, even when some were already infected. The reasons postulated for the high maternal mortality in those days (often between 10 and 20 percent) were numerous, ranging from retained lochia to an act of Divine Providence. It was not until the work of Holmes, Semmelweis, and Pasteur that the etiology of puerperal or childbed fever was demonstrated to the satisfaction of the medical community and that changes were effected in caring for women in labor.

Oliver Wendell Holmes, in 1843, read a paper before the Boston Society for Medical Improvement entitled, "The Contagiousness of Puerperal Fever." In it he demonstrated that at least the epidemic forms of the infection could be traced to inadequate precautions taken by the nurse or physician attending women in labor or women who had just given birth. His work was not well received, nor was that of Ignaz Semmelweis four years later. Semmelweis noted a striking contrast in maternal mortality between women delivered in their homes and those delivered in the Vienna Lying-In Hospital, where he was an assistant. As a result of his own careful investigations, he concluded that childbed fever was essentially a wound infection caused by septic material introduced during vaginal examination. He then required physicians, medical students, and midwives to wash their hands with chlorine water prior to examining women in labor. The mortality dropped dramatically from 10 to 1 percent—yet he, like Holmes, was ridiculed by some of the most prominent men of his time. Many physicians thought it an intellectual insult for them to be expected to believe that the problem could be caused by something invisible to the naked eye. It was not until Pasteur later demonstrated in women with puerperal fever what is now known as *Streptococcus* organisms that Holmes' and Semmelweis' work slowly became accepted and their recommendations adopted.

Modes of Infection

Today, infection is still introduced into the uterus through vaginal examinations, and as the number of examinations during labor increases so does the incidence of infection. Organisms already present in the vagina may be carried to the uterus. The examiner's hands or instruments may become contaminated as a result of droplet infection dispersed by him or other staff members. Personnel working with the mother may be carriers of streptococci and may spread the organism by coughing, sneezing, or just talking. Since the nasopharynx is one of the most common sources of extraneous bacteria brought to the birth canal, all personnel in the delivery room must wear masks that cover the nose and mouth. Anyone with an upper respiratory infection should not be present.

Infection may also result from instruments that are insufficiently sterilized or contaminated prior to use. Bedpans should be cleansed and sterilized after each use. Heat lamps and other pieces of equipment that are taken from one woman to another should first be thoroughly cleansed. Infection may also be caused by bacteria-laden dust carried from one part of a hospital to another via air currents in ventilating ducts. Thus, infectious material from one part of the institution can easily flow and settle on sterilized tables, towels, instruments, and bedclothes.

The woman may also carry infectious organisms on her fingers from various parts of her body to her genitals. Following delivery the birth canal represents a wound for many days. It is vitally important that the woman observe adequate hygiene measures accompanying perineal care, such as cleansing from her vulva to her anus and not back over the area. It is important that perineal pads be sterile and changed frequently, at least every 4 hours. It is also wise to separate any woman with a puerperal infection from other women who have just given birth.

Infection is more likely to occur in women with severe anemia, malnutrition, debilitating or chronic illness, or infection elsewhere in the body. Prolonged labor with exhaustion and dehydration, particularly when accompanied by prolonged rupture of the membranes, traumatic delivery, the use of instruments and intrauterine manipulation, retention of placental fragments, blood clots in the uterus, lacerations, or hemorrhage, are associated with the development of puerperal sepsis.

Analysis of the predisposing factors makes clear the extent to which puerperal sepsis can be prevented by good health care during pregnancy, by sufficient rest and fluids during labor, by minimizing obstetrical trauma, by prevention of hemorrhage, and by careful examination of the uterovaginal tract after delivery, as well as by proper aseptic technique.

Puerperal morbidity is generally diagnosed according to the definition advanced by the Joint Committee on Maternal Welfare in the United States. They define morbidity as a temperature of 38.0° C (100.4° F) or higher occurring on any two of the first 10 days post partum, excluding the first 24 hours. The woman's temperature, according to the Committee, should be taken by mouth at least four times a day. Recently, researchers [4] have questioned the validity of morbidity statistics prepared from these criteria. They note that the majority of women who develop fevers are immediately given antibiotics, causing their temperatures to drop before they can be included in the statistics.

Causative Organisms

Historically, anaerobic *Streptococcus* has been identified as the most common organism causing puerperal morbidity. While a recent report [2] found this to be true of one study population, others [4] reported the gram-negative aerobic rod *Escherichia coli* to be the most common organism. They also found *Peptostreptococcus,* alpha-hemolytic streptococci, *Bacteroides,* enterococci, and coagulase-negative *Staphylococcus* as causative organisms and noted the increasing importance of gram-negative organisms in hospital-acquired infections. Occasionally *Clostridium,* beta-hemolytic streptococci, *Klebsiella, Pseudomonas,* and *Neisseria* are also involved in postpartum sepsis. Mixed flora are common.

Following traumatic delivery, lacerations and contusions are commonly found in the external genitalia. The vulva may become edematous and if the wounds become infected, they are covered with a grayish or greenish exudate and may ulcerate. Infected wounds in the vagina cause the mucous membrane to become swollen and red and, in many instances, to begin sloughing. If the discharge produced is unable to drain properly, the woman may experience high fever, chills, urine retention, dysuria, and pelvic pain.

Cervical lacerations may also become infected; deep lacerations may be the origin of extensive infections such as lymphatic infection, bacteremia, and parametritis. Episiotomy wounds may become infected, with the suture line becoming red and swollen and later containing areas that will slough and ooze serum and pus. The woman may have difficulty voiding as well as local pain, discomfort, and an elevated temperature. The infection is usually treated by removing the sutures and promoting drainage of the exudate. Sitz baths several times a day relieve much of the discomfort.

Sites and Types of Infections

ENDOMETRITIS

Almost all postpartum infections involve the endometrium. The organisms invade the area particularly at the placental site, which takes a longer time to heal than the surrounding endometrium. Blood and lymphatic vessels in the infected area become engorged, and in some instances the necrotic mucosa sloughs. If the lochial discharge is obstructed by the debris or by clots, the woman usually experiences a severe chill and fever until free drainage is established.

In addition to noting an increased pulse and temperature, symptoms that usually appear on the third to fifth day post partum, the nurse should carefully check the woman's uterus and lochial discharge. If she has endometritis, her uterus is usually larger than would be expected for that postdelivery day and it is usually soft. The lochia may be more profuse, bloody, and have a foul odor, depending on the type of infecting organism. The mother's abdomen may also appear distended.

Occasionally the infection spreads from the endometrium to the myometrium, parametrium, fallopian tubes, peritoneum, and blood. Rarely the infection spreads to involve abscess formation in the tubes or ovaries. Mild salpingitis may occur unnoticed and account for secondary infertility.

PELVIC CELLULITIS (PARAMETRITIS)

Infection of the pelvic connective tissue may result from an infected wound in the cervix, vagina, perineum, or lower uterine segment, or as an extension of pelvic thrombophlebitis. The symptoms, which usually occur about the fourth postdelivery day, include chills, high fever, tachycardia, severe local pain in one or both sides of the abdomen, and tenderness on vaginal examination. Initially the fever is high, but as the infection progresses it may become intermittent. On examination, the mother's uterus is observed to be unusually large for that postdelivery day and is sensitive to the touch. As the infection becomes more severe, her uterus becomes fixed. Her pelvic area is warm and soft, with one extremely sensitive spot; the abscess is usually located under this area. If suppuration is present, pointing usually occurs, with the skin over the area becoming red, edematous, and tender. Pointing may also occur in the posterior cul-de-sac, or the abscess can be felt bulging into one of the fornices. When the symptoms of suppuration become apparent, incision and drainage is performed. Most often, however, the infected mass heals by absorption in several weeks.

THROMBOPHLEBITIS

Puerperal infection spreads most commonly along the veins, resulting in thrombophlebitis. The veins most commonly infected are those of the uterine wall and broad ligament. The resulting condition is called *pelvic thrombophlebitis,* while infection of the leg veins is known as *femoral thrombophlebitis.* The vein most commonly involved in pelvic thrombophlebitis is the ovarian. If the left ovarian vein is extensively involved, renal complications may occur because of its junction with the renal vein.

As the inflammatory process in the veins spreads, the thrombus may increase in size in an attempt to wall off the infecting organisms. Occasionally small emboli break loose and lodge in other parts of the body, such as the kidneys, heart valves, and lungs. In the lungs these emboli cause pneumonia, pleurisy, abscesses, infarctions, or, in severe cases, death.

The onset of symptoms of pelvic thrombophlebitis usually occurs during the second week after delivery. The mother generally has repeated severe chills and fever, with her temperature rising to 40.6° C (105° F). Between the episodes she may look and feel well. Specimens of blood for cultures should be taken during the chill to isolate the causative organism.

The signs and symptoms of femoral thrombophlebitis are generally the same as those found during the nonpregnant state.

BACTEREMIA

As a result of infected thrombi breaking loose, usually from the uterine veins, or because of lymphatic spread of bacteria from an endometritis, the mother can become extremely ill. She usually has a severe chill, fever, and rapid respirations. Her skin is pale, her lips and fingers may become cyanotic, and she may soon develop symptoms of peritonitis. Her lochial discharge may increase and have a foul odor. When blood cultures are grown, *Streptococcus* is the organism found most frequently. With treatment the condition rarely lasts more than 10 days.

PERITONITIS

The signs and symptoms of puerperal peritonitis resemble those of surgical peritonitis, except that abdominal rigidity is slight or absent. The mother has chills, high fever, rapid pulse, vomiting, and severe abdominal pain. Paralytic ileus leads to abdominal distension, although severe diarrhea may follow. The mother is treated immediately with antimicrobial agents, gastrointestinal suction, fluid and electrolyte replacement, analgesics, and sedation. Oral feedings are generally resumed when bowel sounds return.

General Treatment

In general puerperal infection is treated by isolating the infected woman to prevent spread of the infection. The number of visitors is minimized and generally nursing the infant is stopped. Supportive therapy is given, including appropriate fluid and electrolyte replacement, blood to combat anemia, and antibiotics to which the organism is sensitive. If the mother is unresponsive to specific antibiotic therapy, septic thrombophlebitis or abscess formation is suspected. When the abscess is found, drainage is usually instituted. If the mother has thrombophlebitis, anticoagulant therapy is begin.

SUBINVOLUTION

Subinvolution is the slowing or stopping of the normal autolytic process of involution. Anything that interferes with myometrial contraction may be a contributing factor, including retention of placental fragments, endometritis, myomas, fibroid tumors, and pelvic infection.

Symptoms of subinvolution are prolonged lochial discharge (after a month or more), followed by prolonged leukorrhea or irregular uterine bleeding and sometimes by profuse hemorrhage. The woman's uterus is larger or softer than would be expected for the given time post partum, and she may have subjective complaints of backache or a sensation of weight in her pelvis.

Treatment with ergonovine maleate (Ergotrate) or methylergonovine maleate (Methergine), 0.2 milligram every 3–4 hours over two to four days, may cause improvement by increasing contractions and thus improving drainage. If there are retained secundines, curettage is indicated and is usually curative. If the patient passes any tissue on her own she should be instructed to save it for her midwife or physician to inspect.

UTERINE DISPLACEMENTS

As soon as the uterus involutes to the point of entry into the pelvic cavity, retroversion may occur, particularly if some degree of subinvolution is present. In the early postpartum period, uterine retrodisplacement may cause lochia to be retained (lochiometra).

Symptoms of retrodisplacement may include backache, sometimes with increased or persistent lochia. Relief in many patients is obtained with bimanual or instrument anteflexion of the uterus, followed by the introduction of a pessary during the third to sixth week post partum. In some cases, knee-chest exercises are also helpful.

RELAXATION OF THE VAGINAL OUTLET AND PROLAPSE OF THE UTERUS

Frequently, improperly repaired lacerations of the perineum may be followed by relaxation of the vaginal outlet. Changes in the pelvic supports during pregnancy and delivery predispose the woman to the development of a cystocele or rectocele, urinary stress incontinence, and a prolapsed uterus. Operative procedures for the correction of these conditions are not done until at least three to six months post partum and are usually postponed until the end of the childbearing period unless urinary stress incontinence becomes a serious problem. Perineal tightening, as mentioned in Chapter 11, is a good prophylactic exercise that can help to maintain the tone of the pelvic supports.

POSTPARTUM HEMATOMAS

Hematomas may develop during the postpartum period in the loose connective tissue beneath the skin that covers the external genitalia (without apparent laceration of the skin), beneath the vaginal mucosa, or in the broad ligaments. They occur once in about every 500–1000 deliveries; it may be several hours before they are noticed.

Vulvar hematomas, particularly those that develop rapidly, may cause excruciating pain, which is often the first symptom to appear. The pain is accompanied by the sudden development of a fluctuant and sensitive tumor of varying size, covered by discolored skin. Vaginal hematomas usually present with symptoms of pressure and inability to void. Hematomas have a varied etiology, including the trauma of a spontaneous labor or forceps application, failure to suture far enough beyond the upper angle of the episiotomy or laceration, or even rough uterine massage.

The prognosis for most women who develop hematomas is favorable. Small hematomas are treated expectantly, as they are absorbed spontaneously. If the pain is severe or the hematoma continues to grow, incision and drainage with ligation of the bleeding points is necessary. Sometimes vaginal packing for 24 hours is useful. Since blood loss is almost always more than the clinical estimate, the mother should be carefully observed for signs of needed blood replacement.

DISORDERS OF THE URINARY TRACT

As noted in Chapter 11, several conditions that may occur following delivery, such as distended bladder, residual urine, and the need for catheterization, predispose the new mother to the development of urinary tract infections. Related symptoms may begin to appear from the third to the twenty-first postpartum day. Symptoms that suggest cystitis include suprapubic or perineal discomfort, dysuria, urinary frequency, and an elevated temperature of around 37.8°–38.3° C (100°–101° F). If the mother has flank pain and higher fever accompanied by chills, pyelitis may be the cause. Following urine culture and sensitivity studies, treatment includes encouraging fluid intake, complete emptying of the bladder, appropriate antibacterial drugs, and if her condition warrants it, bed rest.

OBSTETRIC PARALYSIS

When the fetal head begins to descend into the pelvis or forceps pressure is applied, the mother may complain of intense neuralgia or cramping in one or both legs. In some instances the pain persists after delivery and may be accompanied by muscle paralysis. In this case the fibers of the popliteal nerve may have been injured where they pass over the brim of the pelvis, causing dysfunction of the ankle flexor and toe extensor muscles. (Fortunately, this rarely occurs in the modern practice of obstetrics.) The prognosis for the woman with localized paralysis is good; it is poor if the paralysis is generalized. Generalized paralysis might also be suggestive of a cerebral vascular accident.

A more common but preventable problem is that of footdrop, which may occur when a woman is improperly positioned in stirrups or leg holders. In addition, a neuritic-type pain may also be caused by a separated symphysis pubis or looseness of the sacro-iliac joints. In this instance locomotion may be difficult as well as painful.

PULMONARY EMBOLISM

The greatest danger of a pulmonary embolism in the postpartum period comes from a venous thrombosis. Even though it occurs only once in about 3000–7000 deliveries, it is still a very serious postpartum complication because it is life-threatening. Nurses should be on the alert for significant symptoms: chest pain, even if it is transient, accompanied by shortness of breath, air hunger, tachypnea, or just apprehension. Lung scans are useful diagnostic tools. If the embolus is large, a pulmonary artery embolectomy could be lifesaving.

A pulmonary embolism may also be caused by amniotic fluid in the maternal circulation. After the membranes have ruptured, and particularly just after delivery, amniotic fluid may enter venous sinuses in the uterine wall and travel to the pulmonary vessels. Since the fluid contains vernix and other solid material, it may form small emboli in the lungs and contribute to maternal shock and sudden death. It is also instrumental in producing fibrinogenopenia as a result of intravascular clotting. Amniotic fluid embolism tends to occur in rapid labors in which there are powerful contractions and often is seen in conjunction with the use of oxytocin.

DISORDERS OF THE BREASTS

Mastitis

Mastitis, inflammation of the breast tissue, is sometimes seen during lactation in the postpartum period. Symptoms seldom appear before the end of the first postpartum week and generally not until the third or fourth week. They may include varying degrees of engorgement, chills, increased temperature (usually not above 39.4° C, or 103° F), and increased pulse. The mother's breasts are hard, reddened, and painful.

Mastitis may at first be confined to the areola, with the formation of a subareolar abscess in the underlying milk glands, around the nipple, or in one of the tubercles of Montgomery (Figure 16-1). It may also involve the lactiferous tubules (parenchymatous or glandular mastitis), which is probably the most common form. Further extension of the process involves the connective tissue and the fat around the lobes and lobules (intramammary or phlegmonous mastitis). Cellulitis may be superficial or deep.

The causative organism is most often *Staphylococcus aureus* and the source is almost always the infant's nose and throat. The organism travels through the nipple

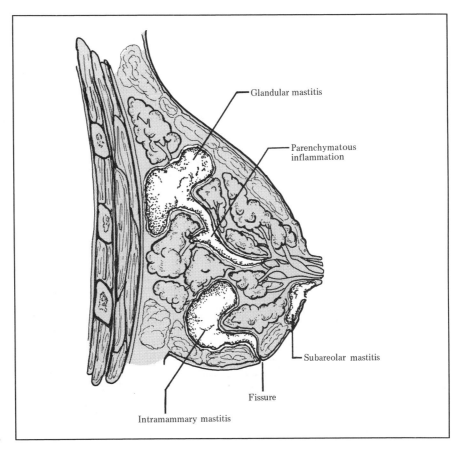

Glandular mastitis

Parenchymatous inflammation

Subareolar mastitis

Fissure

Intramammary mastitis

Figure 16-1. Mastitis.

at the site of a fissure or abrasion (which may be very small), although some believe that the organism may still enter the lactiferous ducts even though the skin is intact. The infant typically becomes a carrier while he is in the nursery, where he comes in contact with personnel who are carriers themselves. Needless to say, the hands of such personnel are a major source of contamination for both the infant and the mother.

Prevention of mastitis may depend on the exclusion of all personnel who are known or suspected *Staphylococcus* carriers from the care of mothers and babies. Nurses are in an excellent position to prevent the development of mastitis by making sure that mothers are aware of the need for cleanliness, i.e., that mothers wash their *own* hands before handling their breasts. In addition, they should know how to prevent injured or fissured nipples—proper cleansing, proper sucking by the infant and the mode of his removal from the breast, and the use of a nipple shield, if indicated. Nurses, of course, should perform a close daily inspection of every infant and isolate those with developing infections of the umbilical cord or skin.

If mastitis is promptly treated within 48 hours (following a culture of the milk), the infection is usually aborted. If the fever persists for more than 48 hours, suppuration usually appears. Physical comfort measures include proper support—a tight breast-binder or bra—and applications of cold or heat to allay the inflammation. Heat is preferred if suppuration is present.

Whether or not actual breast-feeding should be discontinued in the presence of mastitis is a matter of controversy. Advocates of its discontinuation propose that with less stimulation the infection will disappear more quickly and that the mastitis may recur if breast-feeding is continued. Breast-feeding may be painful and the milk may be infected. An infant who harbors the infectious organisms may cause reinfection of the mother or develop a frank infection himself, and so should be closely observed.

On the other hand, if the mother does not stop breast-feeding, she avoids the distention of the breast tissue that occurs when emptying is suddenly discontinued. When lactation is to be continued, breast-feeding may be temporarily stopped and the breasts emptied by artificial means. The milk is usually discarded during the time the mother has a fever. Breast-feeding is resumed within 24 hours after the mother's temperature returns to normal, which is commonly within one to three days unless her recovery is unusually slow.

If a frank abscess forms, its incision and drainage, in addition to antibiotic therapy, is essential for a rapid cure. Healing may require weeks or even months. If this is the case, resumption of breast-feeding is usually considered to be unwise.

Nipple Abnormalities

On rare occasions the nipples are so inverted that the lactiferous ducts open directly into a depression in the center of the areola. Needless to say, this makes breast-feeding extremely difficult, if not impossible. Treatment of inverted nipples is discussed in Chapter 7. Use of a nipple shield may draw them out.

Sore nipples are a common complication of the early weeks of nursing, especially if erosions, blisters, cracks, fissures, or ulcerations develop. The pain that results from breast-feeding with any of these disorders may have an inhibiting effect on secretory function. Primiparas seem to have more problems with sore nipples, especially if they are fair-skinned, older, or if their nipples are deformed.

If nipples are cracked or fissured, infection may easily develop, not only in the mother but also in the baby. If the nipples are bleeding and the baby swallows some blood, he may develop a false melena as a result.

Usually nipple shields and topical ointments are effective in allowing the nipple to heal. If improvement does not follow shortly, the infant should not nurse from the affected breast. Harsh soaps should naturally be avoided, and the nipple should be kept dry and exposed to air.

Secretion Abnormalities

Agalactia, a rare phenomenon, is complete lack of mammary secretion. It may be due to many factors—febrile disorders, ill health, malformation, occlusion or disease of the milk ducts, atrophy or destruction of tissue from mastitis, or insufficient stimulation of the breasts. The infant of a mother with agalactia loses weight and may appear to be in distress.

Overweight women with pendulous breasts may be more likely to have a decreased secretion of milk, since their breasts contain more fat and poorly developed glands [5]. Elderly primiparas may have deficient secretion of milk because of atrophy of the glands.

Polygalactia is an excessive amount of milk secretion. *Galactorrhea* is a constant leakage of milk, bearing no relationship to breast-feeding and persisting after weaning. It, too, occurs rarely and may be associated with a pituitary or hypothalamic dysfunction associated with low estrogen levels and decreased follicle-stimulating hormone. It may also be related to a blockade of the hypothalamic prolactin-inhibiting center by an unknown agent. In some women persistent abnormal or erogenous stimulation of the breasts may be a contributing factor. Galactorrhea may be unilateral or bilateral, slight or profuse. Treatment includes compression of the breasts with a binder and administration of clomiphene, levodopa, or ergot alkaloids on a chronic schedule.

Galactocele

A galactocele is a collection of milk in one or more lobes of the breasts and its symptoms are related to increased pressure. If the galactocele is small, it can be effectively treated by massage; if large, a tight binder is usually effective.

Supernumerary Breasts

One in every few hundred persons has one or more accessory breasts, a condition called *polymastia*. Such breasts, which may have distinct nipples, are sometimes mistaken for pigmented moles. They are commonly situated in pairs (usually two to four) on either side of the midline of the thoracic or abdominal wall, usually below the main breasts. Sometimes they are found in the axillae. Usually they are of no significance during pregnancy, although they may enlarge, secrete milk, and cause discomfort. These changes usually regress after delivery.

EMOTIONAL DISORDERS

The stresses of pregnancy and delivery and the accompanying new responsibilities are precipitating factors in the development of postpartum psychosis in about 1 out of every 1000 new mothers. Although postpartum psychosis is not in itself a distinct clinical entity, its symptoms usually can be identified within six months after delivery, most commonly in the first postpartum month. About half of the patients with postpartum psychosis demonstrate schizophrenic characteristics, while another 40 percent are manic-depressive in behavior. Primiparas and multiparas appear to be affected equally and about one-third of them have probably had a mental illness prior to pregnancy.

In the majority of cases the onset of the psychosis is rather sudden, with a variety of affective symptoms—clouding of consciousness, withdrawal, depression, hostility, suspicion, unreasonable fear, and feelings of inadequacy. The patient may also have hallucinations or delusions regarding the child, her delivery, her mothering role, or her relationship with the baby's father.

Because the early symptoms are very similar to those of the common postpartum "blues," nurses should not be too quick to treat their appearance in a superficial manner, since in some cases they may develop into more serious psychiatric difficulties. The fact that some postpartum psychoses may be prevented by antepartal therapy highlights the importance of the nurse's assessment of the patient's ability to cope with stresses while she is pregnant. Nurses in community settings as well as hospital settings are in a good position to offer support to family members during the crisis period. The adjustments that the family must make are tremendous in scope.

About 20 percent of patients with postpartum psychosis recover within a month. In 40 percent recovery takes longer than six months, and about 15 percent remain chronically ill. For about half of the patients it will remain an isolated event in their lives; the incidence of reccurrence in subsequent pregnancies is about 1 in 7 women.

DRUG ADDICTION

There has been an apparent increase in the number of infants born to addicted mothers in recent years in the United States. The incidence has risen from 1 out of 200 deliveries to 1 out of 50 in some large urban hospitals [1]. Heroin still appears to be the most common addicting agent, but polydrug use involving amphetamines, tranquilizers, barbiturates, cocaine, methadone, and hallucinogens is now a serious problem. The polydrug problem may actually be adding to the number of pregnancies in addicts. Heroin in high concentrations may suppress ovulation through its action on the pituitary, but some authorities [3] think that amphetamines and marijuana may counteract this heroin effect. In addition, unreliable "cuts" of heroin in bags may not be sufficiently potent to suppress ovulation.

A large number of pregnant addicts are in their teenage years and thus fall into a high-risk group. In addition, because of their life-style as addicts, they often have venereal disease, hepatitis, skin infections, malnutrition, or thrombophlebitis. When a multidisciplinary approach is used to provide care for pregnant addicts, the number of prenatal visits rises above the average for all addicts of approximately one per pregnancy [1]. The pregnant addict also faces obstetrical problems common to the addict—preeclampsia, abruptio placentae, premature rupture of membranes, postpartum hemorrhage, and an increased incidence of breech birth.

The problems faced by the pregnant addict are multiple. She usually lacks self-confidence and self-esteem and appears very anxious and depressed. Because she has difficulty with interpersonal relationships, members of the health team caring for her must show patience and understanding when trying to help her. Unless she can establish a trusting relationship with someone on the team at the beginning of her prenatal care, she will not accept and return for care.

In addition to their reluctance to accept prenatal care, addicts commonly arrive at the hospital late in active labor, usually having taken a recent "fix." If labor lasts a long time, these women require higher doses of analgesics than usual. Sometimes a woman's behavior and physical signs lead the nurse to suspect that she is an addict. These include her arrival late in labor with a history of little or no prenatal care, the presence of needle marks on the forearm or attempts to hide them with tattoos or scars, burned fingers or holes in her clothing as a result of smoking when she was "high," cellulitis, thrombophlebitis, skin abscesses, signs of jaundice, pinpoint pupils, or an excessive desire for medication.

In the postpartum period, many experts believe that drugs should be given to prevent withdrawal in order to make the addicted mother's recovery more comfortable [3]. If the mother does not receive drugs, she soon becomes nervous and unable to sleep. Her eyes burn, her nose runs, and she begins to have "gooseflesh" and to perspire. She complains of severe aching in her back, legs, and abdomen, and her muscles begin to twitch. Her blood pressure, temperature, and respiratory rate increase. If she does not receive drugs, she may sign herself out of the hospital and take her infant with her.

Many addicted mothers are concerned about their newborns; their anxiety can be lessened while they remain in the hospital by keeping them continually informed about the baby's progress. They also need much support from the nursing staff in learning adequate mothering practices. It is important to encourage the addicted mother to care for her baby or to assist in their care as much as possible. It is also important to encourage the father of the baby and other family members and friends to visit if they can lend support to the mother.

It is essential to explore with the addicted mother her feelings concerning her infant and her plans for his care. Here, the multidisciplinary team is invaluable in helping the mother to make realistic plans for discharge and postnatal care of both herself and her infant. The option of temporarily placing the infant in foster care or in an institution until she can assume responsibility for him should be presented to her.

REFERENCES

1. Driscoll, J. Metabolic and Endocrine Disturbances. In R. Behrman (Ed.), *Neonatology.* St. Louis: Mosby, 1973.
2. Gibbs, R. S., O'Dell, T. N., MacGregor, R., Schwarz, R. H., and Morton, H. Puerperal endometritis: A prospective microbiologic study *American Journal of Obstetrics and Gynecology* 121:919, 1975.
3. Pierog, S., and Ferrara, A. *Approach to the Medical Care of the Sick Newborn.* St. Louis: Mosby, 1971.
4. Sweet, R. L., and Ledger, W. J. Puerperal infectious morbidity. *American Journal of Obstetrics and Gynecology* 117:1093, 1973.
5. Hellman, L. M., and Pritchard, J. A. *Williams Obstetrics* (14th ed.). New York: Appleton-Century-Crofts, 1971.

FURTHER READING

Fitzpatrick, E., Reeder, S., and Mastroianni, L. *Maternity Nursing.* Philadelphia: Lippincott, 1971.
Gordon, R., Kapostins, E., and Gordon, K. Factors in postpartum emotional adjustment. *Obstetrics and Gynecology* 25:158, 1965.
Greenhill, J. P., and Friedman, E. A. *Biological Principles and Modern Practice of Obstetrics.* Philadelphia: Saunders, 1974.
Jewett, J. F., Reid, D. E., Safon, L. E., and Easterday, C. L. Childbed fever—a continuing entity. *Journal of the American Medical Association* 206:342, 1968.
Kaij, L., and Nilsson, A. Emotional Psychotic Illness Following Childbirth. In J. Howells (Ed.). *Modern Perspectives in Psycho-Obstetrics.* New York: Brunner Mazel, 1972.
Lerch, C. *Maternity Nursing.* St. Louis: Mosby, 1974.
McCormack, W. M., Lee, Y.-H., Lin, J.-S., and Rankin, J. S. Genital mycoplasms in postpartum fever. *Journal of Infectious Diseases* 127:193, 1973.
McLennan, C., and Sandberg, E. *Synopsis of Obstetrics.* St. Louis: Mosby, 1974.
Robinson, D. W. Postpartum ovarian vein thrombophlebitis. *American Journal of Obstetrics and Gynecology* 113:497, 1972.
Sherman, J. *On the Psychology of Women.* Springfield: Thomas, 1971.
White, C. A. and Koontz, F. P. B-hemolytic streptococcus infections in postpartum patients. *Obstetrics and Gynecology* 41:27, 1973.
Ziegel, E., and Van Blarcom, C. *Obstetric Nursing.* New York: Macmillan, 1972.

Chapter 17 Complications of the Newborn

PRETERM AND LOW BIRTH WEIGHT INFANTS

In the past, classifications for newborns were based mainly on the infant's weight at the time of birth (Table 17-1). Recognizing that all newborns weighing 2500 grams or less at birth are not born prematurely, the World Health Organization recommended a new classification. As a result, *low birth weight* is the designation applied to these infants, regardless of the cause of their light weight and the length of their gestation.

Babies are also classified according to gestational age. Those babies who grew at a normal rate in utero, whether or not they are born at term, preterm, or postterm, are referred to as *appropriate for gestational age (AGA)*. If they grew at a retarded rate, they are labeled *small for gestational age (SGA)*, while if the rate of their intrauterine growth was accelerated, they are *large for gestational age (LGA)*. When infants of low birth weight are properly classified, about one-third are SGA (growth retarded) and two-thirds are AGA (preterm).

Assessment of Gestational Age

Because the problems of preterm and low birth weight babies are different, it is important to assess their gestational age and to project the difference in their care and treatment. For instance, an infant weighing over 2500 grams (5.5 pounds) may be assumed to be full term when he is actually LGA and preterm, e.g., the infant of a diabetic mother. Several tools that nurses can easily use have been developed to assess gestational age (Figures 17-1, 17-2; Table 17-2); they are based on the appearance of external characteristics that develop in orderly fashion during gestation and the use of a neurological evaluation. This latter examination is done when the infant is in a resting state. The scores from each part of the evaluation are combined, and the result is plotted on a rating scale, yielding an approximate gestational age.

THE PRETERM INFANT

The characteristics of the truly preterm infant are most noticeable in babies with the shortest gestational age. Factors associated with prematurity are, of course, involved with the onset of premature labor, which may have many causes, including placental malfunction and maternal or fetal disease such as chronic hypertensive disease, preeclampsia, placenta previa, abruptio placentae, cervical incompetence, multiple gestation, or blood incompatibility. Other factors include low socioeco-

421

Table 17-1.
Classifications for
Newborns

Classification	Weight	Gestational Age
Abortus	Under 500 g	20 weeks or under
Immature	500–999 g	21–26/27 weeks
Preterm	1000–2500 g	27–36 weeks
Full-term	Over 2500 g	37–42 weeks
Postterm	—	Over 42 weeks

nomic status, short maternal stature, absence of prenatal care, malnutrition, and a history of previous premature delivery. In the United States, approximately 8 percent of all live births are before term and prematurity still ranks as the leading cause of infant death.

The preterm baby usually weighs from 1000–2500 grams (2.2–5.5 pounds), with a vertex-heel length of under 48 centimeters (19 inches), and a head circumference of 25–31 centimeters (10–12 inches). The baby's head appears large in proportion to the rest of his body. His chest circumference is relatively small—less than 30 centimeters (12 inches), generally 3 centimeters (1½ inches) smaller than his head. The lower his gestational age, the weaker his activity and the less frequent his cry. His loss of weight (10–15 percent) in the first week of extrauterine life is greater than that of the term infant (7–10 percent). As a rule weight is regained more slowly, sometimes not until the third week.

Respiratory System

In general, respirations in the preterm infant are irregular, rapid, and sometimes shallow, with periods of apnea and cyanosis. Periodic breathing (short pauses in respiration) is a common pattern and is differentiated from true apnea. Apnea involves either a given time period without any respirations (15–30 seconds) or a time without respiration after which functional changes in the infant, such as cyanosis, hypotonia, or acidosis, are noted.

The heart rate drops 10–15 seconds after respirations cease and is usually below 100 beats per minute within 30 seconds. No theory completely explains the occurrence of apneic spells, although it is known that changes in the excitatory state of the immature respiratory center can alter breathing remarkably. Therefore, either restraining the extremities of the small, preterm infant and thus changing the sensory input from bones and joints, or increasing the isolette temperature and thus altering skin temperature receptors, will sometimes induce or increase the number of his apneic episodes [7]. Since even short periods of apnea may produce brain

Figure 17-1. Assessing gestational age in the newborn: external criteria. (From L. M. S. Dubowitz, V. Dubowitz, and C. Goldberg, Clinical assessment of gestational age in the newborn infant. J. Pediatr. 77:1, 1970.)

EXTERNAL SIGN	SCORE				
	0	1	2	3	4.
EDEMA	Obvious edema hands and feet; pitting over tibia	No obvious edema hands and feet; pitting over tibia	No edema		
SKIN TEXTURE	Very thin, gelatinous	Thin and smooth	Smooth; medium thickness Rash or superficial peeling	Slight thickening. Superficial cracking and peeling especially hands and feet	Thick and parchment-like; superficial or deep cracking
SKIN COLOR (Infant not crying)	Dark red	Uniformly pink	Pale pink: variable over body	Pale. Only pink over ears, lips, palms or soles	
SKIN OPACITY (trunk)	Numerous veins and venules clearly seen, especially over abdomen	Veins and tributaries seen	A few large vessels clearly seen over abdomen	A few large vessels seen indistinctly over abdomen	No blood vessels seen
LANUGO (Over back)	No lanugo	Abundant; long and thick over whole back	Hair thinning especially over lower back	Small amount of lanugo and bald areas	At least half of back devoid of lanugo
PLANTAR CREASES	No skin creases	Faint red marks over anterior half of sole	Definite red marks over more than anterior half; indentations over less than anterior third	Indentations over more than anterior third	Definite *deep* indentations over more than anterior third
NIPPLE FORMATION	Nipple barely visible; no areola	Nipple well defined; areola smooth and flat diam. $<$ 0.75 cm.	Areola stippled, edge not raised diam. $<$ 0.75 cm.	Areola stippled, edge raised diam. $>$ 0.75 cm.	
BREAST SIZE	No breast tissue palpable	Breast tissue on one or both sides $<$ 0.5 cm. diam.	Breast tissue both sides; one or both 0.5–1.0 cm.	Breast tissue both sides; one or both $>$ 1 cm.	
EAR FORM	Pinna flat & shapeless, little or no incurving of edge	Incurving of part of edge of pinna	Partial incurving whole of upper pinna	Well-defined incurving whole of upper pinna	
EAR FIRMNESS	Pinna soft, easily folded, no recoil	Pinna soft, easily folded, slow recoil	Cartilage to edge of pinna, but soft in places, ready recoil	Pinna firm, Cartilage to edge; instant recoil	
GENITALIA MALE	Neither testis in scrotum	At least one testis high in scrotum	At least one testis right down		
FEMALES (With hips half obducted)	Labia majora widely separated, labia minora protruding	Labia majora almost cover labia minora	Labia majora completely cover labia minora		

(Adapted from Farr et al. *Develop. Med. Child Neurol.* 1966, *8,* 507)
(If score differs on two sides, take the mean).

Table 17-2. Notes on Techniques of Assessment of Neurological Criteria. Source: L. M. S. Dubowitz, V. Dubowitz, and C. Goldberg. Clinical assessment of gestational age in the newborn infant. *Journal of Pediatrics* 77:1, 1970.

Posture   Observed with infant quiet and in supine position. Score 0: arms and legs extended; 1: beginning of flexion of hips and knees, arms extended; 2: stronger flexion of legs, arms extended; 3: arms slightly flexed, legs flexed and abducted; 4: full flexion of arms and legs.

Square Window   The hand is flexed on the forearm between the thumb and index finger of the examiner. Enough pressure is applied to get as full a flexion as possible, and the angle between the hypothenar eminence and the ventral aspect of the forearm is measured and graded according to Figure 17-2A. (Care is taken not to rotate the infant's wrist while doing this maneuver.)

Ankle Dorsiflexion   The foot is dorsiflexed onto the anterior aspect of the leg, with the examiner's thumb on the sole of the foot and other fingers behind the leg. Enough pressure is applied to get as full flexion as possible, and the angle between the dorsum of the foot and the anterior aspect of the leg is measured.

Arm Recoil   With the infant in the supine position, the forearms are first flexed for 5 seconds, then fully extended by pulling on the hands, and then released. The sign is fully positive if the arms return briskly to full flexion (score 2). If the arms return to incomplete flexion or the response is sluggish, it is scored as 1. If they remain extended or are only followed by random movements, the score is 0.

Leg Recoil   With the infant supine, the hips and knees are fully flexed for 5 seconds, then extended by traction on the feet, and released. A maximal response is one of full flexion of the hips and knees (score 2). A partial flexion scores 1, and minimal or no movement scores 0.

Popliteal Angle   With the infant supine and his pelvis flat on the examining couch, the thigh is held in the knee-chest position by the examiner's left index finger and thumb supporting the knee. The leg is then extended by gentle pressure from the examiner's right index finger behind the ankle and the popliteal angle is measured.

Heel To Ear Maneuver   With the baby supine, draw the baby's foot as near to the head as it will go without forcing it. Observe the distance between the foot and the head as well as the degree of extension at the knee. Grade according to Figure 17-2A. Note that the knee is left free and may draw down alongside the abdomen.

Scarf Sign   With the baby supine, take the infant's hand and try to put it around the neck and as far posteriorly as possible around the opposite shoulder. Assist this maneuver by lifting the elbow across the body. See how far the elbow will go across and grade according to illustrations. Score 0: elbow reaches opposite axillary line; 1: elbow between midline and opposite axillary line; 2: elbow reaches midline; 3: elbow will not reach midline.

Head Lag   With the baby lying supine, grasp the hands (or the arms if a very small infant) and pull him slowly towards the sitting position. Observe the position of the head in relation to the trunk and grade accordingly. In a small infant the head may initially be supported by one hand. Score 0: complete lag; 1: partial head control; 2: able to maintain head in line with body; 3: brings head anterior to body.

Ventral Suspension   The infant is suspended in the prone position, with the examiner's hand under the infant's chest (one hand in a small infant; two in a large infant). Observe the degree of extension of the back and the amount of flexion of the arms and legs. Also note the relation of the head to the trunk. Grade according to Figure 17-2A.

damage in very small infants, it is essential that their respirations be carefully monitored.

RESPIRATORY DISTRESS SYNDROME

An infant's lung development depends on the length of gestation. The very young premature baby may have small alveoli and few blood vessels, since there is a great increase in the lung capillary network between 26 and 36 weeks. He often has difficulty in initiating normal respiration, which may result in lung collapse (primary atelectasis). This problem is related to sparsity of pulmonary elastic tissue and general anatomical immaturity of alveoli; weak respiratory muscles and a soft

Figure 17-2. A. Assessing gestational age in the newborn: neurological signs. (See Table 17-2 for explanation of scores.) B. Scores obtained from assessment of external criteria and neurological signs are totaled. The total score is plotted on the graph to obtain the gestational age. (From L. M. S. Dubowitz, V. Dubowitz, and C. Goldberg, Clinical assessment of gestational age in the newborn infant. J. Pediatr. 77:1, 1970.)

NEUROLOGICAL SIGN	SCORE					
	0	1	2	3	4	5
POSTURE						
SQUARE WINDOW	90°	60°	45°	30°	0°	
ANKLE DORSIFLEXION	90°	75°	45°	20°	0°	
ARM RECOIL	180°	90–180°	<90°			
LEG RECOIL	180°	90–180°	<90°			
POPLITEAL ANGLE	180	160°	130°	110°	90°	<90°
HEEL TO EAR						
SCARF SIGN						
HEAD LAG						
VENTRAL SUSPENSION						

A

Figure 17-2 (Continued)

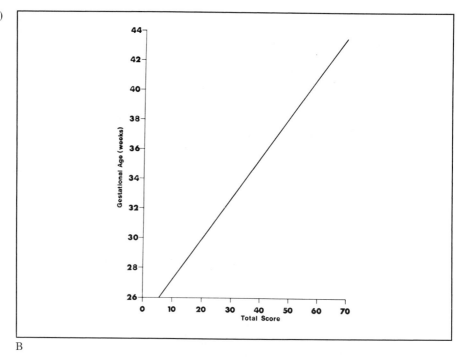

B

yielding thoracic cage, leading to reduced intrathoracic pressure; and a poorly developed respiratory center that requires strong afferent stimuli for response.

In addition to having difficulty in initiating respiration, approximately 10 percent of all preterm babies develop respiratory distress syndrome (RDS), also known as hyaline membrane disease. Its symptoms are evident at birth or shortly thereafter, and the disease course usually lasts three to five days. The infant develops tachypnea, with his respiratory rate usually over 60 breaths per minute. With each inspiration his chest wall retracts, his nares flare, and he may have accompanying respiratory grunting. Soon he may become cyanotic in room air and experience periods of apnea. His general skin color may appear pale due to vasoconstriction. Upon auscultation of his chest, air entry appears diminished. Edema may develop in his extremities because of altered vascular permeability but usually subsides by the fifth day.

In severe cases the infant is extremely hypoactive and flaccid. He develops severe retractions in the first 6 hours and shows no improvement of air exchange after 24 hours. In addition, he remains cyanotic while receiving oxygen. Often he assumes a froglike position with his head turned to one side and his mouth open. After 72 hours, death is unlikely unless the infant encounters further complications, such as pneumonia, pulmonary hemorrhage, or intracranial hemorrhage. In most cases of RDS, retractions begin to improve in approximately 72 hours, and tachypnea, a day or two thereafter.

The etiology of RDS involves deficient or absent pulmonary surfactant, a lipo-protein produced by cells in the alveolar wall. The levels of surfactant increase slowly but remain relatively low during the first six months of gestation. During the last three months, levels of lecithin, the principal component of surfactant, increase rapidly. It is this component that is felt to be insufficient in infants who develop RDS.

Surfactant acts at the air-liquid interface of the alveoli, decreasing surface tension and thus preventing the alveoli from collapsing during expiration. This allows the infant to establish a functional residual capacity. In normal infants, therefore, approximately 25 percent of the alveolar volume remains expanded after expiration; this is not the case with the infant with RDS. An infant with inadequate surfactant and little or no residual capacity requires higher pressures to reinflate his alveoli during the next inspiration.

The resistance within the pulmonary circuit causes reduced blood flow to the alveolar capillaries, and the lungs are therefore ischemic as well as collapsed. As this atelectasis continues, it enhances hypoxia, hypercapnia, and acidosis, which cause an additional increase in pulmonary vasoconstriction and ischemia as well as decreasing surfactant activity. As these events continue, the lung collapse becomes more extensive, requiring more pressure to inflate the infant's lungs and more energy on the infant's part to breathe [8].

Pulmonary vasoconstriction effects further changes in the heart. Normally after birth, as mentioned in Chapter 10, the pulmonary vessels dilate and there is a decrease in the vascular resistance in the lungs. The increased blood flow through the lungs leads to an increased flow and pressure in the left atrium. The pressure in the left atrium, which is higher than that in the right, closes the foramen ovale, eliminating a right-to-left shunt. Pulmonary vasoconstriction reverses this effect and opens the shunt.

In addition, as the infant's arterial Po_2 normally increases, the ductus arteriosis gradually begins to close, thus causing more blood flow to the lung. Hypoxia, which constricts the pulmonary vasculature, also reverses closing of the ductus. It is also believed that hypoxia damages the capillary endothelium, and, when accompanied by high negative intrathoracic pressure, helps to promote transudation of fluid into the alveoli. Fibrin forms a matrix that traps the necrotic alveolar duct epithelium, red blood cells, serum proteins, and so forth. These coalesce to form hyaline membranes that line the alveolar ducts and terminal bronchioles. Unfortunately, the young premature infant lacks the fibrinolysins necessary for dissolution of the membrane. This leads to airway obstruction and further compounds the problem.

The treatment and care of infants with RDS is complex and requires constant observation on the nurse's part. The infant will receive oxygen, but it may be administered in a number of ways. If it flows into an isolette (Figure 17-3), the percentage of oxygen in the infant's environment will be increased. It may be administered via a hood or dome placed over his head, or, in the very ill infant who has been intubated, it may flow through his endotracheal tube. However it is administered, it must be given cautiously, since excessive levels may lead to eye or lung damage. The infant's retina may scar, resulting in blindness (retrolental fibroplasia). The lung tissues may fibrose under excessive oxygen administration, impairing oxygen diffusion from the alveolar lumen to the capillaries.

Figure 17-3. Twin preterm infants receiving oxygen via respirators. (Courtesy of Pennsylvania Hospital, Philadelphia, Pa.)

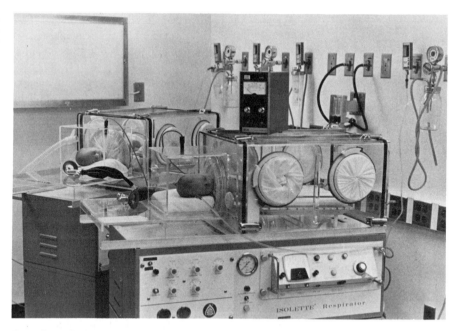

Retrolental Fibroplasia.   In the early 1950s it was discovered that the oxygen used to treat RDS in the premature baby was also the source of another of his major complications, retrolental fibroplasia, caused by inordinately high levels of oxygen in his retinal capillaries. The effect of oxygen on the retinal vessels depends on the length of their exposure to oxygen, the stage of their development, and the oxygen concentration in the arterial blood.

The first stage of reaction involves constriction of retinal vessels. It is felt that the vasoconstrictor effects of short periods of high oxygen are reversible. If vasoconstriction lasts longer than several hours the process may not be reversible, although the point at which this occurs is not known. Severe vasoconstriction is not seen when the retina is fully vascularized. The younger the infant, the less vascularization is present.

The second stage begins within one or two months after oxygen treatment is terminated. At this time there is a proliferation of new blood vessels from the retinal capillaries. They sprout through the retina into the vitreous body. These vessels are often permeable, and hemorrhage and edema sometimes occur. Organization of these hemorrhages can produce pressure on the retina and may result in its detachment. Detachment of the retina is followed by absorption of the vitreous body, pulling together of the retina, and formation of a membrane behind the lens, which ultimately leads to blindness. The process reaches this point in approximately 25 percent of infants with retinal vasospasm during early oxygen therapy. It is important, therefore, to have an ophthalmologist examine these babies periodically and to decrease the oxygen as much as possible if vasospasm is noted [7, 8].

Retinal damage is greatest when the infant's gestational age is less than 36 weeks or when he weighs less than 2000 grams (4.4 pounds). Therefore, the use of oxygen is usually restricted to babies who become cyanotic without it.

In order to prevent both retrolental fibroplasia and lung fibrosis, the percentage of environmental oxygen in the baby's isolette should not exceed 60–70 percent and usually is kept at 35–40 percent. This level is generally checked every hour by using an oxygen analyzer. A more accurate method is to test the infant's Po_2 level. Arterial blood is nearly 100 percent saturated at a Po_2 of 90–100 millimeters of mercury. Cyanosis is usually apparent when the arterial Po_2 falls below 32–42 millimeters of mercury, yet the effects of hypoxemia (pulmonary vasoconstriction and impaired metabolic response to cold stress) occur when the Po_2 is approximately 50 millimeters of mercury. Arterial levels over 100 millimeters of mercury lead to eye and lung impairment, as already mentioned. Therefore, the American Academy of Pediatrics recommends that infants' Po_2 levels be kept between 60–80 millimeters of mercury when they are receiving oxygen for more than brief periods. Arterial blood for testing is usually obtained from the infant's umbilical, temporal, radial, or brachial artery. If the equipment for checking arterial blood samples is not available, the level of oxygen being administered can be decreased gradually by 10 percent over a period of time until cyanosis occurs in the infant. In that case, the oxygen is increased by 10 percent and maintained.

In monitoring the infant's oxygen levels the nurse should keep in mind that as his ventilation improves, his Po_2 level will rise. He therefore needs very close observation. His position is important, since it can maintain or obstruct his airway. The head of his bed may be elevated 10 degrees and his shoulders may be raised. If necessary, his head may be kept in slight hyperextension. In addition to proper positioning, suction should be used as necessary to maintain an open airway.

Infants with RDS usually develop some degree of acidosis. In the early stages respiratory acidosis predominates, but as the infant works harder to breathe, lactic acid levels increase and metabolic acidosis appears. If the acidosis is not corrected, it may lead to pulmonary vasoconstriction, irregular heart beat, depression of myocardial function, dilatation of cerebral vessels that can lead to cerebral hemorrhage, further impairment of surfactant activity, and detachment of bilirubin from albumin, causing kernicterus at low serum bilirubin concentrations. Levels of blood gases and pH are usually used to determine the amount of sodium bicarbonate that will be given to the acidotic infant. A pH of 7.25 or more requires no treatment.

Keeping the infant warm is also essential, since cold stress increases the need for oxygen. In an infant who is already having difficulty maintaining an adequate oxygen level, cold stress can be disastrous. Cold increases the metabolic rate and the production of lactic acid, therefore aggravating hypoxia and acidosis, increasing pulmonary vasoconstriction, and possibly impairing production and activity of surfactant.

Circulatory System

The preterm infant's heart is relatively large at birth compared to his overall body size, and murmurs are not uncommon. Because of immature cardiac conductile tissue, his heart beat may be arrhythmic; therefore, his pulse rate is most accurately obtained by listening to the apical rate for one full minute. His blood pressure is lower than the term infant's (45–60/30–45 millimeters of mercury) and his peripheral circulation is poor.

The proportion of fetal hemoglobin to adult hemoglobin is higher than in the mature baby, and the fetal hemoglobin tends to disappear more slowly. Since fetal hemoglobin releases oxygen to peripheral tissues less readily than the adult type, and since the preterm infant's capillaries may be fewer in number, oxygen perfusion of some of his tissues is marginal, at best. The walls of his blood vessels are known to be very fragile, especially those of the intracranial vessels. This, plus a decrease in several clotting factors (particularly prothrombin), predisposes him not only to bruising but also to hemorrhage, especially in the ventricles of the brain. The precipitate births, breech presentations, and hypoxia associated with premature delivery raise the risks of intracranial bleeding.

The fall in the preterm infant's red blood cell level and hemoglobin concentration is greater and the final rise of these two values is slower than in the full-term infant. This results in a more prolonged physiological anemia in the preterm baby, whose hemoglobin level may drop as low as 6–7 grams per 100 milliliters in four to eight weeks. This is particularly due to a reduced rate of hematopoiesis and the shortened life span of his red blood cells, poor iron stores, and a greater growth rate after birth with a corresponding greater increase in blood volume. The rapid destruction of his immature red cells, together with the immaturity of his liver, predisposes him to hyperbilirubinemia and jaundice.

Nervous System

The development of this system depends on the baby's length of gestation. The young preterm baby lies quietly, and external stimulation elicits weak, uncoordinated, purposeless movements and perhaps a feeble cry. He may first lie in the fetal position but gradually uncurls to lie on his back with his head rolled to one side, hips flexed and abducted, and knees and ankles flexed (frog position) (Figure 17-4). His

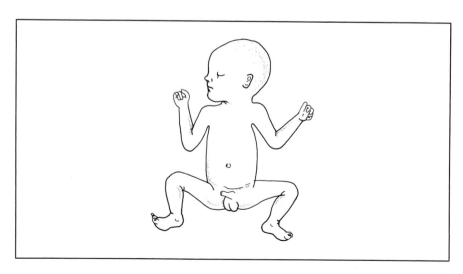

Figure 17-4. Usual position of the preterm infant.

centers for vital functions (respiration and temperature) as well as vital reflexes (cough, swallow, and suck) may be poorly developed. The Moro, tonic neck, Chvostek, and Babinski reflexes are usually present, but tendon reflexes are variable.

Gastrointestinal System

Digestion is rudimentary in an infant of 26–28 weeks' gestation but becomes more effective as his age increases. Even though fat-splitting enzymes are present at birth, the infant fails to absorb 20–40 percent of the saturated fat from his milk feedings. Except for a possible decrease in bile salts, no chemical cause for the poor absorption is obvious. However, unsaturated fats of vegetable origin are better absorbed than animal fats. Both preterm and full-term infants are born with low levels of lipoproteins, which transport fat. These apparently are synthesized in the liver within the first two or three weeks after feeding is begun.

The larger preterm infant has good sucking and swallowing reflexes. Even so, regurgitation may be common, since he is likely to have a limited stomach capacity, a poorly developed cardiac sphincter, and a relatively strong pyloric sphincter. The musculature of his bowel wall is weak and easily distended, so constipation and abdominal distention may be special problems. Normal gastric peristalsis can be seen through his thin abdominal wall.

His liver is relatively large, but its function is poorly developed. Because his liver enzymes are decreased, he is unable to conjugate and excrete bilirubin satisfactorily (tendency to jaundice). Other liver-related problems involve his small glycogen stores (tendency to hypoglycemia), lower serum protein (tendency to edema), decreased blood clotting factors (hemorrhagic disease), and inability to conjugate and detoxify certain drugs. In addition, he has received less than the usual antibody complement from his mother, and his own poor formation of antibody protein predisposes him to infection. He synthesizes IgG poorly and his rate of IgM synthesis is slower than that of the full-term infant.

Genitourinary System

The preterm infant's urine is scanty and infrequent for a few days after birth because of his limited intake. Since tubules continue to be formed during the entire 40 weeks of normal gestation, the baby's ability to excrete sodium and chlorides is compromised, making him more susceptible to electrolyte imbalance, edema, and a more marked and prolonged acidosis. These factors may also affect the excretion of medication he may receive. The preterm baby has more extracellular fluid than the term infant and less renal capacity for concentrating urine, a fact which is of clinical importance when the baby is suffering from diarrhea, vomiting, or other conditions involving loss of water.

Preterm infants have a special tendency to develop inguinal hernias. In girls, the labia minora are not usually covered by the labia majora. In boys, the testes may be in the abdomen, inguinal canal, or scrotum, depending on the infant's gestational age.

Eyes, Ears, Nose, Mouth

The infant's eyes appear prominent and widely spaced. By 24 weeks' gestation, retinal vessels have grown close to the optic nerve. From 24 to 30 weeks no further growth occurs and the fundus is immature. Growth then resumes, so that by 34 weeks the fundus is usually mature [3]. The eyes are most likely to develop retrolental fibroplasia before 34 weeks.

The preterm infant's nose is small and short. His small ears lack cartilage and can be folded with little resistance. His tongue appears large in his mouth and the fat pads in his cheeks are absent. In general, his head looks large and out of proportion to his relatively short neck and extremities and elongated trunk.

Skin, Hair, Nails

The preterm infant's skin is often red and wrinkled, since he usually has little subcutaneous fat. In the smallest babies the nipples are flat, pigmented areas. It is only after 36 weeks' gestation that they rise above the surrounding skin. Engorgement of the breast is rare. The skin on the soles of the feet is likely to be uncreased.

Lanugo is plentiful until 28 weeks; then it decreases in amount. The back, face, and extensor surfaces of the limbs are the most likely to remain covered. The hair on the head is usually soft, short, and scanty. Eyebrows are often absent. The nails are softer than those of the full-term infant but reach to his fingertips as early as 28 weeks' gestation.

Caring for the Preterm Infant

In general, care of the infant is based on providing him with warmth, meticulous physical care, gentleness, precise and careful feeding, and protection from infection. It is also based on the satisfaction of his emotional needs, so necessary for the growth and development of all infants.

FEEDING

There are considerable differences of opinion among competent pediatricians concerning some aspects of feeding premature infants—choice of food, number of calories per pound of body weight, time at which the feedings are started. One food choice, breast milk, has the advantages of easy digestibility and reduced incidence of abdominal distention and regurgitation, in addition to its effectiveness in preventing enteric infections. However, it may lack sufficient protein for the rapid growth of the small preterm infant [16]. Smaller infants may need 4 grams of protein per kilogram of body weight per day, about twice the need of the term baby. The high mineral content of cow's milk may be advantageous, but if water intake is limited or water losses are high, the minerals may not be properly excreted. In general, a basic formula that provides 65 calories per 100 milliliters, with 1.5–1.7% protein, 7% carbohydrate, and 3.5% fat—half of which is polyunsaturated—probably remains the safest recommendation for all preterm infants.

In most instances, 120 calories per kilogram of body weight per day will provide for normal infant growth. The SGA infant has a higher metabolic rate and may require more calories. He may also require a vitamin supplement because of his rapid growth as will the preterm infant because of his poor vitamin stores, although the minimum daily requirement of the rapidly growing preterm infant is not known.

In addition to his poor tolerance of fat, as previously mentioned, the preterm infant often has mechanical difficulties. If he is very small, he may have weak buccal, tongue, and palate muscles. Incomplete nervous system development may result in weak suck and swallow reflexes, so he may have to be gavage-fed. His small stomach capacity sometimes requires that he be fed as little as 5 cubic centimeters at a time to avoid overfeeding. Nurses often use early feedings to judge what the individual infant's volume tolerance is and to make adjustments in his feeding schedule accordingly.

Because the preterm infant tires very quickly, his sucking becomes less efficient, especially if the feeding is prolonged beyond 15 minutes. Sometimes his sucking reflex can be stimulated if the nipple is moved about; this must be done very gently to avoid injuring the mucous membrane in his mouth. If the nipple is pressed down on his tongue or gentle upward pressure is applied under his chin, he often begins sucking with renewed vigor (Figure 17-5).

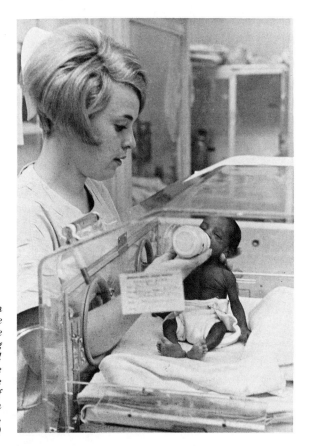

Figure 17-5. Preterm infant bottle-feeding. The nurse stimulates the infant's senses by talking to him, rubbing him, and fondling him even if he must remain in the isolette. (Courtesy of Thomas Jefferson University, Philadelphia, Pa.)

Despite the fact that feeding time is usually the only time a preterm baby is removed from his isolette and can be cuddled in the traditional sense, nurses should remember the importance of other modes of sensory stimulation, such as the sound of a voice and touch, which are just as effective inside the isolette. While the temptation to hold the preterm infant close is hard to resist, nurses will find that the more "comfortable" the baby is, the sooner he will go to sleep and not complete his feeding. Holding him in a semi-erect position away from the body will facilitate both feeding and burping and allow for more direct observation of how he is handling the formula. The nurse may burp the baby in this position with one hand supporting his head and chest, while the other hand gently pats or rubs his back (Figure 17-6). If the baby is burped in the over-the-shoulder manner, he cannot be observed as well. In addition, he is pressed against the bony shoulder, which may be somewhat traumatic, and he is placed dangerously close to the nurse's nasopharynx, a potential source of contamination.

Small infants who cannot suck or swallow or who become cyanotic when fed by bottle are usually fed by gavage (Figure 17-7). A polyethylene French catheter (No. 5 or 8) is used for the feeding and may be indwelling (changed every two to three days) or may be inserted at each feeding and then removed. If the infant is very small, an indwelling nasojejunum tube can be used to provide continuous feedings.

Prepackaged sterile gavage tubes are usually premarked for insertion point, but to be on the safe side they should be remeasured and marked prior to insertion in order to estimate distance into the stomach. If the tube is to be passed through the nose, the distance from the nares to the earlobe and from the earlobe to the xiphoid

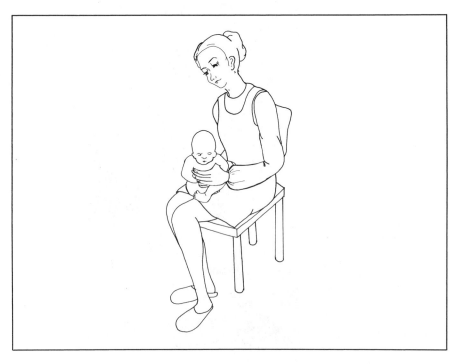

Figure 17-6. Position for burping the infant.

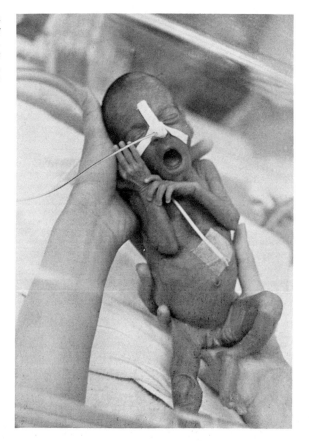

process is marked off. If it is to be passed through the mouth, the distance from the bridge of the nose to the xiphoid process is measured. This method is often preferred, since the narrow nasal passage may be easily injured or infected.

Prior to insertion of the gavage tube or gavage feeding, the infant is positioned on his back, with his shoulders elevated by placing a rolled diaper under them and his neck hyperextended. As the catheter is passed, he is observed for dyspnea and cyanosis (tube in trachea). To determine that this has not occurred, the open end of the gavage tube is placed in a medicine glass containing sterile water. If the tube is in the trachea, air bubbles will appear as the infant exhales.

Another way to test if the tube is in the stomach involves injecting 2 cc of air through the tubing. The flow of air can be heard as a rushing sound when a stethoscope is placed over the infant's stomach.

Before the feeding is begun, a syringe is attached to the feeding tube and is gently aspirated to estimate residual contents of the stomach. If there is residual, it is refed to the baby and the new feeding, reduced by this amount, is poured into the barrel of the syringe and allowed to flow slowly into the infant's stomach. When the catheter is to be removed, it is pinched off, withdrawn, and discarded. The infant is turned on his right side when the feeding is completed.

LOW BIRTH WEIGHT BABIES (SGA)

Low birth weight babies, who are small for gestational age, require as much special care as preterm babies do, since they have been subject to stress in utero. As a result, they are prone to develop a number of conditions neonatally. Most commonly, a baby who is SGA has suffered from severe and prolonged intrauterine malnutrition. This may be caused by any condition resulting in poor placental growth or function (e.g., poor maternal nutrition, preeclampsia, smoking, high-altitude residence, drug addiction, or multiple pregnancy). Chromosomal abnormalities and congenital malformations as well as intrauterine infections may also be contributing factors to intrauterine growth retardation (IUGR).

Intrauterine growth retardation may be of two types. If the stress occurs in the initial stage of growth (as with chromosomal abnormality and congenital malformation), mitosis is impaired, fewer new cells are formed, and the body organs are small and of subnormal weight. Individual cells have a normal amount of cytoplasm. If there is fetal malnutrition later in pregnancy (due to preeclampsia, smoking, or placental insufficiency, for example), the total number of cells will be normal but decreased in size because of lower amounts of cytoplasm. Most cases of IUGR fall into this category. If malnutrition occurs during the period of very rapid brain growth (the last few months of pregnancy), it may be associated with a permanent decrease in the total number of cells. In general, the brain, skeleton, heart, and lungs are least affected by IUGR, while the adrenals, liver, spleen, and thymus are likely to be smaller in size.

Infants who are SGA usually appear thin and wasted, with little subcutaneous tissue. Their skin is wrinkled, loose, often dry, frequently scaling, and commonly meconium-stained. Their umbilical cords may be withered, appearing dull, yellow, and dry. In extreme cases, the trunk (buttocks particularly) and extremities may not have as much musculature as would be expected. Usually the body length is not affected and the head size may be normal, although the hair on the head will be sparse, coarse, and longer than that of the preterm infant. The skull sutures may be wider than normal because of impaired bone growth. Infants who are SGA are usually alert, active, and seem hungry.

These babies are particularly subject to neonatal asphyxia, especially if they have been exposed to chronic intrauterine hypoxia. In utero or at birth they commonly aspirate amniotic fluid, which often contains meconium. With amniotic fluid aspiration, the fluid portion is absorbed by the pulmonary circulation, but the solid particles become lodged in the alveoli and small tubes leading to them. The debris causes mechanical obstruction, while the meconium, if present, is irritating and may cause an inflammation of the bronchial mucosa. Meconium aspiration may be complicated by pneumothorax due to partially blocked, overexpanded areas of the lungs. Pneumonia and pulmonary hemorrhage occur frequently.

The infant who has aspirated meconium may be depressed and require resuscitation. Gasping respirations are sometimes observed; the chest may appear enlarged; respirations are rapid; and rales may or may not be heard. The lungs can remove meconium rapidly and improvement is often marked after 48 hours [7].

Babies who are SGA may also have polycythemia, with a hematocrit of over 60 percent. The cause for this is unknown, although it may be related to hypoxia in utero. No specific congenital abnormalities are associated with SGA neonates. Both preterm and SGA babies are prone to suffer from hypoglycemia and heat loss.

Hypoglycemia

The SGA infant's hypoglycemia is a result of his limited or depleted glycogen stores, and gluconeogenesis in his undergrown liver may be inadequate to support his relatively well-grown brain. The preterm infant is prone to hypoglycemia because of increased energy consumption caused by hypothermia, anoxia, acidosis, or respiratory distress, any of which may exhaust his limited glycogen stores.

In utero, glucose is transferred across the placenta and is the main source of fetal energy. Hepatic gluconeogenesis probably does not occur in utero even though the necessary enzymes are present in the liver at birth. Fat catabolism in utero is not a significant energy source, and plasma free fatty acids exist at low levels.

The placenta begins to accumulate glycogen as early as the eighth week of gestation. As term approaches, glycogen is increasingly stored in the fetal liver and heart and not in the placenta. Such stores are essential to the infant's survival during labor and immediately after birth, but with intrauterine malnutrition or anoxia, they may either fail to accumulate or be utilized before birth [14].

At birth the placental glucose supply is abruptly cut off. At the same time energy demands increase, and the newborn's responses are directed at maintaining blood glucose levels. His system's first reaction is rapid glycogenolysis. Almost all the hepatic glycogen is used in the first 2 or 3 hours after birth. Gluconeogenesis, which begins in the first few hours, becomes increasingly important as a source of glucose for his brain. As the glucose is used, plasma free fatty acids begin to increase.

Newborn blood glucose levels at birth are approximately 60–70 milligrams per 100 milliliters. A rapid decline occurs for the first 2 hours; then the blood level rises to 50–60 milligrams per 100 milliliters at 4–6 hours. However, if the infant's temperature is low, his glucose level is likely to be 40–50 milligrams per 100 milliliters. At 4–6 hours after birth a low birth weight infant will have a glucose level of approximately 40 milligrams per 100 milliliters.

Hypoglycemic infants have blood glucose levels below 30 milligrams per 100 milliliters if they are full-term and below 20 milligrams per 100 milliliters if they are of low birth weight. To be diagnostic these values must appear in two sequential samples taken at least 1 hour apart during the first three days of life. After this, 40 milligrams per 100 milliliters is the diagnostic level. Clinical symptoms usually appear at these levels and are associated with jitteriness, cyanosis, convulsions, apnea, apathy, high-pitched or weak cry, limpness, refusal to feed, or temperature instability. If hypoglycemia is untreated, it may result in central nervous system damage of varying degrees. Treatment consists of careful observation, blood glucose determinations, and intravenous infusion of 50% glucose (1 milliliter per kilogram of body weight) followed by an infusion of 10% glucose. Hypoglycemic infants are fed as soon as possible after birth.

Heat Loss

Both SGA and preterm infants lack the insulating effect of subcutaneous fat, and as a result they are prone to lose heat rapidly. The preterm baby is particularly susceptible due to the poor development of his heat-regulating center and failure of his peripheral responses to heat and cold (sweating and shivering). His sluggish circulation, poor reflex control of skin capillaries, feeble respirations with poor oxygen consumption, muscular inactivity, and poor food intake are all contributing factors.

Temperature maintenance is even more difficult in a cool environment for the small preterm infant whose caloric intake is already limited by a small stomach capacity. Since fewer calories are required for maintenance of body temperature if the baby is kept in a warmer environment, he is placed in an incubator (isolette) where the environmental temperature can be regulated to keep his body temperature in the range 35.6°–37.2° C (96°–99° F).

While isolettes are expensive equipment, they supply correct heat, humidity, and concentration of oxygen to suit individual babies as well as save nursing time. They also allow easier observation of the baby from a distance. On the other hand, they allow the naked infant to lose heat by radiation, and their humidity reservoirs are probably one of the greatest sources of bacterial growth in the nursery. For this reason, the water is changed frequently or the reservoir is kept empty. Isolettes are kept scrupulously clean and the infant is moved to a new one at least every three days. Careful monitoring by an observant nurse is just as essential for infants in isolettes as for those in open cribs, and the same precautions for their safety and freedom from infection must be taken.

Currently temperature-control isolettes are being used frequently. These can provide a more sensitive temperature regulation, since their heating element is activated by a probe placed on the infant's anterior abdominal wall. Skin temperature is considered to be a more reliable index than rectal temperature, because the latter only increases or decreases when the infant's own thermostatic mechanism is failing. Unfortunately, an infant can become overheated in an isolette, particularly if it is placed in direct sunlight or if the servo-control temperature probe slips off his skin. Therefore, it is important that the infant's body temperature be adequately monitored.

Hypocalcemia

Hypocalcemia is often an additional problem of preterm infants as well as of those babies subjected to an abnormal intrauterine environment (e.g., maternal diabetes or hyperparathyroidism) or suffering from a postnatal infection. In fetal life the plasma levels of glucose and calcium are regulated by placental exchange. Perhaps as a result, the baby's regulatory mechanisms for both these substances are somewhat immature. He shows rapid changes in his plasma glucose, as already noted, and in his plasma calcium during the first days after birth, with a delay of one or two weeks before the levels characteristic of maturity are reached.

In utero, the fetus accumulates most of his calcium during the last trimester, so that 75 percent of the calcium in a full-term infant is acquired after the twenty-eighth week of gestation. Fetal calcium concentration is higher than the maternal concentration, and fetal calcification proceeds normally despite poor maternal nutrition and even placental insufficiency and fetal malnutrition. Therefore, SGA babies normally have adequate calcium stores at birth. The true preterm infant, however, has missed most of his intrauterine calcium accumulation and is born relatively calcium-deficient. In addition, the baby's immature kidney cannot reabsorb sufficient calcium from the tubules and responds poorly to parathyroid hormone, thereby causing retention of phosphate. As a result, the calcium level decreases and the phosphorus level increases during the first days after birth [14].

Certain factors besides the degree of prematurity and calcium deficiency in the bones tend to predispose the newborn to hypocalcemia. If the infant has been stressed due to obstetrical trauma or asphyxia, the endogenous corticosteroid his body releases will tend to decrease his serum calcium. If his acidosis is treated with bicarbonate, the ionized fraction of serum calcium will be decreased as a result. If his diet is low in calcium and high in phosphorus, the risk of hypocalcemia is increased. Cow's milk has a particularly high phosphorus level and a low calcium-to-phosphorus ratio, and the low dose of vitamin D in some commercial formulas encourages calcium transport into the bone and could potentiate a resulting hypocalcemia. If the infant has received an exchange transfusion with citrated blood, the ionized calcium level is likely to be decreased, whether or not calcium gluconate is given to him.

Symptoms of hypocalcemia are nonspecific in the newborn. Twitching, jitteriness, and convulsions are most frequent, followed by cyanosis and vomiting. Chvostek's and Trousseau's signs, which are present in older children with hypocalcemia, occur in only 20 percent of hypocalcemic neonates. Chvostek's sign in particular is not very reliable, since it is present in many normal newborns.

Hypocalcemia, defined as calcium levels below 7–7.5 milligrams per 100 milliliters, peaks on the first day after birth and again at around five or six days, particularly in infants being given cows' milk formula. After seven to ten days, most infants achieve a calcemia level of 9 milligrams per 100 milliliters. The incidence of hypocalcemia is said to be highest in late winter and early spring, presumably due to the increased maternal parathyroid activity to compensate for lack of sunlight and decreased vitamin D.

Treatment consists of a slow intravenous injection of calcium gluconate followed by a calcium preparation added to the formula. Unless the hypocalcemia results in convulsions, which are an immediate threat to life, there is usually no structural damage to the central nervous system associated with it.

Sequelae of Low Birth Weight

Preterm infants are likely to have lower average heights and weights than full-term babies of the same age during the first one or two years of life unless allowances are made for the length of gestation. A number of infants will take longer than that to reach average growth and development norms, and a few will never reach them, perhaps due to genetic causes or socioeconomic factors. Preterm infants are notoriously late within this time period in reaching developmental milestones—smiling, sitting without support, standing, walking, talking, and bladder control. Again, this developmental lag is largely eliminated if age is calculated from the estimated date of confinement. SGA babies are more likely to be mentally retarded than preterm infants because of the intrauterine anoxia to which they were subjected.

Other sequelae of premature birth have been itemized [1]. They include reduced intellectual ability, neurological deficits (spastic diplegia), vision and hearing difficulties, and a greater risk of infectious disease in the first year of life. The majority of premature infants are remarkably well adjusted and normal in behavior, although a short attention span, lack of confidence, and emotional instability were noted in some studies. Some of these findings may be the result of damage to the central nervous system, but others may result from an overprotective or rejecting attitude of the parents toward the child or may be due to the innate personality characteristics of the individual.

POSTMATURITY

An infant is postmature if he is born during or after the forty-second week of gestation. By this definition, approximately 12 percent of all pregnancies are prolonged. The postmature infant may be appropriately sized but quite often he is SGA because of a decrease in placental function. In this case he may actually have a wasted appearance. Vernix is virtually absent from his loose skin, which becomes dry, cracked, and parchment-like soon after birth. His subcutaneous fat is likely to be decreased so that his body appears thin and long. Frequently his long nails, skin, and cord are meconium-stained. Usually he has a profuse amount of long scalp hair. He appears alert and wide-eyed, indicating chronic intrauterine hypoxia. As a result of this, perinatal mortality is higher for postmature infants than for full-term infants [8].

Approximately 75–85 percent of the deaths among postmature babies occur during the stress of labor. Often the infant's oxygen supply was marginal for days before delivery. When postmaturity is suspected, maternal urinary estriol determinations and oxytocin challenge tests are often used as an index of fetal well-being and placental function so that measures may be taken to deliver the baby before the stress becomes too great.

HEMOLYTIC DISORDERS

Hemolytic disease in the newborn is a result of fetal erythrocyte antigens' gaining access to the maternal circulation. The mother's body responds by producing antibodies, which may then cross the placenta, attach themselves to fetal cells bearing the antigen, and cause these cells to be removed from the fetal circulation; they are subsequently destroyed. Stevenson [12] noted that at least 50 genetically determined erythrocyte agglutinogens exist, and that maternal-fetal incompatibility for one or more of these antigens probably occurs in all pregnancies. Fortunately, not all agglutinogens are sufficiently antigenic to result in clinically significant isoimmunization. The Rh and ABO antigens evoke a strong response and therefore are the most important.

Rh Incompatibility

What is commonly referred to as the Rh (rhesus) antigen is found on the erythrocytes of 85 percent of all Caucasians, approximately 95 percent of all black people, and virtually all Orientals. Rh is really not one antigen but a group of six antigens designated as C, D, E, c, d, e. Because of the strong antigenicity of D, individuals are classified as Rh-negative or Rh-positive according to whether or not they possess this particular antigen.

In order for hemolytic disease to become a problem for the fetus or infant, the fetus must possess the antigen (Rh +) on his erythrocytes while his mother does not (Rh −). The father of the baby must be either homozygous for the gene (DD) or heterozygous (Dd) in order for the infant to inherit the antigen. The fetal antigen in turn must reach the maternal circulation and produce an antibody response. Fetal transfusion of 0.5 milliliter or more will produce primary maternal sensitization, while after this, smaller amounts will evoke an antibody response. In addition to occurring with a pregnancy, sensitization may also follow an abortion or an improperly matched blood transfusion.

In order for the fetus to be affected, the maternal antibody must cross the placenta. In Rh immunization, the IgG fraction of these antibodies is readily transferred to the fetus, attaching to his Rh-positive erythrocytes. The red blood cells are then removed from his circulation—primarily by the spleen—and destroyed. With the destruction of many of his erythrocytes, the fetus becomes anemic. The excessive bilirubin resulting from the erythrocyte breakdown leaves him with hyperbilirubinemia. If the anemia is severe, the fetus or infant may have cardiac failure and generalized edema. In an effort to compensate for the anemia, hematopoietic tissue in the fetus' liver and spleen becomes active, partially explaining why these organs become enlarged.

If the fetus is severely affected (hydrops fetalis), his hematopoietic tissue cannot compensate for the anemia. He may be stillborn, or, if born alive, suffer from severe anemia, generalized edema, and cardiac failure.

In most cases, however, the fetus or infant is not so severely compromised but must still cope with hyperbilirubinemia. With rapid hemoglobin breakdown, the rate of bilirubin production exceeds the capacity of the infant's liver to conjugate it. Normally, the bilirubin is transported via albumin to the liver, where hepatic cells conjugate it with glucuronic acid, changing it to a water-soluble form. The conjugated form (direct bilirubin) again attaches to albumin for transport through the circulation and excretion by the kidneys. With very rapid breakdown of the erythrocytes, excessive amounts of unconjugated bilirubin (indirect bilirubin) accumulate in the blood, rapidly attaching to the albumin for transport. Once the albumin binding sites are saturated, the excess unconjugated bilirubin remains free. This fraction is fat-soluble and diffuses across vascular membranes into tissues, especially those of the brain. Bilirubin deposits in the brain (kernicterus) produce irreversible damage.

Usually on the first prenatal visit a woman's blood type and Rh factor are determined. If she is Rh-negative, a serum screening test for antibodies is done. Even if no antibodies are detected, the screening may be repeated at monthly intervals throughout the pregnancy.

Since the intensity of the disease is likely to be greater with rising serum titers, generally the higher the titer, the more dangerous the outcome for the infant. Chances for the infant's survival have been reported to be excellent if the mother's titer is 1:64 or less; however, when it rises above this, chances of his survival decrease [6]. The use of antibody titers to accurately predict fetal outcome is limited. Antibodies may not rise significantly in some severe cases, and occasionally a mother's titer may rise even though she carries an Rh-negative fetus. While some physicians still feel that serum antibody titers are of value in predicting fetal prognosis, many now feel that they serve only to indicate whether or not the mother is sensitized. Since the bilirubin levels rise in the amniotic fluid of an affected fetus, amniocentesis is now used more frequently to determine fetal prognosis.

Since the mother must have prior sensitization with antibody formation in order for the fetus to be affected, first pregnancies are usually not associated with problems. If an Rh-negative primigravida has previously become sensitized, perhaps by incompatible blood transfusion, an amniocentesis will be performed at approximately 28 weeks' gestation. For women who have shown moderate to severe sensitization previously, the procedure is performed earlier.

Amniotic fluid is analyzed for the breakdown products produced during erythrocyte destruction, mainly bilirubin. The amount of blood pigments in the amniotic fluid closely parallels the severity of the hemolytic process. When analyzed using a spectrophotometer, a spectral absorption curve is obtained by plotting optical density against the wavelength of visible light spectrum. The breakdown products of hemoglobin absorb monochromatic light at a wavelength range of 400–500 millimicrons, with the cumulative peak seen at 450 millimicrons. Using this technique researchers have developed a number of graphs that are used to predict the severity of the hemolytic disease. The graph proposed by Liley (Figure 17-8) contains three zones: Zone A indicates mild or no hemolytic disease; zone B, moderate disease; and zone C, severe disease. A moderately affected fetus (zone B) has a good chance of survival if labor is induced at 35–37 weeks of gestation, or if delivery by cesarean section is performed at 36–37 weeks if induction of labor fails. A severely affected fetus (zone C) may require delivery as early as 33 weeks if death is to be avoided [10]. Those fetuses severely affected prior to a time of viability may be transfused in utero to prevent fetal death.

In utero transfusion is indicated when the fetus is severely affected (Liley's zone C) and will die prior to 32–34 weeks of pregnancy if not transfused. A minimum of 5 hours prior to transfusion, 10–15 milliliters of a radiopaque contrast medium is injected into the amniotic fluid. The fetus swallows the medium, thus providing an outline of his intestines on x-ray 5–24 hours later. Using local anesthesia, the physician passes an open lumen needle through the mother's abdominal and uterine walls into the fetal abdominal cavity. After further x-rays to confirm the position of the needle, polyethylene tubing is threaded through the needle into the fetal abdomen and the needle is removed. With a three-way stopcock attached to the catheter,

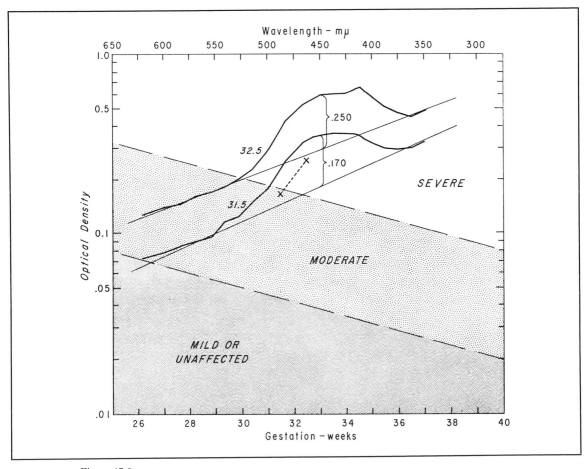

Wavelength – mµ

Figure 17-8.
Spectophotometric analysis of amniotic fluid of an erythroblastotic fetus taken at 31.5 and 32.5 weeks' gestation. Analysis indicates progression from moderate to severe disease. The infant will be delivered if mature; if not, he may receive an intrauterine transfusion. (From S. G. Babson and R. Benson. Management of High-Risk Pregnancy and Intensive Care of the Neonate. St. Louis: Mosby, 1971.)

50–150 milliliters of packed red cells are injected into the fetus over a two-hour period. The packed red cells are from freshly drawn O-negative blood that is compatible with the mother's blood. The amount injected depends on the estimated fetal weight. Since the fetus is now being maintained on transfused blood, transfusions may be repeated every 7–10 days until a total of about 350 milliliters is given or until the fetus is believed to have a good chance of survival if delivered.

The erythrocytes are absorbed from the fetal peritoneal cavity, elevating the fetal hemoglobin and preventing cardiac failure and generalized edema. The fetus who is already hydroptic, as evidenced by thickening of the scalp on x-ray, does not benefit from the procedure, and it is felt that it should be reserved for fetuses that are not so severely affected. The incidence of maternal complications from the procedure is 2–3 percent from hemorrhage, infection, and further sensitization because of damaged placenta. Fetal loss is 10–15 percent due to cardiac failure (overload), infection, serum jaundice, and needle trauma.

At birth, a sample of cord blood from infants of Rh-negative mothers is routinely sent to the laboratory. Samples of anticoagulated blood are used for hemoglobin and hematocrit measurements, reticulocyte count, white blood cell count, and blood smears. Clotted blood samples are used for blood typing, Coombs' test, and measurements of serum bilirubin. The umbilical cord is clamped as early as possible during delivery to avoid the infant's receiving extra antibodies and erythrocytes from the placenta. Should he receive them, these extra erythrocytes place an added strain on his liver's conjugating system when they are broken down. The umbilical cord is usually left about 10 centimeters (4 inches) long to facilitate introduction of umbilical catheters in case exchange transfusions become necessary in the next few days.

The infant is carefully observed for signs of pallor, jaundice, and an enlarged liver and spleen. The jaundice, which commonly appears during the first 24 hours, may be evident in the sclera, umbilical cord, skin, and mucous membrane. With increasing jaundice, the infant may appear lethargic and feed poorly, and his activity and muscle tone may decrease. As the bilirubin levels climb, signs of central nervous system irritability develop; the infant has a high-pitched cry, muscle spasticity, retraction of the head, and later, convulsions.

In order to avoid central nervous system involvement, serum bilirubin levels are carefully monitored. Generally infants do not exhibit signs of kernicterus if bilirubin levels remain below 18–20 milligrams per 100 milliliters of blood. However, the pre-term infant whose liver is especially immature may develop symptoms at levels as low as 9 milligrams per 100 milliliters of blood [2].

The amount of free bilirubin may be increased if hypoxia, acidosis, hypothermia, or hypoglycemia occurs. In acidosis the binding of albumin is impaired. In hypothermia and hypoglycemia, the level of nonesterified fatty acids increases, and the acids then compete with bilirubin for the albumin-binding sites. Low albumin levels increase the danger of kernicterus. Sulfonamides and salicylates compete with bilirubin for protein-binding sites, and caffeine sodium benzoate uncouples bilirubin from albumin. To determine the infant's albumin binding capacity, HBABA 2-(4-hydroxybenzeneazo) benzoic acid determinations may be done [15]. If the binding capacity is high, the infant should be able to handle increased amounts of bilirubin.

Infants who are born with a positive Coombs' test, a cord hemoglobin of 14 grams per 100 milliliters of blood or less, and a cord unconjugated bilirubin level of 4.5 milligrams per 100 milliliters of blood or more need exchange transfusion. Infants whose bilirubin levels indicate a rise of more than 0.5 milligram per 100 milliliters of blood per hour during the first 48 hours of life or whose bilirubin levels are projected to exceed 20 milligrams per 100 milliliters, need treatment [10]. O-negative compatible blood, 500 milliliters, is used for exchange transfusion. It is preferable to have freshly drawn blood, since 110 milliliters of acid citrate dextrose added to a pint of blood to preserve it lowers the albumin and erythrocyte volume. It also contributes to the production of postexchange hypoglycemia by stimulating insulin secretion.

While receiving an exchange transfusion, the infant is placed in an incubator or on a working surface with a radiant overhead heater so that his temperature is carefully maintained. A piece of plastic tubing is placed in his umbilical vein. The other end of the tubing contains an adaptor (Tuohy) and two stopcocks. One stopcock is connected to a bag of blood and the other to a bottle for collecting the waste blood. Five to 20 milliliters of blood is injected into the infant at a time, depending on his size and condition, and the same amount is withdrawn and discarded after each injection. His apical rate is monitored continuously and his respirations and skin color are meticulously observed. A pacifier can be used during the procedure to keep the infant from crying. After transfusion of each 100 milliliters of blood, 0.5–1 milliliter of 10% calcium gluconate solution is given intravenously to prevent hypocalcemia. At least 500 milliliters of blood should be used for each exchange transfusion to ensure removal of 90 percent of the infant's erythrocytes and Rh antibodies (Figure 17-9).

While the exchange transfusion corrects the anemia, decreases the bilirubin level, and removes Rh antibodies, the procedure is not without complications. Mortality has been reported to be as high as 5 percent, but a significant portion of these deaths were of already moribund, hydropic, and kernicteric infants. Complications from the procedure include air or thrombotic emboli; sepsis, hypothermia, bradycardia, or cardiac arrest from low pH of donor blood; heart failure from hypervolemia or hypovolemia; and hypocalcemia from citrate binding.

An alternate way to reduce increased bilirubin levels is by the use of phototherapy (Figure 17-10). Although it does not eliminate the need to perform exchange transfusions on all infants, it does eliminate the need for some and reduces the number of transfusions needed for others [9]. Light therapy can reduce serum levels of uncon-

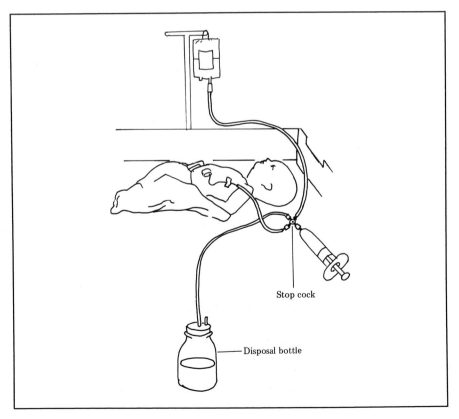

Stop cock

Disposal bottle

Figure 17-9. Infant receiving an exchange transfusion.

Figure 17-10. Infant receiving phototherapy. The infants eyes are well protected from the light rays, which may cause retinal damage. (Courtesy of Thomas Jefferson University, Philadelphia, Pa.)

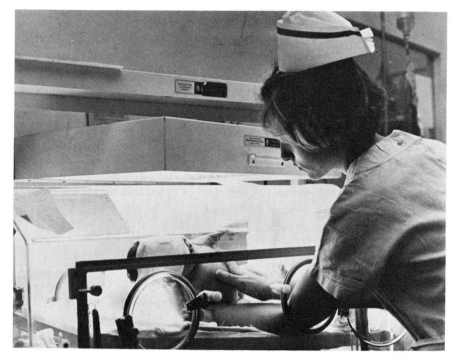

Figure 17-10. Infant receiving phototherapy. The infants eyes are well protected from the light rays, which may cause retinal damage. (Courtesy of Thomas Jefferson University, Philadelphia, Pa.)

jugated bilirubin by as much as 25–50 percent. Bilirubin is photo-oxidized to biliverdin, then to secondary yellow pigments, and finally to colorless, presumably nontoxic compounds [1]. The exact intensity of illumination to be used in phototherapy is inexact, but the general recommendation is continuous exposure of the naked infant to 200–400 footcandles of fluorescent white light, daylight, or light from blue bulbs. The average decrease of bilirubin should be 3–4 milligrams of serum indirect bilirubin in 8–12 hours.

To prevent retinal damage, the eyes should be protected from the light rays by the use of cotton and gauze pads, with a head bandage to keep them in place. It is essential that the bandage cover the eyes but keep the eyeballs free of pressure. It is also essential that the infant's bilirubin and hemoglobin levels be carefully monitored, for the changes in skin color may mask increasing levels of bilirubin and anemia. Loose stools, rashes, and changes in activity are common side effects of light therapy. Overheating may also occur as a result of heat production from the light. Since little is known about the long-term effects of light therapy, it should not be used prophylactically or indiscriminately.

In women who have not yet become sensitized, Rh sensitivity can be prevented by the use of Rh_0 (D) immune globulin (RhoGAM), which confers passive immunity to the woman by neutralizing the Rh-positive antigen. When given within 72 hours after delivery it neutralizes and later destroys the Rh-positive antigen of the fetal erythrocytes that have entered the mother's circulation during delivery. Her own immune system is therefore not activated. The globulin will remain for several months, and during that period she will have positive antibody titers which gradually decrease in potency. The immunization must be repeated after each delivery or abortion of an Rh-positive fetus. RhoGAM is not effective for and should not be given to a woman who is already sensitized. Therefore, mothers must have a negative Coombs' test prior to its administration. Crossmatching is also done to ensure compatibility of the anti-D preparation and the mother's own erythrocytes.

While hemolytic disease most commonly occurs in response to the Rh D antigen, it can also occur in response to c(hr), C (rh), E (rh), and e(hr), or in response to the ABO blood-group antigens.

ABO Incompatibility

While ABO incompatability occurs more often than Rh incompatibility during pregnancies, its clinical problems are far less severe. Antibodies formed against A and B antigens are of two immunoglobulin fractions. A naturally occurring type (IgM) is formed in response to a variety of antigenic stimuli (e.g., food proteins). This type does not cross the placental barrier. The second type, an immune one (IgG), does cross the barrier. Mothers with type-O blood usually produce anti-A and anti-B antibodies of the IgG type that pass through the placenta to the fetus, causing hemolysis of the fetal erythrocytes if fetal blood type is A, B, or AB.

Mothers with type A or B blood produce anti-B or anti-A antibodies of the IgM variety. It is believed that certain amounts of immune types (IgG) of anti-A or anti-B antibody may exist at all times in the circulation of type-O mothers and therefore may cross the placenta during a woman's first pregnancy. This explains why the firstborn children represent 40–50 percent of the cases of ABO disease. The next born is usually affected less than the first. The reasons for this are unknown. Most cases of ABO incompatability occur with a woman whose blood type is O, while her fetus' blood type is A or B.

The infant with ABO incompatability may become jaundiced within the first 24 hours after birth, but his anemia is usually not as severe as that seen with Rh incompatability. There is usually no pallor or cardiovascular stress in the infant. After birth, antibody may be detected by the Coombs' test. Treatment is the same as that for the infant with hyperbilirubinemia due to Rh; however, exchange transfusion is rarely necessary.

NEONATAL INFECTIONS

Asymptomatic maternal infection usually precedes fetal infection, which occurs antepartally or intrapartally. Modes of transmission are through infected amniotic fluid, from the maternal bloodstream across the placenta, or from direct contact with infected maternal tissue in the birth canal. Physical signs are unique in their subtlety and lack of specificity. Although antibiotics are the mainstay of therapy for infections in the newborn, supportive therapy is also essential to meet normal infant needs. It includes the maintenance of body temperature, the administration of oxygen as indicated, and administration of fluids to maintain normal fluid, electrolyte, and acid-base balance, as well as the interaction necessary for the foundation of a basic trust relationship.

Bacterial Infections

Bacterial agents are responsible for three major clinical disorders—pneumonia, septicemia, and meningitis. Gram-negative rods cause 75–85 percent of bacterial infections and *Escherichia coli* is the predominant organism. *Pseudomonas aeruginosa,* often found growing on nursery equipment, is the next common causative organism. The remaining 15–25 percent of major infections are caused most often by gram-positive cocci, of which streptococci and staphylococci predominate.

Bacterial infections may be acquired in utero, during the infant's descent through the birth canal or after birth in the delivery room or nursery. Most are of the ascending type, resulting in amniotic fluid infection following passage of bacteria from the perineum, vagina, or both through a ruptured amniotic membrane. Sometimes, however, the organisms pass through an intact membrane. From the amniotic fluid they gain entry to the fetus, primarily through the oral cavity, and move to the lungs, gastrointestinal tract, and middle ear, although their presence in the amniotic fluid does not necessarily mean that the fetus will become infected. Since early rupture of membranes predisposes the fetus to exposure to intrauterine infection, it is better if delivery can be accomplished within 24 hours of the rupture. If an infection is suspected in the newborn, the best sites for specimen collections for culture are the throat, axillae, inguinal folds, or external auditory canals, preferably 1–2 hours after birth [8].

In general, if the infection is manifested during the first 48 hours, it is likely to have been congenitally acquired (most likely caused by coliforms and group-B streptococci) and is best treated with kanamycin or gentamicin and ampicillin. Onset at a later age is usually related to hospital-acquired organisms (*Staphylococcus* and *Pseudomonas*). The best treatment in this case is a combination of polymyxin and nafcillin or gentamicin and nafcillin.

PNEUMONIA

Pneumonia is the most common of the serious neonatal infections and has been given as a cause of death in 10–20 percent of autopsies. The peak incidence is during the second and third days after birth. Congenital pneumonia is commonly associated with obstetrical abnormalities such as premature rupture of membranes, uncomplicated premature delivery, prolonged labor, and maternal infection. The bacteria most frequently involved are *E. coli* and other enteric organisms, staphylococci, and group-B streptococci. Symptoms, which are evident at birth or within 48 hours after birth, include rapid, shallow respirations, slight retractions, apnea, pallor or cyanosis, and flaccidity. Crepitant rales are sometimes detectable. Body temperature is likely to be elevated in a full-term infant, whereas a preterm baby may have a subnormal temperature.

If the infection is acquired postnatally, *Pseudomonas* is the most common cause along with penicillin-resistant staphylococci and enteric organisms. Clinical signs appearing 48 hours after birth or later include tachypnea and poor feeding or aspiration during feeding. Recovery is more common from this type of pneumonia than from the congenitally acquired variety [8].

SEPTICEMIA

Septicemia is a generalized infection that is characterized by growth of bacteria in the infant's bloodstream. Presently, coliform organisms are the most frequent cause. Early symptoms are vague and nonspecific—loss of appetite, inactivity, loss of weight, vomiting, diarrhea, abdominal distention, abnormal respirations, jaundice, or skin lesions. Meningitis occurs in about one-third of these infants. Septicemia is usually diagnosed from a blood culture, although centrifuged spinal fluid or urine is sometimes used. When the identity of the causative organism is unknown, kanamycin (Kantrex), or gentamicin (Garamycin), and ampicillin may be given immediately. The use of antibiotics has decreased mortality from septicemia from 90 percent to a range of 13–45 percent [8].

MENINGITIS

Almost half of the cases of meningitis in children occur during the first year of life, with the highest incidence occurring in the neonatal period, most frequently in preterm and male infants. Causative organisms are the same as those for septicemia, and the systemic symptoms are similar. Fullness of the anterior fontanelle is the most specific sign, while neck stiffness (Kernig's sign) is rare in the neonate. Opisthotonos may be seen in about 25 percent of infected infants, and coma and convulsions, in about 50 percent.

Diagnosis of meningitis is confirmed by abnormalities in the spinal fluid. Treatment is the same as for septicemia. Fatality rates from meningitis are high—60–75 percent—and the majority of survivors have some form of central nervous system handicap [8].

DIARRHEA

Diarrhea is another important bacterial infection most frequently caused by *E. coli,* although *Salmonella, Shigella,* and *Staphylococcus* are sometimes involved. *E. coli* and *Salmonella* infections produce a stool that is green and slimy, while *Shigella* infections produce watery stools that lack odor and have blood-tinged mucus in them. Early symptoms of the infection are loss of appetite, weight loss, and listlessness—all of which may precede diarrhea by one or two days. *Shigella* infections tend to start explosively. As diarrhea continues, the infant becomes dehydrated and acidotic (metabolic acidosis), and the process is more rapid if vomiting is also present. Milder forms of infectious diarrhea are not unusual.

Diarrheal stools should be cultured as soon as they appear. Neomycin or polymyxin is commonly administered orally before the results of the culture are returned. Diarrhea can become epidemic in a nursery, since the organisms are easily transferred from baby to baby, particularly from unwashed hands of personnel and from gowns; therefore, scrupulous aseptic technique is absolutely essential. In addition, any abnormal stools in infants should be reported, so that isolation precautions may be taken if necessary.

Because these babies may not be given to their mothers to be fed, it is important that nurses keep the parents informed about their baby's status. Since the changes in the appearance of an infant who has diarrhea can be quite startling and anxiety-provoking, the parents will need extra support in coping with this additional stress.

OMPHALITIS

Omphalitis, infection of the umbilical stump, causes the umbilical area to become edematous and red, with a purulent exudate (in mild forms there usually is no exudate). Cultures of the blood and umbilicus should be done. Since omphalitis may herald septicemia, treatment for this infection should be initiated immediately.

SYPHILIS

Untreated syphilis during pregnancy is a major cause of abortion, fetal death in utero, and premature labor and delivery. If the maternal infection is treated before the fifth month of pregnancy, it is unlikely that the fetus will be affected; it is believed that the placental membrane only becomes permeable to *Treponema pallidum* after that time. In addition, since penicillin crosses the placenta, treatment of the mother almost always successfully treats the fetus also. As a screening device, a serologic test for syphilis (STS) is commonly included in the examination a mother receives at her first prenatal visit. Penicillin is also the treatment of choice for the neonate who shows signs of rhinitis, skin eruptions of the copper-colored macular variety, and x-ray evidence of osteochondritis or periostitis.

Rhinitis (snuffles), caused by a swelling of the nasal mucous membrane, is one of the most frequent signs of congenital syphilis. It tends to make breathing and sucking difficult and is accompanied by a profuse nasal discharge that is extremely irritating to the skin it contacts. Skin lesions may appear on all or part of the infant's body. The palms of his hands and soles of his feet are commonly affected, becoming erythematous, swollen, and peeling. Fissures may appear in all directions about the mouth, anus, and vulva. Infection of the central nervous system occurs in approximately one-third of all syphilitic infants, and a large proportion of such babies have splenomegaly.

Symptoms in early infancy correspond to secondary stages of syphilis in the adult. If he is untreated, the child will show other manifestations of disease later, such as condylomas, peg-shaped and notched (Hutchinson's) incisor teeth, nerve deafness, pupillary abnormalities, tabes, paralysis, and dementia.

Diagnosis of syphilis in the newborn is made on detection of spirochetes in the nasal discharge, open skin ulcers, and a positive *Treponema pallidum* inhibition test (TPI). The TPI test offers more conclusive evidence of true infection than the STS, which may react positively to maternal antibodies that have been transmitted across the placenta to the infant. Usually these antibodies disappear within three or four months.

Since the nasal discharge and exudate from skin lesions is potentially contagious, it is wise to observe good isolation technique, including the use of gloves when working with the infected infant. Although the need for additional therapy beyond the initial treatment is remote, generally it is agreed that children should be followed for one or two years after treatment.

SKIN INFECTION—IMPETIGO

Impetigo contagiosa is a bacterial skin infection caused by streptococci or staphylococci that invade the superficial layers of the skin. It tends to spread from one spot to another and is easily transmitted to other persons by direct or indirect contact, so isolation precautions are essential. The skin vesicles, which are most likely to develop in body folds, creases, and moist surfaces, contain purulent material and rupture easily, with the exudate forming a crust that eventually drops off. Because of continued auto-inoculation, the lesions may persist for several weeks. When the infection occurs in the newborn (pemphigus neonatorum), large blisters form over the skin.

Antibiotic ointments are usually quite effective in the treatment of impetigo; they are applied at least twice daily to areas that cannot be protected by a dressing. Before application of the ointment, crusts of the lesions are removed by washing them gently with warm saline solution.

Viral Infections

Viral infections in the newborn occur less frequently than bacterial ones. Generally they are transmitted from the mother, but they may be acquired after birth. Many of the infants who survive these infections are left with varying degrees of damage to the central nervous system. The most common viral infections are caused by rubella, cytomegalovirus, and herpesvirus.

CONGENITAL RUBELLA SYNDROME

Rubella causes a chronic infection of the fetus and neonate that begins in the first trimester of pregnancy and may persist for months after birth. Some infants may harbor the virus for as long as three months or more, and if pregnant women who are not immunized are exposed to them, they run the risk of becoming infected themselves.

It is estimated that about 10–20 percent of pregnant women are susceptible to rubella. A history of having or not having had the infection is often unreliable, since the clinical signs mimic other viral infections and in many cases infected older children and adults are asymptomatic. Serology is the best diagnostic method, and among the various serologic procedures, the test for hemagglutination inhibition (HI) is the most sensitive one. The presence of HI antibody in serum indicates immunity to rubella. A minimum fourfold rise in titer is necessary to diagnose the infection. Since the HI test is not easy to perform, it should be done by properly trained personnel. It would be disastrous to erroneously tell a susceptible pregnant woman that she is immune, or vice versa.

Because the teratogenic effect of rubella occurs almost exclusively during the first trimester of pregnancy, the exposed pregnant woman should find out as soon as possible whether or not she is immune to the infection. A sample of her serum should be collected immediately for rubella HI titer, and if results are strongly positive, no further test is necessary. If the antibody titer is low or if the original test is sero-negative, a second sample is tested three weeks later. A fourfold rise or more in HI titer or its initial appearance signifies recent infection and the possibility of damage to the fetus.

In general, maternal infection in the first month of pregnancy causes infection and congenital malformations in 33–50 percent of exposed fetuses; in the second month, 25 percent; and in the third month, 9 percent. If the mother becomes in-fected in her fourth month, only about 4 percent of the fetuses are affected, primar-ily by permanent hearing impairment. The chief clinical signs of congenital infec-tion are hypoplastic intrauterine growth retardation, congenital heart disease, and cataracts. The most common cardiac malformations are patent ductus arteriosus and narrowing of the peripheral pulmonary arteries. In a few cases there may be severe myocardial degeneration. Cataracts, which may be unilateral or bilateral, are usually present at birth but sometimes do not appear for a few days or weeks. Mi-crophthalmia and glaucoma are other eye abnormalities that may develop.

Thrombocytopenia and petechiae occur in 40–80 percent of infected infants. Hepatosplenomegaly is common, and hyperbilirubinemia due to hemolysis is fre-quent. Sometimes rubella hepatitis develops, and pneumonia is not uncommon. Neurological abnormalities, which are present in a few neonates, most often appear later in infancy.

The diagnosis of congenital rubella is indicated by the combination of cataracts and congenital heart disease in the neonate. Although elevated IgM levels are not always detectable at birth, serologic diagnosis is possible by demonstrating the rubella antibody in the serum immunoglobulin M (IgM) [8].

The best method of treatment is prevention, by having all women of childbearing age vaccinated against the infection. If a woman is diagnosed as having rubella during early pregnancy, therapeutic abortion is an alternative for some parents to consider if they do not want to take the chance of having an abnormal infant. Since infected babies can communicate the virus to others, the immune status of female nursery personnel of childbearing age should be determined at the time of their employment. If they are susceptible, they should be vaccinated.

CYTOMEGALOVIRUS INFECTION

Congenital infection caused by the cytomegalovirus may be transmitted from asymptomatic mothers across the placenta or by the ascending cervical route. The results of a congenital infection range from extensive tissue damage that is incompatible with life, particularly if the infection has occurred early in preg-nancy, to survival with serious brain damage or survival with a total absence of sequelae.

An infant who has this infection is often SGA and hypoplastic. The principal tissues and organs affected are the blood, brain, and liver. Hemolysis leads to anemia and hyperbilirubinemia, and thrombocytopenia with petechiae and ecchymoses occurs frequently. Hepatosplenomegaly is common. Encephalitis with signs ranging from lethargy to hyperactivity and convulsions may result. Microcephaly may be present at birth, and 10–20 percent of symptomatic infants will have chorioretinitis.

Diagnosis involves recovery of the virus from the urine, elevated IgM levels, and identification of cytomegalovirus antibodies within the serum IgM fraction. Of the antiviral drugs used in treatment of this infection, none as yet have been proved particularly effective [8].

HERPESVIRUS INFECTION

About 95 percent of neonatal infections with the herpesvirus are due to type 2, which causes most infections involving the cervix, vagina, and external genitalia. (Type 1 causes lip lesions in older children and adults and skin lesions above the waist.) The infant is infected either when the organism ascends into the uterus or by direct contact during his passage through the birth canal, in a manner similar to infection by gonorrhea. Infection by the transplacental route is rare.

Neonatal herpesvirus infection presents a wide array of clinical signs. One variety of the infection is usually fatal to almost all affected infants; it involves the adrenals, liver, brain, blood, and lung. Symptoms, which are present at birth or by three or four weeks of age, include fever, hepatosplenomegaly, hepatitis with jaundice, a bleeding tendency, and neurological abnormalities. Vesicular skin lesions indicative of the disease are seen in about one-third of the infected infants. They appear occasionally in clusters and are thinly spread over the entire body.

Other, more localized varieties of neonatal herpesvirus infection are less severe, resulting in death in about 25 percent of the cases. The central nervous system, eyes, and skin are most commonly affected, either singly or together. Over one-half of the infants who survive have residual neurological or visual damage. Clinical signs include convulsions, abnormal muscle tone, opisthotonos, bulging fontanelle, and lethargy or coma. Eye signs include conjunctivitis, chorioretinitis, and a cloudy cornea (keratitis). Sometimes skin lesions are the only manifestation of the infection.

When there are no skin lesions, diagnosis is often difficult, since the symptoms are otherwise nonspecific and very similar to those of septicemia. The most reliable diagnostic procedures are cultures of the virus from the baby's skin lesions and throat and identification of herpes antibodies in the serum IgM fraction. Systemic treatment with idoxuridine has been used with success in some infants and with failure in others. Research is being done to determine its effectiveness [8].

Protozoan Infection

Toxoplasmosis, the most common protozoan infection, is transmitted to the fetus transplacentally, particularly during the second and third trimesters. The mother, who may be asymptomatic, usually contracts the organism from eating raw or poorly cooked meat or by contact with infected animals. Signs, which appear at birth or soon after, include neurological abnormalities such as convulsions, coma, hypotonia, microcephaly, or hydrocephalus. The infected infant may also have intracranial calcifications, chorioretinitis, microphthalmia, hepatosplenomegaly, jaundice, petechiae, ecchymoses (thrombocytopenia), and pallor (anemia). The fatality rate is about 12 percent; neurological disorders in survivors are common. Toxoplasmosis is diagnosed by demonstration of specific antibodies in serum IgM [8]. More information is needed on the potential value of therapy for pregnant women and newborns who are diagnosed as having toxoplasmosis.

DRUG ADDICTION

While the addicted mother faces multiple problems, approximately 50 percent of the live-born infants of mothers who use "hard" drugs experience symptoms of neonatal addiction. Maternal use of 6–12 milligrams of heroin daily will usually result in withdrawal symptoms in the newborn. In addition, many newborns, half in some populations, have birth weights of less than 2500 grams (5.5 pounds). A significant portion of these babies (40 percent in some populations) are full-term infants who are SGA. The perinatal mortality in these groups ranges from 15 to 20 percent [1, 4, 10], with the infants succumbing to respiratory difficulties, intracranial hemorrhage, inadequate hydration, electrolyte imbalance, and congenital anomalies. Recent studies show a mortality of 3–4.5 percent in rigorously treated infants [5].

The higher the daily dose of narcotic, the longer the mother has had her habit, and the closer to delivery she had her last "fix," the greater the chances are that her infant will have withdrawal symptoms. Most infants (60 percent) show withdrawal symptoms within 24 hours, practically all within four days. Rarely, an infant will show symptoms 7–10 days after birth. Excitement of the autonomic nervous system and gastrointestinal and respiratory distress are the most common signs of withdrawal in the newborn (Table 17-3). Two complications that addicted infants appear to be spared are RDS and jaundice. Heroin and phenobarbital are believed to increase bilirubin glucoronyl transferase activity, thus decreasing the incidence of jaundice. Heroin, thought to be an important enzyme inducer, also is reported to speed maturation of pulmonary function [13]. If the health care team is not aware of the mother's addiction, neonatal diagnosis may present a problem, since many of these signs are the same as those found with sepsis, hypocalcemia, hypoglycemia, and cerebral hemorrhage (Figure 17-11).

Once symptoms appear, treatment with chlorpromazine, phenobarbital, diazepam, methadone, or paregoric is begun (Table 17-4). In addition to drug therapy, the infant is given supportive treatment. Because of his increased activity, his caloric requirements are increased. Small frequent feedings of a concentrated formula may be given, since larger feedings may not be retained. In the very ill infant, parenteral feeding may be necessary to prevent aspiration and dehydration. With adequate therapy, the infant will decrease crying and activity, begin sleeping between feedings, maintain a normal temperature, and begin to gain weight.

In attempting to combat the problems of addicted mothers, health care professionals have organized methadone maintenance programs for them. Mothers who participate in these programs generally receive better prenatal care, and as a rule their newborns fare better than those of the street addict. The infants' hospital stays are shorter, and the mothers have shown improved attention to child care.

Table 17-3. Common Signs and Care of Addicted Infants

Infant Behavior	Intervention
Hypertonicity	Observe body prominences for skin breakdown Use sheepskin Change position frequently Check temperature because of increased activity; if it is elevated, decrease environmental temperature
Tachypnea	Watch for signs of progressive respiratory distress Hyperextend head to assure patent airway Maintain in semi-Fowler's position Maintain warmth
Sneezing and nasal stuffiness	Observe for respiratory distress Suction as necessary Feed slowly, allowing for periods of rest as necessary
Poor feeding	Observe sucking quality Feed small amounts frequently
Inability to sleep	Observe character of sleeping pattern Reduce environmental stimuli Swaddle Feed frequently
Fist sucking	Observe fingers and hands for skin breakdown Keep skin area clean Apply mittens
Regurgitation, vomiting, or diarrhea	Observe for character, occurrence, or precipitating factor (medication, handling) Observe for fluid and electrolyte balance Maintain side-lying position to prevent aspiration Give good skin care Maintain fluid balance
Tremors or convulsions	Observe character, location, frequency, and any predisposing factor Decrease environmental stimuli Maintain airway Prevent self-trauma Frequent skin care and position changes
High-pitched cry	Note character, duration, or other reasons for cry Decrease environmental stimuli Feed frequently Swaddle tightly in blankets Hold close to nurse's body

Source: L. P. Finnegan and B. A. Macnew. Care of the addicted infant. *American Journal of Nursing* 74:685, 1974. Copyright April, 1974, The American Journal of Nursing Company. Reproduced by permission.

Table 17-4. Drugs Used in Neonatal Addiction

Drug	Dosage and Administration
Chlorpromazine	1–2 mg/kg/day, IM, for 2–4 days; may then be given orally for about 7 days in lesser doses
Phenobarbital	8–10 mg/kg/day, IM, for 2–3 days; may then be given orally for about 7 days in lesser doses
Paregoric (for gastrointestinal symptoms)	3–5 drops every 3 hours until infant appears drowsy or encounters respiratory depression; dosage is tapered slowly over 7 days

Source: S. Pierog and A. Ferrara. *Approach to the Medical Care of the Sick Newborn.* St. Louis: Mosby, 1971.

Figure 17-11. Common withdrawal signs of an addicted newborn. A. Normal newborn head lag. B. Hypertonicity of newborn addict. C. Standing position of normal newborn. D. Newborn addict supports his own weight with little help. E. Startle reflex in normal newborn. F. Tremors of addicted newborn.

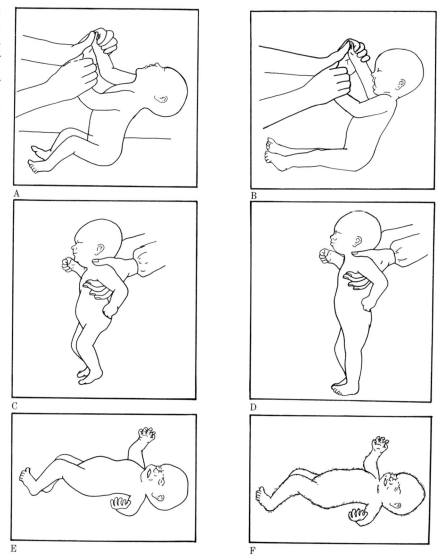

Symptoms in these babies may not appear until the end of the first day, and on rare occasions may not appear until the first or second week of life.

There have also been attempts at drug withdrawal during pregnancy or attempts to extend the intervals between doses in late pregnancy. When this was attempted, mothers reported violent fetal kicking, which was interpreted by the medical team to be signs of fetal withdrawal. There appeared to be no damage to the fetus, but some authorities now advocate no withdrawal attempts after the seventh month of pregnancy [12].

Infants addicted to barbiturates usually are full-term and are of adequate weight. They have a later onset of withdrawal signs (6½ hours to seven days), and the signs last longer than those of the heroin-addicted infant. Infants whose mothers were on barbiturates for medical reasons tend to have symptoms that last for briefer periods than babies whose mothers were addicted.

DISORDERS OF METABOLISM

Infant of the Diabetic Mother

Infants of diabetic mothers are routinely subjected to stresses not normally encountered by other newborns. There is an increased incidence of intrauterine deaths and premature deliveries. In addition to facing the problems encountered by the preterm infant, these infants are frequently large for gestational age and appear plethoric and cushingoid. They are also subject to hypoglycemia, hypocalcemia, electrolyte imbalance, respiratory distress syndrome, hyperbilirubinemia, and possibly a greater incidence of congenital anomalies. The overall survival rate of these infants is 80–90 percent.

The LGA infant of the mother with uncontrolled diabetes was formerly thought to be edematous. These babies are now thought to be macrosomic, with an increased number of total body cells. The reasons for this are not totally clear, but it may be due to increased insulin levels in the fetus, resulting in an increase in protein synthesis. Hyperadrenocorticism may also play a part. Other theories hold that the fetus' hyperinsulinism and hyperglycemia in utero lead to excessive growth and deposition of fat, thus accounting for his large size. Another theory is that the infant's large size is due to pituitary growth hormone.

These infants in utero also have hypertrophy and hyperplasia of the beta cells in the islets of Langerhans and are in a state of hyperinsulinism, perhaps due to the mother's hyperglycemia. At birth, their hyperinsulinism causes their blood sugar levels to drop rapidly, especially during the first 2–3 hours after birth. Hypocalcemia frequently accompanies the hypoglycemia. The reasons for this are not fully understood.

In caring for the infant of a diabetic mother the nurse should observe the baby carefully, especially for signs of hypoglycemia, RDS, and hyperbilirubinemia. The infant should be kept warm in an incubator. Tests for blood glucose levels should be done every hour for the first 6–8 hours. Early feedings of 5–15% glucose should be started, often within an hour of birth, and should be given every 2 hours for approximately three times. Formula is then given if tolerated. If hypoglycemia is present (serum glucose level below 30 milligrams per 100 milliliters), a parenteral glucose infusion of 10–15% dextrose in water should be started, usually in the umbilical vein.

The frequent incidence of respiratory distress in these infants may be due to asphyxia in utero because of placental insufficiency or to the fact that many are preterm infants often delivered by cesarian section. Approximately 50 percent of infants of diabetic mothers develop tachypnea soon after birth, unassociated with RDS.

It has been reported by many authorities that infants of diabetic mothers also have a higher incidence of congenital anomalies. This issue has been disputed in reports presented to the World Congress on Obstetrics and Gynecology [11].

Phenylketonuria

Phenylketonuria (PKU) is inherited as an autosomal recessive disorder. An infant receives an abnormal gene from each of his heterozygous parents. It occurs in approximately one in 10,000–20,000 births and is more common in Caucasians from Northern Europe and the United States.

The basic defect in PKU is deficient amounts of the liver enzyme phenylalanine hydroxylase, which converts phenylalanine to tyrosine. In carriers, enough enzyme is present to prevent high concentrations of phenylalanine and its metabolites, which are formed from alternate pathways, from accumulating in the blood, urine, sweat, cerebral spinal fluid, and tissues. The infant who is homozygous for the gene is defenseless. When normal levels of phenylalanine (1–4 milligrams per milliliter) are exceeded as the newborn feeds during the first few weeks of life, a metabolite of phenylalanine, phenylpyruvic acid, can be detected in the urine. The urine can be tested with Phenistix (paper impregnated with ferric salt) or a few drops of 5% ferric chloride placed on a wet diaper. The diaper will turn green in the presence of phenylpyruvic acid. These tests, however, are not felt to be reliable until the infant is 4–6 weeks of age. Earlier diagnosis can be made if increased levels of phenylalanine are found in the infant's blood three to four days after birth. The blood test (Guthrie test) is performed using blood from a heel prick. Many states now require a routine blood screening for PKU just prior to the newborn's discharge from the hospital.

Infants with the defect may become severely mentally retarded. The exact cause of this is unknown, but it has been attributed to a neurotoxic agent that has an inhibitory effect on development before myelinization in the central nervous system is complete. It has also been postulated that brain damage may already have begun by the time the phenylpyruvic acid is detected in the urine. The children may also have seizures, become hyperactive, and exhibit erratic and unpredictable behavior. Untreated infants also fail to thrive and suffer from skin rashes, vomiting, and irritability. The decreased tyrosine leads to a decreased melanin production and reduced pigment in skin, hair, and eyes, explaining in part why the majority of these infants have fair skin, blonde hair, and blue eyes.

Treatment is aimed at eliminating foods from the infant's diet that are high in phenylalanine. Therapy with exogenous enzyme has been of no value. The diet is begun in infancy and maintained during the period of rapid myelinization until the baby is approximately 4 years old, to avoid damage to the central nervous system.

Since virtually all vegetable and animal protein contains phenylalanine, the infant is placed on a special protein formula (Lofenalac) that contains essential amino acids but is low in phenylalanine. During pregnancy, mothers with PKU should also be placed on diets with decreased levels of phenylalanine, since phenylalanine will cross the placenta and may cause mental retardation in infants who are themselves only carriers of the gene.

Galactosemia

This disorder is transmitted as an autosomal recessive trait and is not common, occurring in approximately 1 in 35,000 births.

Lactose (milk sugar) is normally broken down in the digestive tract into galactose, which is absorbed and converted to glucose in the liver. When the enzyme galactose 1-phosphate uridyl transferase is absent, galactose accumulates in blood and tissues. Affected infants appear normal at birth but within a few days begin to vomit, have diarrhea, lose weight, become jaundiced and drowsy, and have an enlarged liver.

Diagnosis is made on the finding of increased levels of galactose in the blood or urine and/or low levels or absence of galactose 1-phosphate uridyl transferase in red blood cells. Carriers of the disease have decreased levels of the enzyme in their erythrocytes.

Treatment is aimed at eliminating all milk and galactose-containing foods from the diet. Nutramigen and soybean preparations such as Sobee or Mull-Soy are substituted. Untreated infants who survive develop irreversible cataracts and mental retardation.

CHROMOSOMAL ABNORMALITIES

Trisomy 21 Syndrome

Trisomy 21 syndrome is also known as trisomy G syndrome, mongolism, or Down's syndrome. In approximately 95 percent of all cases, trisomy 21 syndrome is due to meiotic nondisjunction of one of the G-group chromosomes, usually in the maternal gamete. The infant thus inherits an extra chromosome in this group and a total cell complement of 47 chromosomes.

The incidence of this type of nondisjunction increases with advancing maternal age. The frequency in young mothers is approximately 1 in 1000–2000 births; at 35 years of age, 1 in 300 births; and at 45 years of age, 1 in 30–50 births. Many authorities believe that the ova of women over 30 have a greater chance of mechanical error when they proceed through both meiotic divisions than the ova of younger women.

A smaller number of cases of Down's syndrome are due to translocation, in which chromosome 21 attaches to another chromosome, often chromosome 22 or one of the D group. Advanced maternal age is not a factor in these cases, and in fact the parents are usually younger, one of them possibly being a carrier of the disorder. The parent in this case appears normal and has 45 chromosomes. The chance of this couple's producing another affected child is significant. Theoretically, each pregnancy carries a 33 percent chance of recurrence.

An even smaller percentage of children with Down's syndrome may be due to mosaicism, in which the child has a mixture of two cell types, one with 46 chromosomes and the other with 47.

Down's syndrome is usually diagnosed at birth. The infant has hypotonic muscles, hypermobility of the joints, short broad hands with stubby fingers, a transverse palmar crease (simian line), a small round head with low-set ears, a flattened occiput, and a small mouth with a protruding tongue (Figure 17-12). As the child grows, he is usually of short stature, has some degree of mental retardation, and is susceptible to many respiratory diseases. Infants with Down's syndrome often have asso-

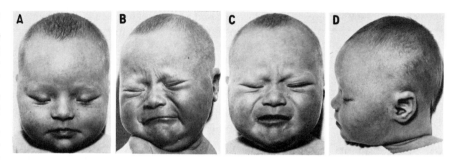

Figure 17-12. Neonate with Down's syndrome. A. Note upward slant of the eyes and epicanthal folds. B. Characteristic grimace. C. Relative broadening of the face. D. Fat pad at the back of the neck and helical distortion of the ear. (From E. L. Potter and J. M. Craig. Pathology of the Fetus and Infant [3rd ed.]. Copyright © 1975 by Year Book Medical Publishers, Inc., Chicago. Used by permission.)

ciated cardiac, renal, and gastrointestinal defects. While male children with the disorder are believed to be sterile, female children may reproduce and have a 50 percent chance of having an infant similarly affected.

Trisomy 18 Syndrome

Trisomy 18 syndrome (E syndrome) occurs in approximately 1 in 5000 births and is far more frequent in females than in males. It is easily recognizable at birth due to the infant's facial features, which include low-set ears, a prominent occiput, wide-spaced eyes, and micrognathia. The infant also has rocker-bottom feet and a characteristic overlapping of his index finger over the third finger. Usually these infants, fail to thrive and die at an early age.

BIRTH INJURY

The most common and serious form of birth injury is *intracranial injury*. Prolonged labor, difficult delivery requiring use of forceps, precipitate delivery and breech extraction are likely to result in a sudden change in the shape of the skull rather than the gradual molding process that takes place throughout a normal labor. Intracranial hemorrhage results.

The edema or hemorrhage accompanying intracranial injury leads to a compromise in the blood supply to various portions of the brain, which may suffer temporary or permanent damage. Large hemorrhages occur most commonly in the falx cerebri, which separates the two halves of the cerebrum or in the tentorium cerebelli, which divides the cerebellum from the cerebrum. In the preterm infant, the vessels of the choroid plexus may be injured, resulting in a hemorrhage into the ventricular system of the brain.

The infant with intracranial injury is abnormally sleepy and difficult to arouse; he has little spontaneous movement, a depressed or absent Moro reflex, and poor sucking and/or swallowing reflexes. If his intracranial pressure is high, his respirations may be slow, grunting, irregular, and periodic. Bradycardia exists and his fontanelle bulges. There may be spasticity of his muscles, twitching, or even generalized convulsions. He may have an elevated or subnormal body temperature and his cry, although weak, is likely to be sharp and shrill.

Prognosis, of course, varies with the severity of the injury. Mortality is high when large or vital areas of the brain are affected, and infants who survive are likely to be mentally retarded or have spastic paralysis.

General supportive measures are used in treatment. If convulsions occur, phenobarbital is usually given. Vitamin K may be given to minimize bleeding. Infants are handled gently and sparingly. Sometimes a spinal tap or subdural tap in the area of the fontanelle may relieve some intracranial pressure. The best treatment is prevention through careful obstetrical management of the mother.

Three other common birth injuries, previously discussed in Chapter 13, are *caput succedaneum, cephalhematoma,* and *facial nerve paralysis.* A fourth is *brachial palsy.* When the nerve fibers running from the neck through the shoulder and toward the arm are injured during obstetrical maneuvers, a partial paralysis of the arm results. Most often this involves the muscles of the upper arm and not those of the hand and fingers. The infant holds his arm at his side with his elbow extended and the hand rotated inward (Figure 17-13). If the nerve fibers have not broken, recovery is usually rapid and complete within a few weeks. If the nerve fibers are broken, recovery depends on their regeneration, which may take from two to three months or may never occur. During this time the muscles of the shoulder are exercised gently to prevent contractures from forming.

Sometimes *fractures* occur during birth, most often of the clavicle when the shoulder is extracted. No special management is required for this, since it usually heals rapidly without producing much pain or disability. Breaks of an extremity (humerus, femur) are rare and are usually apparent from their abnormal appearance. They heal well when immobilized in the correct position by splints or slings. Since parents may be fearful of hurting the baby by handling him, they should be instructed in his care and encouraged to give him adequate love and attention.

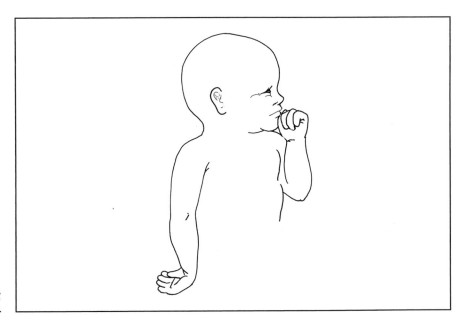

Figure 17-13. Brachial palsy.

CONGENITAL MALFORMATIONS

Malformations of the fetus range from very small defects, such as supernumerary digits, to those that are incompatible with life. The incidence of congenital malformations may be affected by maternal race (more common in Caucasians than in blacks except for supernumerary digits), age (more frequent in infants of mothers over 35—mongolism, central nervous system malformations), parity (anencephalus and spina bifida are more common with first births and those after the sixth), and fetal sex (the majority of anencephalics are female).

In general, if a woman has given birth to a malformed child previously, there is an increased likelihood of subsequent malformed infants. Since congenital malformations are often multiple, the presence of one deformity may mean that another is present as well. Current theory indicates that both genetic and environmental factors play a part in the etiology of most congenital anomalies.

Central Nervous System

The nervous system of the newborn is immature anatomically, chemically, and physiologically. In the preterm infant there is little myelination, and polysynaptic connections are just beginning to form. Neurological function is largely at the brain stem and spinal cord level. The primitive reflexes represent primitive released neuronal function, largely uninhibited by higher cerebral control. Deep tendon reflexes are normally symmetrical; patellar, biceps, and triceps are the most easily elicited.

The three most common congenital anomalies of the central nervous system involve either abnormal size of the head or defects in closure of the bony spine. They are anencephalus, hydrocephalus, and spina bifida.

Anencephalus, the most common cause of gross hydramnios, is a malformation characterized by complete or partial absence of the pituitary gland, brain, and overlying skull. The condition is incompatible with life. The face is very prominent as a result of the absence of the skull, the eyes often protrude markedly from their sockets, and the tongue hangs from the mouth. About 70 percent of anencephalics are female. It is believed that both genetic and environmental factors play a part in the etiology of this defect. Diagnosis, which is suggested by the inability to palpate a fetal head abdominally, is confirmed by x-ray. Increased amounts of alpha-fetoproteins, formed in the fetal liver, are found in the amniotic fluid of fetuses with anencephaly, probably because of leakage of their cerebrospinal fluid.

Hydrocephalus involves an excessive accumulation of cerebrospinal fluid in the ventricles of the brain with resulting enlargement of the cranium. It accounts for about 12 percent of all malformations found at birth, and about 33 percent of the time it is associated with spina bifida, although other defects are also common. It is often the result of meningitis, head trauma, or subdural hematoma in the newborn.

The volume of the fluid is usually 500–1500 milliliters, and since the head in utero is often too large to enter the pelvis, breech presentations are common. Cephalopelvic disproportion is the rule, and dystocia is the result, with uterine rupture a definite risk. Hydrocephalus is suspected if, on abdominal and vaginal examination, the floating fetal head feels unusually broad or if during labor the head remains high despite a normal pelvis and good contractions. Diagnosis may be confirmed by x-ray or ultrasonic cephalometry.

Often the disorder is not manifested until several weeks after birth, when the head rapidly begins to increase in size—sometimes 2.5 centimeters (1 inch) or more a month—and signs of increased intracranial pressure appear in the infant. For most babies surgical intervention provides the only hope of relief.

In cases of *spina bifida,* the posterior portion of the bony canal containing the spinal cord is completely or partially absent because of failure of the vertebral laminae to develop or to fuse. This defect is relatively common, particularly in the lumbar or sacral region.

Sometimes the meninges protrude through the defect to form an external cystic tumor (meningocele) that contains cerebrospinal fluid and is present at birth. Occasionally the cord as well as the meninges protrudes (myelomeningocele). The prognosis is generally not good, since hydrocephalus often occurs following surgical repair. In addition, there may be residual rectal or bladder paralysis, with spasticity and deformity of the legs.

Circulatory System—Congenital Heart Disease

The most common causes of death in pediatric referral hospitals, excluding problems specifically related to prematurity, are congenital heart defects, despite the fact that there has been rapid advancement in their diagnosis and management. Most of these deaths occur in the neonatal period, particularly during the first two weeks after birth.

About 70 percent of newborns with fatal heart defects will have one of the following five structural defects because of errors of embryogenesis in the first two months of gestation: hypoplastic left ventricle syndrome (hypoplasia of left ventricle, aortic atresia, or mitral atresia), complicated coarctation of the aorta, transposition of the great arteries, hypoplastic right ventricle syndrome (with pulmonary arterial atresia or stenosis), or severe tetralogy of Fallot. Statistically, the low-risk cardiac newborn is likely to have a simple left-to-right shunt lesion—commonly a ventricular septal defect. Atrial septal defect and patent ductus arteriosus are less common but are still important.

Signs and symptoms of various defects vary with the type and severity. In general, the cardinal signs are cyanosis, respiratory distress, systemic venous congestion (hepatosplenomegaly), and diminished cardiac output. A heart murmur is not usually a presenting sign. Tachypnea is a sign of cardiorespiratory difficulty, and when little respiratory effort is associated with it, congenital heart disease is suggested as the cause. Marked respiratory effort, especially with grunting, suggests lung disease, but there may be much overlap in these two areas. Other observations may include reluctance to feed, easy exhaustion, or changes in color (pallor, grayishness, or cyanosis).

The diagnosis may be made from history, physical findings, x-ray, and electrocardiogram results. Sometimes cardiac catheterization or angiography supplies confirmation. When these infants remain in the newborn nursery while diagnosis is being completed, the staff should take special precautions to prevent infection and unnecessary stresses. Signs such as cyanosis and respiratory distress may be treated symptomatically by the use of oxygen administration and positioning. Frequent small feedings will avoid the possibility of gastric distention and increased pressure on the diaphragm and heart. In the presence of heart failure, digitalis is often prescribed.

Musculoskeletal System

Clubfoot (talipes equinovarus) is relatively common, occurring in about 1 in 1000 births. It involves extension and inversion of the foot so that the tarsal bones are displaced and the foot cannot be passively restored to normal position. This defect may occur alone or in association with spinal or central nervous system anomalies (particularly spina bifida) or oligohydramnios. There is some evidence that there may be an underlying genetic defect in the formation of connective tissue. Plaster boots applied to the feet in the correcting position are used to remedy the defect.

Talipes calcaneovalgus and *metatarsus varus* are milder deformities that may be treated by passive manipulation of the foot in the opposite direction and maintenance of the correct position for a minute at a time. This is done frequently during the day, and parents may be taught to continue the exercise at home.

Congenital dislocated hip, as discussed in Chapter 13, is a fairly common malformation that is six times more frequent in girls than in boys. X-rays reveal lateral displacement of the upper end of the femur and poor development of the acetabulum on that side. A dislocated hip is treated by maintaining abduction of the hips during the early months of life, usually by cast application. Frequently, when an infant in the newborn nursery is discovered to have a dislocated hip the application of a triple layer of diapers will maintain the recommended abduction.

In addition to the skeletal fractures already discussed, injury to the sternocleidomastoid muscle may occur during delivery, particularly if the presentation is breech. The damaged muscle is less elastic and does not elongate at a normal rate during growth, with the result that the child's head is gradually turned to one side, producing *torticollis* or *wry neck.* Surgery can be used to correct the muscle contraction. If the initial injury was slight, healing is usually spontaneous.

Gastrointestinal Disorders

CLEFT LIP AND CLEFT PALATE

Cleft lip occurs in approximately 1 in 800 births and results when the embryo's lateral and medial nasal processes fail to fuse between the fifth and eighth week of intrauterine life. The incomplete cleft may be little more than a notch in the lip, or it may extend up into the nostril. The incidence is higher in families with a history of the defect. The deformity may also occur in infants whose mothers had rubella in the first trimester of pregnancy.

Should the palatal processes fail to fuse (usually one month later than the nasal processes), the infant is born with a cleft palate. More than 40 percent of the time these two defects occur in conjunction with one another.

Corrective treatment for these disorders is surgery. The cleft lip is usually repaired as soon as the infant can tolerate surgery. The cleft palate is usually not closed until 1½–2½ years of age.

Prior to closure of a moderate to severely affected cleft lip, feeding is a problem since the infant cannot create a vacuum in his mouth which enables him to suck. A soft nipple with a large hole, a specialized nipple such as a Breck feeder, or a rubber-tipped medicine dropper may be used to feed him. His parents should be supported and encouraged to feed him and helped to see their infant's assets.

ESOPHAGEAL ATRESIA

Esophageal atresia is a serious anomaly and most commonly involves the upper (proximal) end of the esophagus, which ends in a blind pouch, while the lower end is connected to the trachea by a fistulous tract. The infant may also have associated cardiac defects and anal atresia.

As the infant swallows fluid and mucus, the pouch fills and soon overflows. The infant froths and drools and may aspirate the material into his trachea, resulting in pneumonia. Frequent suctioning is necessary to keep his nasopharynx clear of secretions; otherwise, he becomes cyanotic and experiences respiratory distress. He should be kept in an incubator with humidity to keep the secretions liquified. He should also be kept warm and precautions should be taken to keep him free from infection. A gastrostomy may be performed to provide for his nutrition.

The condition is usually diagnosed by x-ray after a catheter is passed through the infant's nose into his trachea. The x-ray shows the catheter coiled on itself in the blind pouch. Treatment consists of surgical anastamosis of the esophageal segments. If there is too large a gap between the segments, the upper segment may be brought to the skin surface, a gastrostomy performed, and later a colon transplant used to join the segments.

PYLORIC STENOSIS

Pyloric stenosis is not actually a congenital malformation but is a common functional anomaly present at or soon after birth. The musculature of the pyloric sphincter hypertrophies, thus hindering the passage of stomach contents into the duodenum. It occurs in approximately 1 in 350 births, and about 80 percent of the affected infants are male. It is far more common in Caucasians than in blacks or Orientals and is more common in firstborn children.

Although the anomaly may be present at birth, symptoms usually begin at 2–3 weeks of age when the infant begins vomiting. The vomiting, which occurs during or shortly after feeding, becomes progressively more marked and projectile in character. If the infant is untreated, the probability of death is high. Surgical relief of the obstruction consists of longitudinal splitting of the pyloric muscle (Ramstedt's operation).

IMPERFORATE ANUS

During the eighth week of embryonic life the membrane separating the rectum from the anus is normally absorbed. When this does not occur, imperforate anus results.

The infant is unable to pass stool and abdominal distention occurs. If the anal opening is blocked by a thin membrane, perforation of it may be all the treatment that is necessary. When there is a distance between the anal dimple and the end of the colon, surgical repair includes either a temporary colostomy or joining of the colon to the anal dimple by an abdominal perineal operation. Whatever procedure is used, following surgery the infant is positioned on his side and turned frequently to prevent tension on the suture line. Skin care is very important postoperatively to prevent skin breakdown and subsequent infection. An aluminum paste or zinc oxide ointment may be applied to the skin for this purpose.

Genitourinary Disorders

UNDESCENDED TESTICLES

Usually testicles descend into the scrotum in the eighth month of fetal life. If only one has descended, the scrotal sac appears uneven; if both have failed to descend, the sac appears small. Newborns with undescended testicles may be preterm infants.

Descent may be spontaneous during the first few weeks of life or up to the age of puberty. Correction is necessary prior to puberty, since the undescended testis is at a higher temperature in the abdomen and the sperm-forming cells may degenerate because of this. Some physicians use testosterone during the preschool years to stimulate descent if there is no mechanical obstruction such as a hernia. Surgical intervention (orchidopexy) may be performed during infancy or the school years. It is usually avoided during the preschool years because of the child's fear of bodily intrusion.

HYDROCELE

A hydrocele is an accumulation of fluid around the testis or along the spermatic cord. It appears as a swollen, oval, translucent sac. The fluid is gradually absorbed.

PHIMOSIS

In phimosis the foreskin of the male infant has a very narrow orifice. It does not obstruct the flow of urine but may cause some straining during urination. It also prevents proper cleaning of the penis, since retraction of the foreskin is impossible. Treatment consists of circumcision or stretching the foreskin with a hemostat.

PARENTAL REACTIONS TO PROBLEM NEWBORNS

The image of the expected baby represents self and loved ones to the prospective parents. In most instances it is likely that there will be some discrepancy between the parents' fantasized ideal child and the actual child; coming to an acceptance of that discrepancy is one of the developmental tasks of parenthood. When the discrepancy is great, as in the birth of a defective child or when the parents' wishes are too unrealistic, a problem may develop in the establishment of a healthy parent-child relationship. The parents' reactions, of course, are shaped by the type and degree of defect and their own past experiences with parents and siblings, as well as by the acceptance and emotional support that the two partners give each other and that is given by other important people in their environment.

If the expected ideal child is defective, parents' goals, fantasies, and idealizations have to be modified in relation to reality. This adaptation takes the form of grief work—a readjusting to the real situation and a redefinition of relationships to compensate for the unexpected. Grief over the loss leads to mourning, with the sadness, withdrawal, resentment, and self-blame inherent in the mourning process. Nurses who are aware of these developments will have an increased understanding of the impact of disappointment, the feeling of helplessness, and the sense of failure that these parents are experiencing, and will be able to help them to eventually begin to build on the strengths in the situation.

In a culture that emphasizes success, a defective child presents an extremely stressful situation. If a parent views the child as an extension of self, he may consider the defective child as proof of a defect within himself. Therefore, the parent may be a person whose ego is threatened and can be expected to build up strong defenses against the pain that comes with recognition of a child's anomaly. Parents may develop excessive concern about the child, which suggests that they perceive him as a defective child—not merely a child with a defect. This can prolong dependent ties instead of helping the child in the process of gradual separation, which is so necessary for the development of his emotional autonomy.

Some parents may feel that with enough love the child will be "whole," and in lavishing love and attention on him they may fail to relate adequately to other members of the family. At the other extreme, some parents and family members show an intolerance of the child and an almost irresistible urge to deny their relationship to him. Just as the infant's imperfection has an effect upon his total family, the ways in which they react to him and accept him affect his total personality development.

Parents often react initially by feeling shock, hurt, disappointment, and a helpless resentment at the revelation that they have a child who is not perfect. Since the baby is regarded as part of themselves, their efforts toward rehabilitation are motivated not only by reality but also by a desire for restitution for the child and themselves. As soon as most parents are able to master the expression of acute grief, they tend to regard as unacceptable any negative feelings they have toward the baby. This frequently leads to a denial of difficulties and a hiding of anxieties.

Denial of the defect is often reflected in the parents' "shopping around" for a more acceptable diagnosis, hostility toward professional workers, overprotection of the child, or projection of difficulties onto other people or circumstances. The depression sometimes associated with recognition of the handicap may result in denial of the fact that the defective child has the same needs as any other child and that with help he can often develop a degree of independence and social acceptability as well as a sense of achievement. The parents' acceptance of a referral for special help is often accompanied by a feeling of inadequacy, since, if one denies a problem, he need not seek or accept help related to it.

Lack of opportunity to discuss the diagnosis can create a situation in which parents feel overwhelmed and unable to gauge the reality of their child's retarded development. Denial then serves to forestall anxiety and depression.

A repetitive aspect of the mourning process in the parents' reactions—the need to grieve about the loss—indicates the need for repeated opportunities to review the situation. The nurse's availability to them and encouragement of a trusting environment can make this task easier and more completely accomplished. Guilt feelings commonly enter into the mourning process. Parents ask, "Where did I fail? Was it someone else's fault? Why me?" Expressions of guilt take many forms—anger, aggression, hostility—and demonstrate how important the child's appearance and wholeness really are. Parents search for the cause of the malformation, and since explanations do not always relieve anxieties, they often resort to fantasies. Mothers recall significant fears that they had during pregnancy and may blame the defect on procedures that were performed before or during pregnancy or delivery, or on the obstetrician and medical personnel. In addition, parents may have fears about subsequent pregnancies or about their ability to give adequate care to this baby or may feel the need to prove that they are "good" parents.

The father of a defective child sometimes changes his work habits, working day and night, following the birth. It is suggested that this may illustrate his desire to prove himself as an adequate man, partner, and father. Another practical interpretation involves the financial burden and need for money that a child with special problems might represent. The extra time spent at work is also time spent away from the home situation, which is a constant reminder of the child's defect.

In the hospital the mother sometimes shows a vagueness or detachment when she is at the point of verbalizing her loss but is not realistically able to feel it. She wants someone to care about her, share her grief, and guide her in the acceptance of her loss, and so she turns to the nurse.

Nurses grieve over the parents' loss but do not always realize this. They often attempt to deny their feelings and respond by acting in a formalized, stiff, uncaring way, only reinforcing the loneliness the parents are experiencing. As long as nurses are unable to accept their own grief in a realistic context, they will have little alternative but to inhibit the expression of grief in the parents. The hospital is the place for crying for many parents—for getting it out of their systems. They need a nurse who will stand by, letting them cry, and letting them feel that it is good for them to cry. The initial mourning period is not the time to accentuate the positive nor to tell parents that they have other perfect children or time to have more. This baby is the important one at that moment, not the ones they have already or could have in the future.

It is of value to review pertinent hospital regulations and routines. In situations in which parents are not permitted to see their defective baby immediately because the staff wants to spare them the pain, consideration should be given to whether or not the parents are really being done a service. Are the nurses in reality sparing themselves the difficulties inherent in giving the parents support at this time? Is it a good idea to isolate the mother from other mothers with healthy newborns, whether it is by room placement itself or by confinement to her own room when babies are out of the nursery? It is often assumed that she prefers to be alone, but she is rarely asked if this is so, an apparent direct violation of respect for her individuality. Again, such practices spare the feelings of the nursing staff and do not put their adequacy to the test.

It is essential for the nurse to gauge the parents' mourning reaction in order to know how and when to help them take an active role in planning the child's care. If the parents' mourning reaction is not understood and if the care of the child is carried out without their active participation or they are kept separated from him, their mourning may resolve into a persistent depressed, self-reproachful state. But if their own needs for support are met, they will be able to look realistically at the needs of the child. It is essential that nurses demonstrate that they value the infant by giving him complete and expert care. Sometimes this is all that is needed to open the channels of communication for the parents to express their disappointment and grief and to begin to recognize the strengths and normal aspects of the child. Accurate listening and observation should alert the nurse to the parents' needs. If the parents begin to feel that they are doing the best possible for the infant with the resources they have, their thinking usually changes from despair and guilt to more positive feelings. As they participate in the care of the child, they can be helped to accept what cannot be changed, find satisfaction in improvement, and prepare to appreciate what the child offers.

In an atmosphere of trust and confidence, parents should be able to express their critical questions to members of the health care team who can describe what is known or not known regarding the defective child. It is important that staff members do not give parents unrealistic hope for the future and that they tell the parents *together* about the prognosis, especially if it is poor, since neither one is in any better condition to accept the news. Communication between parents and nursery personnel and between nursery personnel and staff on the postpartum unit is essential if the parents are to receive the support they need.

If the baby is stillborn or dies in the neonatal period, parents react similarly. Initial responses commonly involve disbelief and shock, anger, inadequacy, and guilt, especially if the pregnancy was not wanted. The last phases of the mourning process—resolution and idealization—take the longest (six months to a year), as thoughts of the loss become replaced with other interests and relationships. At the time of the baby's death it is felt that the couple should be told together so that they may give each other mutual support. Sometimes, even if they have communicated well before the birth of the baby, they have such strong feelings after the infant's death that they are unable to share them. Since this can only hinder the resolution of grieving, they should be encouraged to talk together about their loss. It is felt that parents will have a better chance of successful grieving if they have seen the child, especially if he was abnormal. If they do not, they will have to mourn on the basis of fantasy, and the fantasized abnormality may be far worse than the actual defect.

Again, in the hospital setting, it is most often nurses upon whom parents rely for acceptance, support, and encouragement. If the nurses are aware of their own feelings of grief and helplessness in the situation, they will be able to work more effectively with the parents.

Parents' reactions to premature birth have been reported to revolve around four psychological tasks that they must accomplish. The first is anticipatory grief, or preparing for the infant's death. Their anxieties are increased at this time, not only concerning whether or not the baby will live, but, if it does, whether or not it will be deformed or mentally retarded. The second task is realization and acceptance of the mother's failure to carry the infant to term. This phase is often accompanied by guilt feelings that one or both parents might have done something to cause the premature labor.

The third task is the resumption of the process of relating to the infant. The support required here is very similar to that needed by parents of children with defects. Nurses can establish a supportive relationship by talking with the parents together, by finding out what they believe is going to happen or what they know about the infant's problem. What the baby and his equipment will look like and why it is necessary should be discussed before the parents are taken to the nursery to see him. Whenever possible, the parents should be permitted to scrub, gown, and enter the nursery and to touch, hold, or feed the baby. Extended visiting hours for them should be made available.

While the parents are there, nurses should describe their infant's individual behavioral characteristics, since this helps to emphasize his individuality, that he is somebody "special" from the very beginning. They might again describe the infant's equipment and what is being done for him, staying by the parents' side to answer their questions. If the baby is under the bili-light, turning it off and removing his eye patches for a brief period will allow the parents to establish eye contact with him, to get the feeling that the baby is really theirs.

The final task the parents must accomplish is that of learning the special needs of the baby. They need to develop confidence in their ability to care for the infant; feeding will be one of the first experiences on which they can base this feeling. Efforts of nursing personnel should be directed toward reassuring and guiding parents so that their attempts to feed and care for their baby meet with success. Since the parents usually must go home without the baby, it is important that they be encouraged to return to the nursery to visit and feed the baby, or to call whenever they wish for information on his condition.

Public health or visiting nurses and hospital home-care coordinators should be involved in the planning of care for the family as soon as possible after the birth of the child. In this way a relationship is established between the parents and the nurse, who can provide continued guidance once the family is together in the home following the infant's discharge.

REFERENCES

1. Babson, S. G., and Benson, R. *Management of High-Risk Pregnancy and Intensive Care of the Neonate*. St. Louis: Mosby, 1971.
2. Brain damage in newborn may be due to kernicterus. *Journal of the American Medical Association* 212:45, 1970.
3. Crosse, V. M. *The Pre Term Baby and Other Babies with Low Birth Weight*. Edinburgh: Churchill Livingstone, 1971.
4. Driscoll. J. Metabolic and Endocrine Disturbances. In R. Behrman (Ed.), *Neonatology*. St. Louis: Mosby, 1973.

5. Finnegan, L., and Macnew, B. Care of the addicted infant. *American Journal of Nursing* 74:685, 1974.
6. Hellman, L. M., and Pritchard, J. A. *Williams Obstetrics* (14th ed.). New York: Appleton-Century-Crofts, 1971.
7. Klaus, M., and Fanaroff, A. Respiratory Problems. In M. Klaus and A. Fanaroff (Eds.), *Care of the High-Risk Neonate*. Philadelphia: Saunders, 1973.
8. Korones, S. B. *High-Risk Newborn Infants*. St. Louis: Mosby, 1976.
9. Lucey, J., Ferreiro, M., and Hewitt, J. Prevention of hyperbilirubinemia of prematurity by phototherapy. *Pediatrics* 41:1047, 1968.
10. Pierog, S., and Ferrara, A. *Approach to the Medical Care of the Sick Newborn*. St. Louis: Mosby, 1971.
11. Pregnancy and diabetes: How risky? *Journal of the American Medical Association* 212:1287, 1970.
12. Stevenson, R. *The Fetus and Newly Born Infant*. St. Louis: Mosby, 1973.
13. Sweet, A. Classification of the Low Birth Weight Infant. In M. Klaus and A. Fanaroff (Eds.), *Care of the High-Risk Neonate*. Philadelphia: Saunders, 1973.
14. Wald, M. Problems in Chemical Adaptation. In M. Klaus and A. Fanaroff (Eds.), *Care of the High-Risk Neonate*. Philadelphia: Saunders, 1973.
15. Waters, W. J. The reserve albumin binding capacity as a criterion for exchange transfusion. *Pediatrics* 70:185, 1967.
16. Williams, S. R. *Essentials of Nutrition and Diet Therapy*. St. Louis: Mosby, 1974.

FURTHER READING

Banks, M. J. Reactions of a Family to a Malformed Infant. *American Nurses' Association Clinical Sessions*. New York: Appleton-Century-Crofts, 1967.
Blake, F., Wright, F. H., and Waechter, E. *Nursing Care of Children*. Philadelphia: Lippincott, 1970.
Clausen, J., Flook, M., Ford, B., Green, M., and Popiel, E. *Maternity Nursing Today*. New York: McGraw-Hill, 1973.
Marx, J. L. Cytomegalovirus: A major cause of birth defects. *Science* 190:1184, December 19, 1975.
Owens, C. Parents' response to premature birth. *American Journal of Nursing* 60:1113, 1960.
Owens, C. Parents' reactions to defective babies. *American Journal of Nursing* 64:83, 1964.
Seitz, P., and Warrick, L. Perinatal death: the grieving mother. *American Journal of Nursing* 74:2028, 1974.
Solnit, A., and Stark, M. Mourning and the birth of a defective child. *Psychoanalytic Study of the Child* 16:523, 1961.

Appendix Certificate and Master's Degree Programs in Nurse-Midwifery in the United States

CERTIFICATE PROGRAMS

Frontier School of Midwifery and Family Nursing
Wendover
Leslie County, Kentucky   41775

United States Air Force
Nurse Midwifery Program
Malcolm Grow USAF Medical Center
Andrews Air Force Base, Maryland 20331

University of Minnesota
School of Nursing
3313 Powell Hall
Minneapolis, Minnesota   55455

College of Medicine and Dentistry of New Jersey
School of Allied Health Professions
Nurse-Midwifery Program
100 Bergen Street
Newark, New Jersey   07103

State University of New York
College of Health Related Professions
Nurse-Midwifery Program, Box 1216
450 Clarkson Avenue
Brooklyn, New York   11203

Medical University of South Carolina
Nurse-Midwifery Program, College of Nursing
80 Barre Street
Charleston, S.C.   29401

Meharry Medical College
Nurse-Midwifery Program
Department of Nursing Education
Box 14
Nashville, Tennessee   37208

Georgetown University School of Nursing
3700 Reservoir Road, N.W.
Washington, D.C.   20007

MASTER'S DEGREE PROGRAMS

Yale University School of Nursing
Graduate Program in Maternal and Newborn Nursing and Nurse-Midwifery
38 South Street
New Haven, Connecticut   06510

The University of Illinois at the Medical Center
College of Nursing, Department of Maternal Child Nursing
Nurse-Midwifery Program
P.O. Box 6998
Chicago, Illinois   60680

University of Kentucky
College of Nursing
Albert B. Chandler Medical Center
Lexington, Kentucky   40506

The Johns Hopkins University
School of Hygiene and Public Health
Nurse-Midwifery Program
615 North Wolfe Street
Baltimore, Maryland   21205

University of Mississippi
Nurse Midwifery Program
2500 North State Street
Jackson, Mississippi   39216

St. Louis University
Department of Nursing
Graduate Program in Nurse-Midwifery
1401 South Grand Boulevard
St. Louis, Missouri   63104

Columbia University Graduate Program in Maternity Nursing
   and Nurse Midwifery
Department of Nursing, Faculty of Medicine
Columbia-Presbyterian Medical Center
622 West 168th Street
New York, New York   10032

University of Utah
College of Nursing, Graduate Major in Maternal and Newborn
   Nursing and Nurse Midwifery
25 South Medical Drive
Salt Lake City, Utah   84112

Index

Bradycardia, 84
  fetal, 207, 208, 215, 241
  puerperal, 260
Brain, fetal, 127, 129
Brassiere, maternity, 150, 264
Braxton-Hicks contractions, 142, 184, 203
Breast pump, 265, 328
Breast-feeding, 253, 323–329. *See also* Breasts,
        during puerperium
  baby's sucking manner, 302, 325–326
  bubbling the baby, 329
  drugs affecting, 328–329
  lactation, 262
  rooting reflex, 302, 325
  technique, 325–326, 327–328
Breasts. *See also* Breast-feeding; Nipples of
        breasts
  anatomy, 31–32
  artificial methods of emptying, 264–265,
        328
  cracked or fissured nipples, 265, 328, 416
  manual expression of milk or colostrum,
        264–265, 326–327
    lactation, 262
    let-down reflex, 326–327
    milk secretion, 324
    support, 150, 264
  mastitis, 268, 295, 415–416
    during puerperium, 264–265, 415–416
  during pregnancy, 147–150, 164
  during puerperium, 262–265
    colostrum secretion, 148, 263, 324
    disorders of, 415–418
    engorgement of, 264–265, 326, 328
  self-examination of, 149–150, 268
  size of, 31–32, 35
  supernumerary, 417–418
Breathing
  of mother
    during labor, 186, 203
    during pregnancy, 153–154
  of newborn, 293, 296–297
Breck feeder, 465
Breech presentation, 192, 193, 196, 198, 216,
        285, 287
  delivery of baby in, 386–390
Brow presentation, 192, 390–391
Brown fat, newborn, 223
Bubbling of newborn, 329
Bulbocavernous muscle, 22
Bulbourethral gland, 22, 43, 45, 48

Calcium gluconate, 355
Candida albicans, 54, 145, 295
Caput succedaneum, 285, 291, 383, 384, 391,
        461
Carcinoma, endometrial, and IUDs, 64
Cardiac complications, in pregnancy,
        116–117
Cardiac output
  during labor, 368

  during pregnancy, 154
  during puerperium, 260
Cardiovascular system
  during pregnancy, 154–156
  during puerperium, 260
Carriage, during pregnancy, 143, 160, 185
Carunculae hymenalis, 256
Cascara, 328
Castration, 72
Cataracts, congenital, 293
Catecholamines, 162
Catheterization, postpartum, 262
Cell division, 40, 46, 107
Center for Disease control, U.S., 7
Central nervous system, 30, 162
  malformations of, congenital, 462–463
  effect of progesterone on, 36
Centriole, 46
Centrosome, 41
Cephalic presentation, 192, 198
Cephalohematomas, 291–292, 461
Cerebral edema, newborn, 291
Cervical caps, 55–56
Cervix, 25, 27, 48
  dilation of, 198, 204, 212, 215, 236, 239
  disorders of, in infertility, 73
  hormonal effects on, 36
  effacement of, 210–212, 239
  incompetent, 73, 338
  mucus, 39
  mucus plug in, during pregnancy, 144, 203
  during pregnancy, 144
  during puerperium, 255
Cesarean section, 1, 74, 236, 398–401
  effects on newborn, 401
  indications for, 399
  postoperative care, 400
  preoperative preparation, 399–400
  types, 399
Chadwick's sign, 145
Chest, newborn, 295–297
Child adoption. *See* Adoption
Childbirth. *See also* Labor
  education for. *See* Education for
        childbirth
  during emergency, management of,
        232–236
  family concept in, 8–9
  in the home, 8–9, 95, 235
  mortality. *See* Mortality
Children
  adoption of. *See* Adoption
  reasons for having, 87–88
  sexual development, 13–15
Chill, postpartum, 232, 261
Chimerism, blood, 359–360
Chloasma, 7, 151
Chloroform, 1
Chlorpromazine, 454
Choanal atresia, 293
Cholestasis, 153